MAN'S
BODY

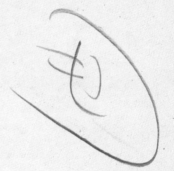

MAN'S BODY

–

AN OWNER'S MANUAL

Compiled by
The Diagram Group

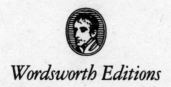

Wordsworth Editions

This edition published 1998 by Wordsworth Editions Ltd.
Cumberland House, Crib Street, Ware, Hertfordshire SG12 9ET.

ISBN 1-84022-024-4

Printed and bound in Great Britain by Mackays of Chatham PLC.

MAN'S BODY

Editorial director:	Margaret Doyle
Editors:	Nancy Bailey, Ben Barkow, Jefferson Cann, Louise Clairmonte, Carole Dease, Kathryn Dunn, Bridget Giles, Catherine Groom, David Heidenstam, Jane Johnson, Susan Leith, Howard Loxton, Helen Varley, Julie Vosburgh
Contributors:	Rosie Boycott, Minakshi Compton, Trevor Day, David Lambert, Ruth Midgley, Irene Stanton, Susan Sturrock
Medical consultants and contributors:	Dr. Katherine Anderson MB, BS, DRCOG, MRCP Paul D. Blumenthal, MD, MPH Francis Scott Key Medical Center, Baltimore, MD Robert Youngson, MD
Research:	Ruth Berenbaum, Cornelius Cardew, Matthew Smout
Design Director:	Richard Hummerstone
Designers:	Darren Bennett, Robin Crane, Roger Kohn, Philip Patenall
Illustrators:	Jeff Alger, Allison Blythe, James Dallas, Robert Galvin, Peter Golding, Brian Hewson, Susan Kinsey, Pavel Kostal, Kathleen McDougall, Graham Rosewarne,
DTP operators:	Mark Carry, Lee Lawrence, Raul Lopez, Garreth Plumb, Philip Richardson

Foreword

The male body is a mystery to its owner. The purpose of this book is to unravel some of the mystery.

Its standpoint is that of the ordinary man. Medical science and its language are complex; and so are the functions and malfunctions of the male body. MAN'S BODY sets out to make a wide range of information and practical guidance clear and concise.

The editors have brought together both international statistical evidence and the insights of recognized specialists; and all this material has been presented to a panel of practicing physicians for their reveiw and commentary.

The words 'average' and 'typical' are often used in MAN'S BODY. They are reference points – statistical figures based on scientific surveys. They should not be made the basis of any judgment, except matter of fact ones. They refer to what is or what happens; not to what is best or what should be.

The editors, researchers, and artists of MAN' BODY hope that this book will help toward a fuller enjoyment of their body and their life.

Contents

GROWTH AND DEVELOPMENT

1

Sex Determination

Sexual Reproduction

Some creatures – such as the amoeba – reproduce by just splitting in two. That may be convenient! But the resulting offspring are very predictable. One amoeba can produce endless replications: but the youngest will still be identical tothe first. Sexual reproduction, in contrast, gives almost infinite variety, for the offsprings' characteristics are a jumbled mixture from both parents' family trees. Some have certain talents, and some manage to combine many talents: all of which helps a species as complex as man to survive in a demanding world.

Sexual Inheritance

Every cell in the human body contains a 'blueprint' of information, on the basis of which it was constructed. This information is contained in 23 pairs of chromosomes, which lie in the nucleus of the cell. The chromosomes determine the output of protein, the basic building unit: which proteins the cell manufactures, when and how. This in turn determines the cell's characteristics and activities.

When a cell divides to make the body grow, the pairs of chromosomes double up before the division. This means both new cells still get 23 pairs, and still get every piece of information that the old cell had. But when the body produces cells for sexual reproduction, it divides cells without doubling their chromosomes first. The pairs separate and each sexual cell gets only 23 single chromosomes, one of each pair. So each of these cells has only half the information that goes into a normal cell. The sperm is the male example of such a cell, and the ovum is the female example. When the two unite, the new fertilized cell, from which the offspring grows, contains 23 pairs of chromosomes again – each parent having contributed half.

Male or Female?

Of the 23 pairs of chromosomes in a body cell, 22 are always matching pairs – each chromosome in the pair is similar. Women also have their 23rd pair identical: they are both called X chromosomes. But men, instead, have two chromosomes that do not match. One is an X, as in women, the other is different, and is called a Y chromosome. The Y chromosome contains the code that determines the male sex. The XX combination occurs in, and produces, a female; the XY combination, a male.

When the female cell splits for sexual reproduction, the sexual cell that results contains one chromosome from each of the 23 pairs – including one X chromosome.

When the male cell splits for sexual reproduction, the sexual cell contains one chromosome from each of the 22 identical pairs, plus either the X or Y – but not both. Which it is determines the offspring's sex. If it is an X, it forms a pair with the female's X – a female child occurs. If it is a Y, it gives the XY non-pair that is typical of, and forms, a man. More males are conceived than females–but males die off at a faster rate, even in the womb.

There are more male stillbirths than female stillbirths, and the earlier in the term of pregnancy the stillbirth occurs, the more likely it is to be male. At four months, there are about two male stillbirths for every female; at full term it is more like 1.5 to 1. As a result, the ratio of fetus males to females declines, until at full term, in advanced societies, it is about 105 or 106 males for every 100 females.

Fertilization to produce a male.
(White arrow shows other cells produced which degenerate.)

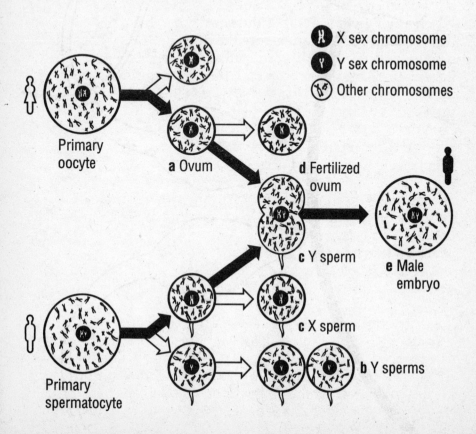

X sex chromosome
Y sex chromosome
Other chromosomes

Primary oocyte

a Ovum

d Fertilized ovum

c Y sperm

e Male embryo

c X sperm

b Y sperms

Primary spermatocyte

Moment of Fertilization

On the left, below we show the edge of a female ovum – magnified about 50,000 times. (The ovum varies a great deal in size; but despite its minuteness, it is always by far the largest cell that the body produces.) We also show three spermatozoa, magnified by the same amount. The ovum has just been fertilized by the topmost spermatozoon. Immediately this has passed through, the ovum's outer wall hardens, to prevent any more from entering.

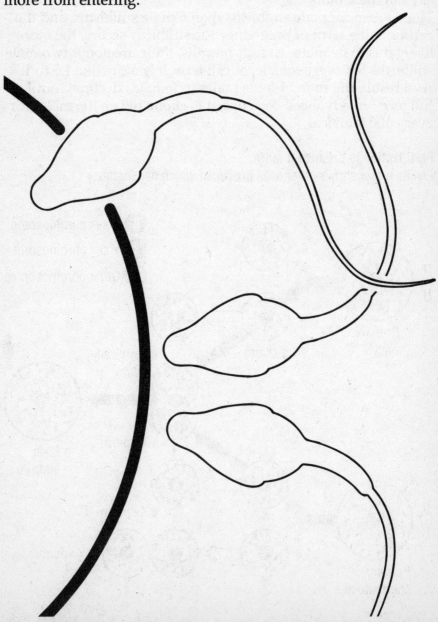

Sex Differentiation

External

Until the 8th week after conception, male and female fetuses still appear exactly the same. One week later – when the fetus is still only 1¼in (3cm) long and weighs 0.07oz (2g) – the external membrane has vanished from the genitals of the female fetus, giving entrance to a primitive vagina. Meanwhile, in the male, one end of the genital folds has begun to lengthen into a rudimentary penis. By the 11th week, the contrasting shapes of the external genitals are established.

Internal

Inside the fetus the process is more complex and drawn out. In the undifferentiated fetus there are two tube systems: the Müllerian and the Wolffian ducts. But in the female, between the 7th and 9th weeks, the Wolffian tubes almost disappear, while the lower Müllerian tubes combine to form the vagina. Then, more slowly, through to the 34th week, the undifferentiated sex glands (gonads) turn into primitive ovaries, and the upper Müllerian tubes become the Fallopian tubes. In the male, in contrast, it is the Müllerian tubes that disappear. The gonads migrate to the scrotum to become testes, and the Wolffian tubes each develop into a vas deferens.

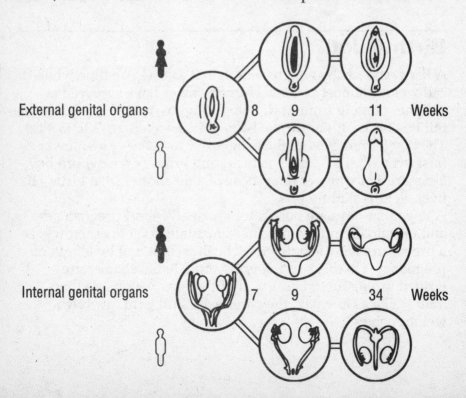

External genital organs   8   9   11   Weeks

Internal genital organs   7   9   34   Weeks

The Growing Fetus

Human development in the womb is faster than at any time
after birth. The drawings show the change in proportion of an
average fetus in 4-week stages. As the fetus grows it moves
and changes position in the womb.

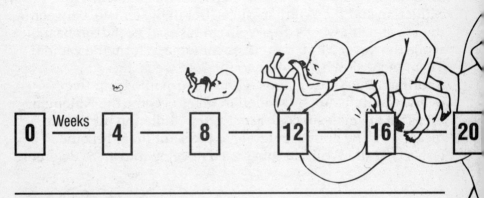

| 0 | Weeks 4 | 8 | 12 | 16 | 20 |

Birthweight

A kangaroo's baby weighs less than 0.05oz (1g), a blue whale's
calf weighs almost 10 tons. Human babies have survived at
weights ranging from under 2lb (0.9kg) to over 29lb (13.15kg) –
but it is far healthier for the baby to be an average 7½lb (3.4kg).
The boy's average is slightly higher (7½ – 3.4kg), girls' lower
(just over 7lb – 3.17kg). The heart and lungs of a newborn boy
are marginally bigger than those of a newborn girl at birth. His
liver weighs slightly less.

A few more boys are born after unusually short pregnancies
and marginally more girls after unusually long ones. However,
a premature baby is defined by birth weight, not by length of
pregnancy. On this basis, slightly more female babies are
termed 'premature', because slightly more weigh less than
5½lb (2.5kg). However, they are really 'full term low birth
weight babies.'

1

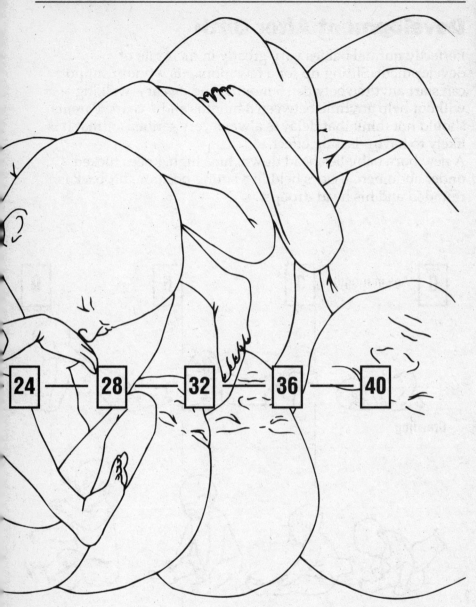

24 — 28 — 32 — 36 — 40

Underweight or overweight, babies that deviate far from the average are less likely to survive. Babies of average weight have a death rate of under 2%; babies weighing 6 or 9lb (2.72 or 4.08kg) 3%, and babies weighing 4½lb or 10¼ lb (2.04 or 4.76kg) a 10% death rate. Those far below average who do survive are more likely to be handicapped.

Development After Birth

Perfectly normal babies vary greatly in their rate of development. Sitting up for a few moments without support can start anytime between 5 months and a year – walking without help anytime between 8 months and 4 years. Parents should not think that delay is always very serious, or that it is likely to have a lasting effect.

A new born baby lies head down, hips high, knees tucked under abdomen. If he is held in a sitting position, his back is rounded and his head droops.

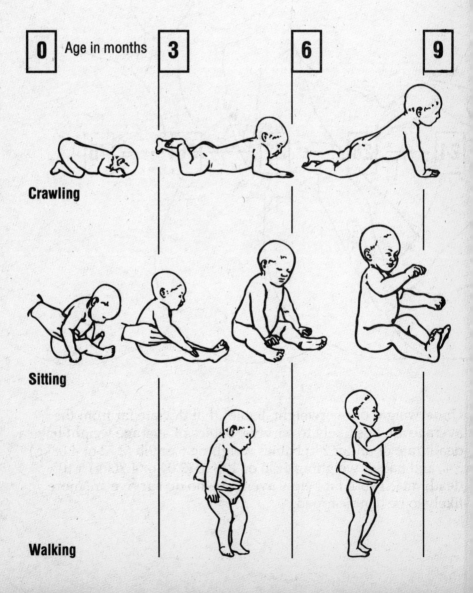

| 0 | Age in months | 3 | 6 | 9 |

Crawling

Sitting

Walking

Between one and three months, he begins to lift his chin off the ground for a moment, and lift his head for a moment if held sitting. But if held standing, he sags at the knees and hips. By about six months, he can support himself on his arms, sitting, and can bear his own weight if held standing. Between eight and ten months, he begins to be able to crawl on hands and knees, to sit and lean forward without support, and to hold himself upright. At a year he can creep like a bear, on hands and feet, turn around as he sits, and walk with one hand held. At 13 months, he can walk alone.

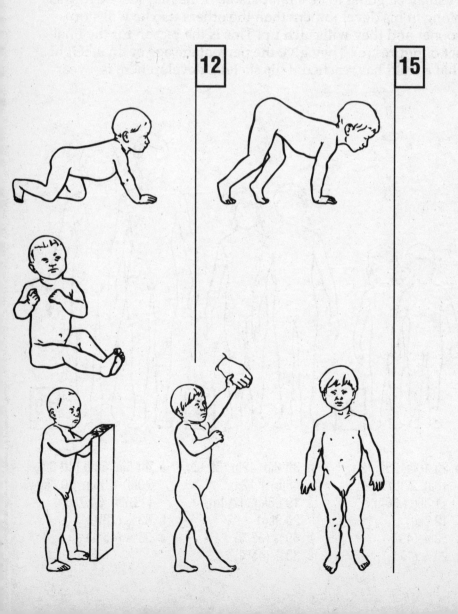

Growth, Height and Weight

The first set of figures (**a**) give typical heights and weights for each age (figures for girls in brackets). The next set (**b**) tells you how much of his final adult height a boy is likely to have achieved at each age, eg 78% at age 10. The third set (**c**), so you can calculate, from his actual height, how tall a boy will be as an adult, eg a boy 4ft 8in (142.24cm) at 10 is likely to be almost 6ft (182.88cm).

Such predictions are averages only. In fact there are two reasons why a child may be taller than average at a given age. He may be going to be a tall person, or he may just be further along in his development than the others – so he will stop sooner and they will catch up. This is the reason for the final set of figures (**c**). They give the percentage age of final height that a child has reached if his skeletal development is a year

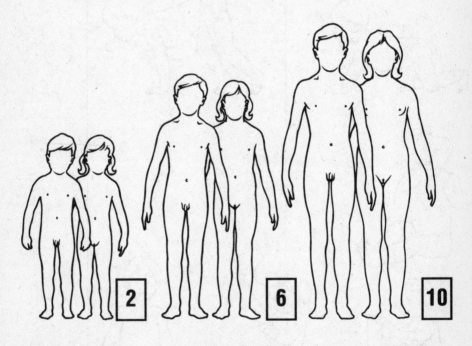

a 2ft 10in, 25lb (2ft
   10in, 27lb) .86m,
   11.3kg (.86m,
   12.2kg)
b 53% (49%)
c 20% (17%)

a 3ft 8in, 42lb (3ft 9in,
   46lb) 1.12m,
   19.05kg (1.14m,
   20.9kg)
b 69% (65%)
c 33% (45%)

a 4ft 5in, 68lb (4ft 6in,
   70lb) 1.35m, 30.8kg
   (1.37m, 31.7kg)
b 83% (78%)
c 53% (45%)

ahead (first figure), or a year behind (second figure), the average. For example, a 10 year old boy of advanced development will have grown 79.7% of his final height – he has not much further to go. The same age boy with slow development has only grown 76.4% of his final height. So these figures give a more accurate prediction if the child's physical development is not average. Scientists use X-rays of bone formation to determine skeleton age – but you can get a rough idea by noting the child's development of permanent teeth. Compare the ages his teeth appear with the ages on pp 188-191. If they appear at the earlier age, his development is advanced; if at the later age, slow; if between, average.

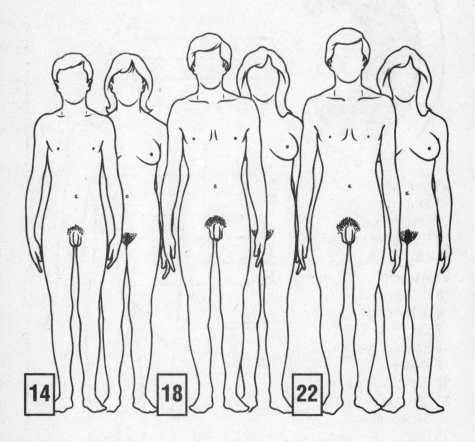

14

18

22

a 5ft 2in, 109lb (5ft 3in, 108lb) 1.57m, 49.4kg (1.60m, 49kg)

b 97% (91%)

c 85% (70%)

a 5 ft 4in, 125lb (5ft 8in, 143lb) 1.63m, 56.7kg (1.75m, 64.9kg)

b 100% (99%)

c 98% (92%)

a 5ft 4in, 128lb (5ft 9in, 155lb) 1.63m, 58.1kg (1.75m, 70.3kg)

b 100% (100%)

c 100% (100%)

Embryo and Adult

The growing embryo of a human being only a few days old, already has three distinct layers of cells: ectoderm, mesoderm and endoderm. These will go to form different parts of the finished body.

Changing proportions

At eight weeks, the body's main divisions are already formed.

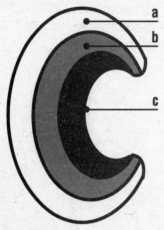

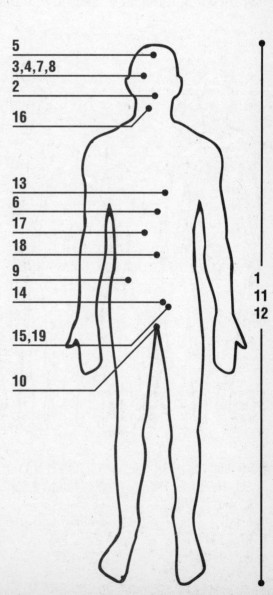

a Ectoderm
1 Skin
2 Lining of mouth
3 Conjuctiva and cornea
4 Lens

b Mesoderm
5 Brain
6 Spinal cord
7 Eye
8 Sclera of eye
9 Kidney
10 Reproductive organs
11 Cartilage and bone
12 Skeletal muscle
13 Heart
14 Uterus
15 Outer wall of gut

c Endoderm
16 Thyroid
17 Liver
18 Pancreas
19 Inner wall of gut

1

But the proportions are very different to those of an adult, or
even a baby. Only the trunk will stay constant, at three-eighths
of body length. The head, instead of forming half the body
length as at eight weeks in the womb, will be just one-fourth at
birth, and one-seventh at 25 years old. And the legs will shoot
up, from one-eight of body length, to three-eighths, and then
one-half in the adult. Compare too how long the trunk is, and
how wide the shoulders, against the head's dimensions in the
illustration below.

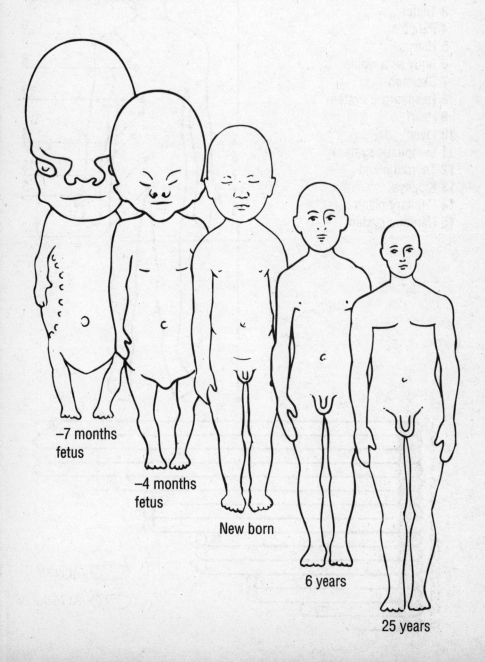

−7 months
fetus

−4 months
fetus

New born

6 years

25 years

Growth of Parts

At birth, some parts of our body still have much further to grow than others. For example, the nervous system (15) will only increase about 5 times in size, while the muscles (1) will increase 40 times.

1 Muscle
2 External genital organs
3 Testes
4 Pancreas
5 Uterus
6 Body as a whole
7 Skeleton
8 Respiratory system
9 Heart
10 Liver
11 Lymphatic system
12 Thyroid gland
13 Kidneys
14 Pituitary gland
15 Nervous system

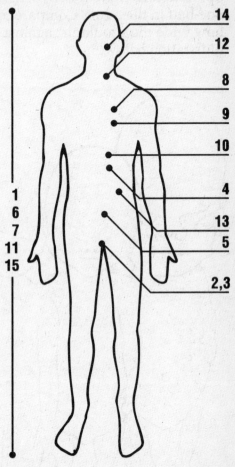

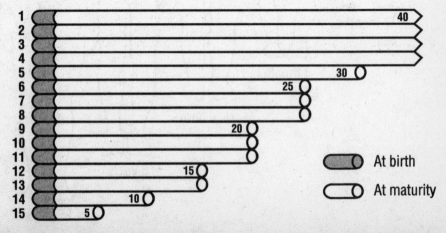

Rate of Growth of Parts

This graph shows how fast the different parts of the body
grow. Slowest are the genitals: testes, epididymides (tubes in
which spermatazoa are stored), seminal vesicles, prostate and
other sexual organs. Next in speed is the body as a whole – its
skeleton, muscles, external dimensions, blood volume and
many of its internal organs. Fastest – at first – is the central
nervous system (brain and spinal cord) and many of the
dimensions of the head. And fastest of all, for a while, is the
lymph system – only to shrink back down again. This is the
only part of the body to grow to much larger than its final size.

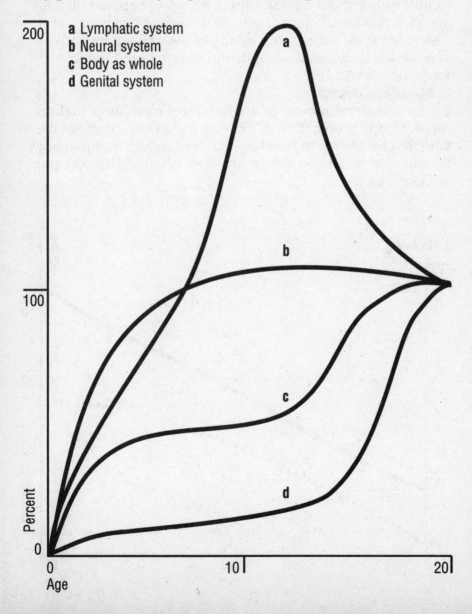

a Lymphatic system
b Neural system
c Body as whole
d Genital system

Milestones in Development

1 Throwing

Increase in throwing distance is mainly marked by development of an overarm throw. This coincides with changes in feet position to allow greater body rotation. A right-handed child uses a weight shift from rear left foot to leading right foot on delivery. In an adolescent, the shift is from rear right foot to leading left.

2 Sprinting

A simplified run begins by about 18 months, but true running (with a moment of no body support) does not appear till the age of 3. Adult running pattern is established by about 5 or 6. Thereafter speed of running is largely determined by body size, which increases the length and the strength (and so frequency) of stride.

3 Standing Jump

This shows development of the standing broad jump – taking off and landing on both feet. (The running jump confuses the situation by adding in running abilities.) Achievement in boys continues at an almost steady rate throughout childhood and adolescence.

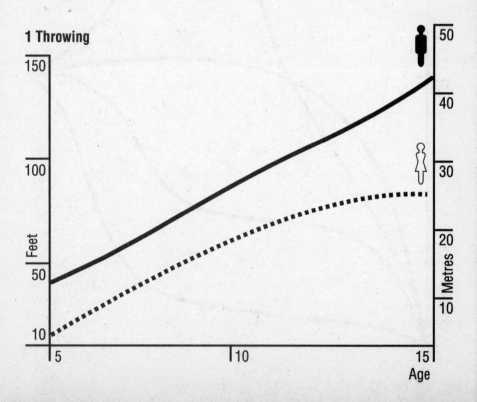

1 Throwing

2 Sprinting

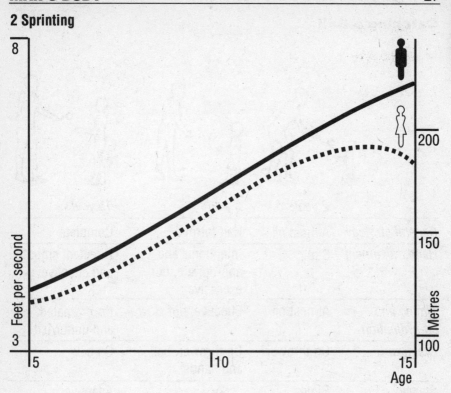

3 Standing Jump

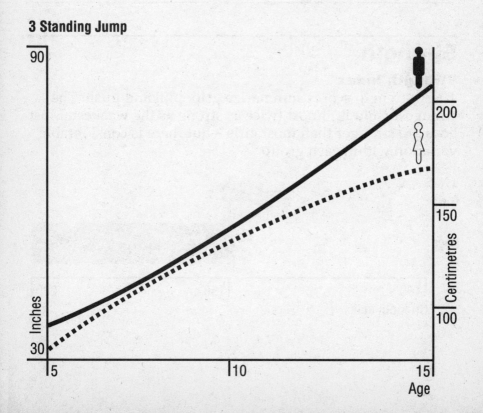

Catching a Ball

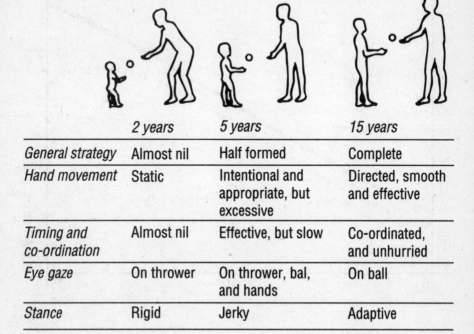

	2 years	5 years	15 years
General strategy	Almost nil	Half formed	Complete
Hand movement	Static	Intentional and appropriate, but excessive	Directed, smooth and effective
Timing and co-ordination	Almost nil	Effective, but slow	Co-ordinated, and unhurried
Eye gaze	On thrower	On thrower, bal, and hands	On ball
Stance	Rigid	Jerky	Adaptive

Strength

Strength Index

These strength scores summarize grip, pull and push. The strongest child is almost twice as strong as the weakest. Most boys are stronger than most girls – but there is considerable variation within each group.

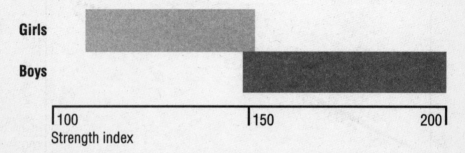

Girls

Boys

100   150   200

Strength index

Muscular strength

Here we show how different aspects of strength develop with age. The main determinant of strength is body size. This is not surprising, since muscle is 40% of body weight. But body weight only accounts for 30 to 35% of strength variation, and height for only another 10%. Age in itself (independent of growth) also shows some effect – perhaps because of developments in the centers of motor control. But strength also varies with build.

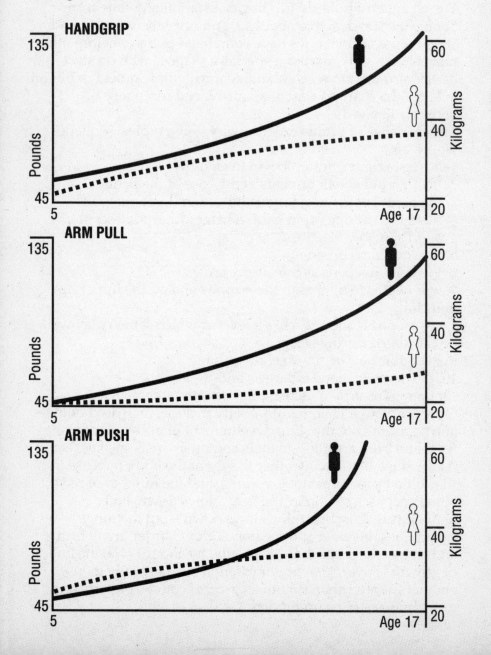

Puberty

Puberty is the time when boys and girls become able to conceive a child. In a boy, the testes start producing sperm. (In a girl, ova begin to mature, and menstruation occurs.) But this sexual fact is tied in with many other changes, affecting almost every part of the body – as well as with the long period of psychological change, leading up to adulthood, that we call adolescence.

Physical Development

The changes of puberty in a boy can start at any time from about 10 years of age to about 15, and finish between 14 and 18. So some normal boys have completed puberty before other normal ones have started (especially as those who do start earlier also tend to reach sexual maturity more quickly). But on average the changes start at about 12, and reach a peak between 13 and 14.

The sequence of events can also vary, but a typical sequence would be:

1. the testes and scrotum begin to enlarge;
2. the first pubic hair appears at the base of the penis;
3. the penis begins to enlarge; and, about the same time
4. there is a sudden rapid gain in height (the 'adolescent growth spurt');
5. the shoulders broaden;
6. the voice deepens as the larynx grows;
7. hair begins to appear in the armpits and on the upper lips and chin;
8. sperm production reaches a level at which semen may well be ejaculated during sleep;
9. the pubic hair begins to show color;
10. the prostate gland enlarges; and
11. there is a sudden increase in strength.

Other particular changes of puberty include: increased oiliness and coarseness of the skin; development of body odor for the first time from armpits, genitals and other areas such as feet. At the same time, many other tissues of the body increase in size, blood pressure, blood volume, and the number of red blood corpuscles, all rise, the heart slows down; body temperature falls; breathing slows down – but the lungs' capabilities increase; and the bones grow harder, more brittle, and change in proportion. Typically, by about $17^3/4$, the bulk of growth is over. Height, for example, usually only gains another 2% after that. (In other cases, of course, puberty and growth may still be under way.)

1

The hormones involved

The changes of puberty are produced by hormones – chemicals manufactured in certain organs of the body called glands. Hormones travel round the body in the bloodstream and affect how cells in other parts of the body work and develop. The signal to produce the hormones of puberty comes from the hypothalamus, a gland in the brain.

The signal apparently has to wait until the hypothalamus has matured to a certain point. But when it appears, it acts on the pituitary, an important gland at the base of the brain, and this begins to produce two hormones called FSH and LH. (Their full names, 'follicle-stimulating hormone' and 'luteinizing hormone', refer to their role in the female body, where they are also the trigger hormones of puberty – though more LH is produced in men.) The two hormones act, in a boy, on the testes. After about a year, while their level builds up, LH stimulation results in the testes producing testosterone, the main masculinizing hormone of puberty. Testosterone makes the penis grow, pubic hair develop, and so on. Meanwhile FSH stimulates the testes to start producing sperm. To keep a limit on the level of sexual activity, both LH and FSH are under what is called 'negative feedback control.' That is, the effects they have hinder their own production, so their level falls, until their very absence creates the conditions in which they can reappear. For example, LH stimulates testosterone production, which reacts back on the hypothalamus. As a result, the hypothalamus sends out a message cutting back

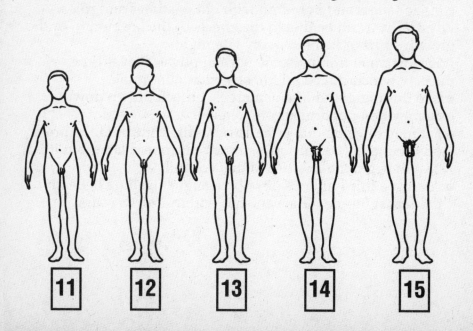

| **11** | **12** | **13** | **14** | **15** |

LH production. As LH is then no longer stimulating testosterone production, the testosterone level falls – allowing LH to start to be made again. (With FSH, the control mechanism is probably not the testosterone level.)

Influences on timing

In this century, the age of the onset of puberty in the western world has fallen steadily. The reasons are not fully understood. Rising standards of living and better health may be reasons. The age of puberty, however, is also determined by inherited family traits, nutrition level, general living conditions and physical and psychological state (mental disturbance and long childhood illness can each delay puberty).

Physical problems

Puberty can fail to occur, in rare cases, because of hormonal imbalance. Also certain disorders become more common after puberty: acute myeloid leukemia, bone cancer – and, less seriously, short-sightedness.

But many of the so-called physical problems of puberty are really only psychologically significant. Very early or late development, skin troubles and increased body odor, are all embarrassments rather than serious physical problems.

A common but temporary problem can be extreme lethargy – which is both physical and psychological in cause and effects.

Psychologically, it can be due to the great psychic changes going on at this time, which can result in anxiety, self-consciousness and boredom with old pastimes and roles. Physically, it can be due to the effects of the hormones, or the growth spurt or just too many late nights.

It is worth mentioning some normal physical events of puberty which can be misconstrued as abnormal

- The thyroid gland often enlarges, but should go down again when puberty is completed.
- Fat may develop due to faulty appetite control in the brain (not to glands or gluttony). It may disappear later, but it is best to begin the practice of diet control.
- Almost a third of boys develop a slight swelling beneath the breast nipple. This vanishes within 1 to 1½ years.

Adult Height Range

The range of the normal is fairly narrow; the range of the possible is fairly wide. A convenient example is height. Of every 100 men, 95 are between 5ft 4in (162cm) and 6ft 2in (187cm).

Average man (in USA)
Height: just over 5ft 9in (175cm)
Weight: almost 162lb (73.5kg)
Chest: 38³/4in round (98.5cm)
Waist: 31³/4in (80.6cm)
Hips: 37³/4in (95.9cm)

Male heights and weights
(*= comparable statistics for females)

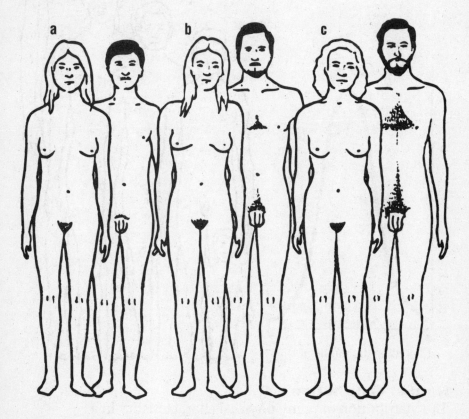

a 5ft 6in, 141lb
(167.64cm, 63.95kg)
*5ft 2in, 114lb
(157.48cm, 51.71kg)

b 5ft 10in, 156lbs
(177.8cm, 70.76kg)
*5ft 6in, 130lb
(167.64cm, 58.96kg)

c 6ft 2in, 174lb
(187.96cm, 78.92kg)
*5ft 10in, 144lbs
(177.8cm, 65.31kg)

Extremes

- the tallest man who has ever lived, whose height has been verified, was 8ft 11.1in (272cm) at death (age 22)
- the shortest man who has ever lived measured 26½ inches at death (age 19).

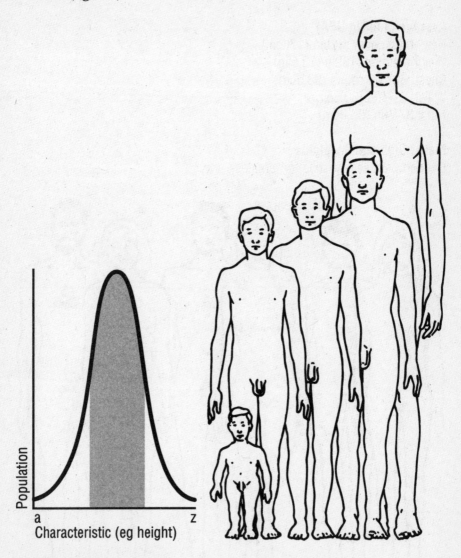

Characteristic (eg height)

Normal distribution

The distribution of many physical characteristics in a population can be summarized in a curve called the 'normal distribution' curve, shown above. The range of the characteristic goes all the way from a to z, and there are examples in the population at every point in between. But there are very few people at either of the extremes and very many in the central area.

Make-up of the Body

- Of every 100 men, 95 weigh between 127 (57.60kg) and 209lb (94.80kg). For women the figures are 95 (43.09kg) and 195lb (88.45kg).
- Of the average 162lb (73.48kg) man, about 43% of body weight is muscle, 14% is fat, 14% bone and marrow, 12% is internal organs, 9% is connective tissue and skin, and 8% is blood.
- Of the average 162lb (73.48kg) man, 47% of the weight is in the trunk and neck, 34% in the legs, 12% in the arms, and 7% in the head.
- The average man, broken down into his elements, consists of 65% oxygen, 18.5% carbon, 9.5% hydrogen, 3.3% nitrogen, 1.5% calcium, 1% phosphorus and 0.35% or less each of potassium, sulphur, chlorine, sodium and magnesium, with traces of iron, iodine, zinc, fluorine and other elements. This gives him enough water to fill a 10-gallon (45.46 litres) barrel, enough fat for 7 bars of soap, enough phosphorus for 2200 match heads, and enough iron for a 3in (7.62cm) nail.

Build

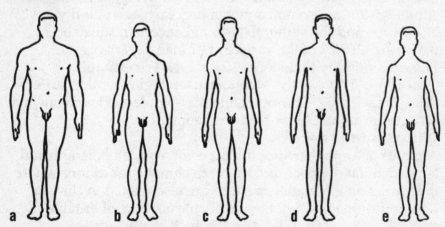

a A typical shot-putter or weightlifter. Such athletes are taller and heavier than any others, with large arms relative to their legs.

b A typical 100m or 200m sprinter – relatively short and muscular, with short legs relative to his body and large limb muscles.

c A typical modern highjumper – less ectomorph than in the past because modern Olympic heights need muscle power too. .

d A typical traditional highjumper: a fairly extreme ectomorph, with very long legs relative to his body.

e Average man.

Ethnic Differences

These days, no one is comfortable with the word 'race'; it has been too much a part of man's inhumanity to man. But patterns of ethnic variation exist, and there are fairly consistent differences in the physical characteristics of different peoples. Three great ethnic groups – Caucasian, Mongoloid and Negro – account for almost all the world's population. But sometimes the differences within each group are as large as those between them. Take, for example, skin color: Negro skin colors range from near-black to sallow; Mongoloids from yellowish to flat white to deep bronze; and Caucasians from fair and pinkish to dark brown.

Height is another extreme variable. Height relates partly to ethnic factors, but little to overall ethnic group – with certain notable exceptions, such as the Pygmy peoples of Central Africa. Average heights for a sample selection of people reveal a jumbled sequence of Negro, Caucasian, and Mongoloid characteristics (for example, Negro peoples are both shortest and tallest). Even within a people, other genetic and environmental variations prevent consistency: for example, height, being less totally inherited, can be determined more by environment than by ethnic criteria. Within a people, the ethnologist may also note much more, such as similarity in blood type and the ability to taste or eat certain substances, which are all part of the variety of human experience.

The susceptibility to diseases also varies. For example, Caucasians native to the Mediterranean region tend to suffer from Thalassemia – a form of anemia – while sickle cell anemia is common among black-skinned people.

Climatic influences

Animals of a species differ in coat color, size, limb, length and location of fat deposits, according to climatic conditions where they live. Some human variations are also related to climate. The environment did not make people acquire inheritable characteristics – but it did decide which characteristics flourished. Those people who flourished bred among themselves, and passed on these features. An inheritor who moves to a different environment carries the inherited characteristics with him and will pass the dominant ones on to his offspring.

Skin color is a well-known example. The extra melanin in dark skins gives added protection against the sun. People who live where there is little strong sunlight have pale skin, which enables vitamin D to be synthesized by the body from sunlight absorbed through the skin (see p168). Yellow skin contains a dense keratin layer that reflects light well in deserts or snow. Dark eye color and the thick, folded eyelids of Mongoloid peoples also protects against harmful radiation in sunlight. Negroid hair protects the scalp from heat, while allowing sweat loss from the neck. Straight hair, grown long, protects against the cold. Noses typically vary with air humidity. In dry conditions they are longer and narrower in order to moisten the inhaled air as much as possible. But the flat Mongoloid face developed as protection against the cold: the nose is not prominent, so it is less susceptible to frostbite. Peoples such as the Inuit, who live in the Arctic Circle, have developed facial fat as further protection against the cold.

Other features, not all inherited, that vary with climate, include average weight, which is greater the colder it is. For instance, the average Inuit man is considerably heavier than the average Spanish man. Body shape also varies: two bodies that weigh the same can have very different surface areas. Body area is larger the hotter it is, for a large area gives more skin from which to sweat and to radiate heat. Metabolic rate varies in the same way. A typical European has a 'thermal equilibrium' of 77°F (25°C) with the surrounding temperature. This means that at that temperature, naked, standing still, he shows no tendency to get hotter or colder. The Inuit's metabolic rate is 15 to 30% higher than the European's giving him a lower thermal equilibrium. Indians, Brazilians and Australians have a metabolic rate 10% lower than that of a European.

Man and woman

This shows how some characteristics of the typical man and woman compare.

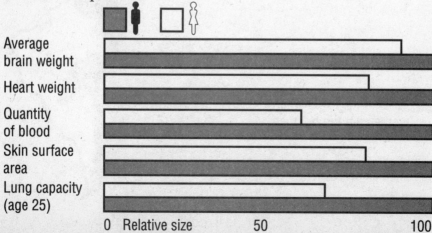

	Man	Woman

- Average brain weight
- Heart weight
- Quantity of blood
- Skin surface area
- Lung capacity (age 25)

0   Relative size   50   100

The age pattern

In most societies, more men than women are born. The ratio is generally about 105 male babies for every 100 female. But, in modern America and western European society, more males than females die at each age before old age is reached (except perhaps for a brief period during childhood). In other words, female life expectancy is longer. So the older one is, the more women of that age group there are for every 100 men. Parity between the sexes is usually reached between the ages of 30 and 40. After this, female predominance grows steadily, until at 95 a man is outnumbered 4 to 1.

Worldwide distribution

Worldwide, there are just over 100 women for every 100 men. But this ratio varies widely from country to country. In most of

Female–male ratios

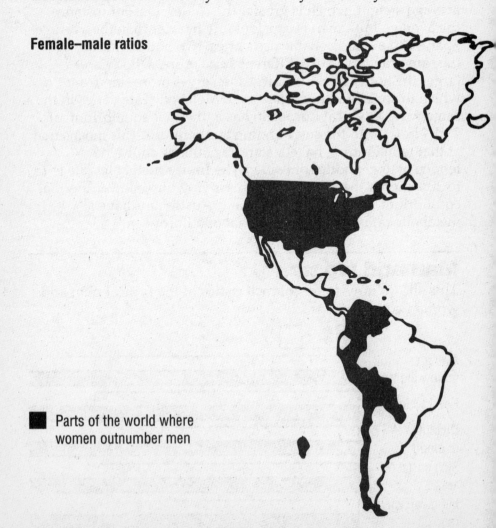

■ Parts of the world where women outnumber men

Asia and the Middle East and large parts of Africa, men
predominate; in the United States and western Europe,
women. In general, in less developed parts of the world, lack
of contraception and medical facilities increases the maternal
death rate in childbirth. Also the lower status still given to
women may still mean that more effort is made to save a male
child. Yet some less developed countries still show a female
predominance.

A male predominance can also arise because of immigration,
as in Alaska. Men are the first to go to new countries in search
of their fortune. As standards rise, the numbers of women
catch up. In the United States female predominance was not
reached until the census of 1950.

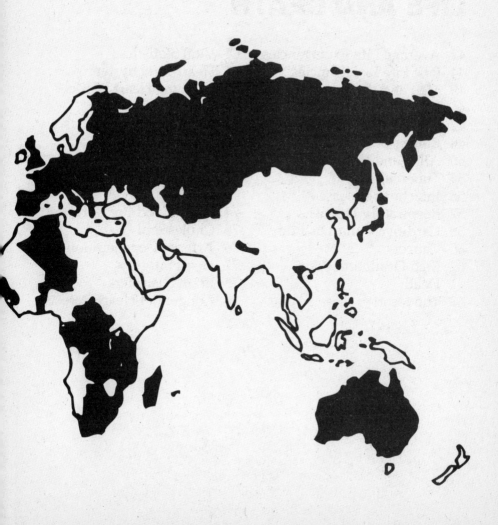

LIFE AND DEATH

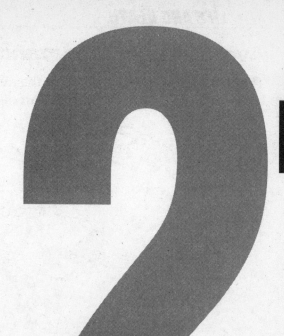

2

Average Life Expectancies

The maps show countries where the average life expectancy at birth for a child born in the first half of the 1990s is within the

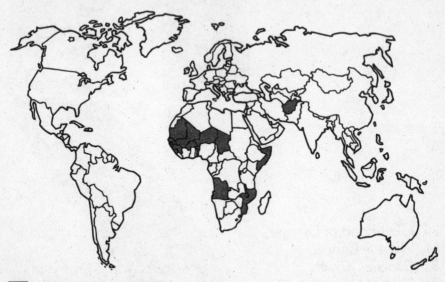

■ **Under 50 years (11%)**
Some of the developing countries in Africa have the lowest average life expectancy figures. The shortest life expectancy figure is for Sierra Leone, where men live on average until 45, women until 43.

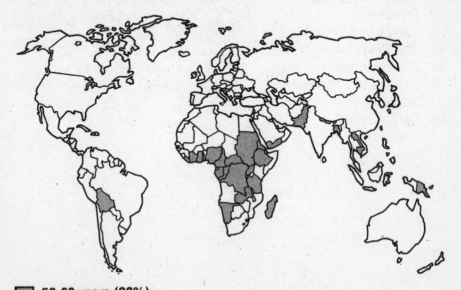

■ **50-60 years (28%)**
Included in this group is much of the rest of Africa and a few Asian countries.

age limits stated below each one. The percentage figure given
with each group shows what proportion of total world
population born in countries belonging to the different groups.

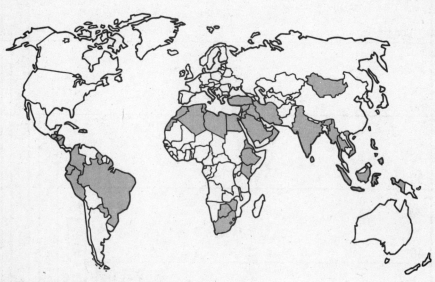

60-70 years (32%)
This group is the largest in terms of total population. It includes India
and most of South East Asia.

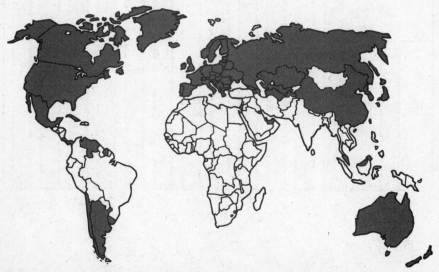

70+ years (29%)
North America, all European countries, and China are in this group.
Norway, Denmark, Sweden, Iceland and the Netherlands all have high
average life expectancy figures. The highest is Japan: women 82, men 79.

Past Life Expectancies

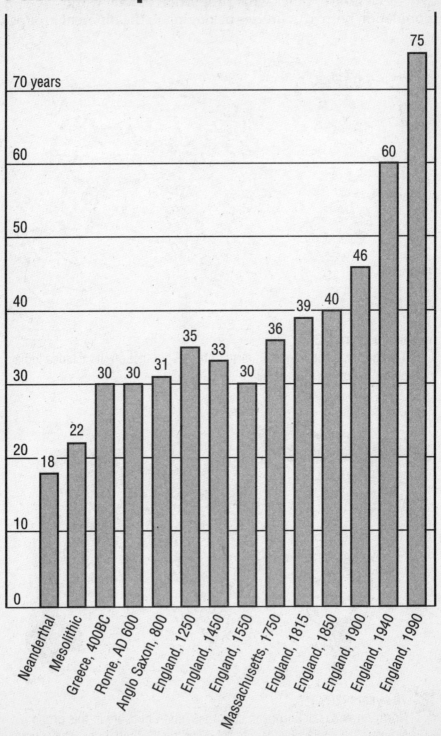

Men and Women

On average, women live longer than men in most countries of the world. (In the selection below Nepal, Bhutan and Bangladesh are the only exceptions.) But no one is quite sure why women live longer. It may be some factor in their physical constitution. Alternatively, it may be the consequence of the different types of work that men and women, at present, tend to do.

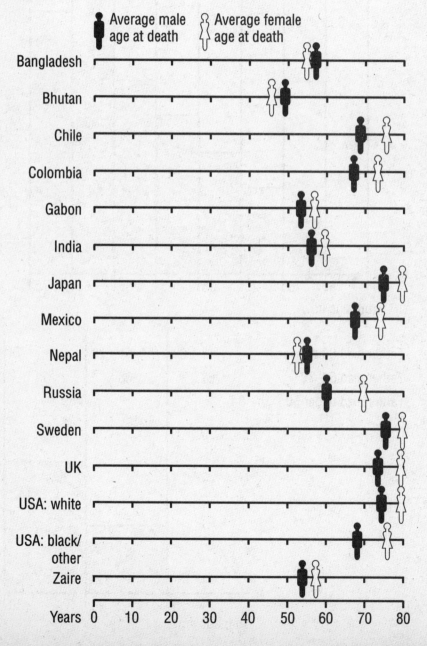

Average male age at death / Average female age at death

Bangladesh
Bhutan
Chile
Colombia
Gabon
India
Japan
Mexico
Nepal
Russia
Sweden
UK
USA: white
USA: black/other
Zaire

Years 0 10 20 30 40 50 60 70 80

How Long Will I Live?

Look at the bottom of this first table, and find your age now.
Then look up the column – the number at the top is the age
men can expect to live to. But you are likely to live longer if
your father also lived to an old age – as the second table shows.

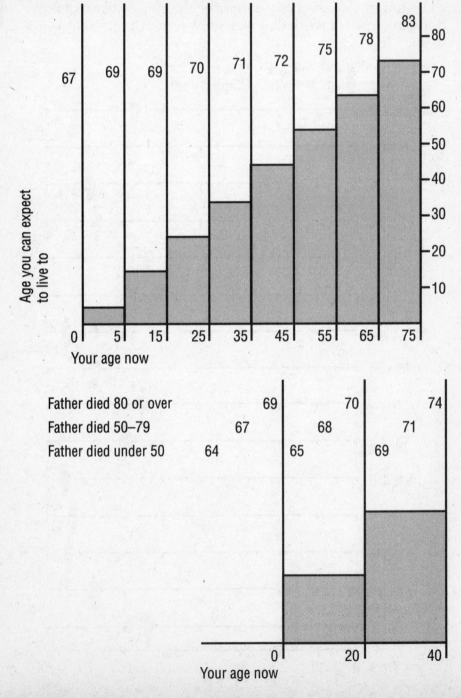

67	69	69	70	71	72	75	78	83

Age you can expect to live to

Your age now: 0 5 15 25 35 45 55 65 75

	Your age now 0	Your age now 20	Your age now 40
Father died 80 or over	69	70	74
Father died 50–79	67	68	71
Father died under 50	64	65	69

Your age now

Survival Patterns

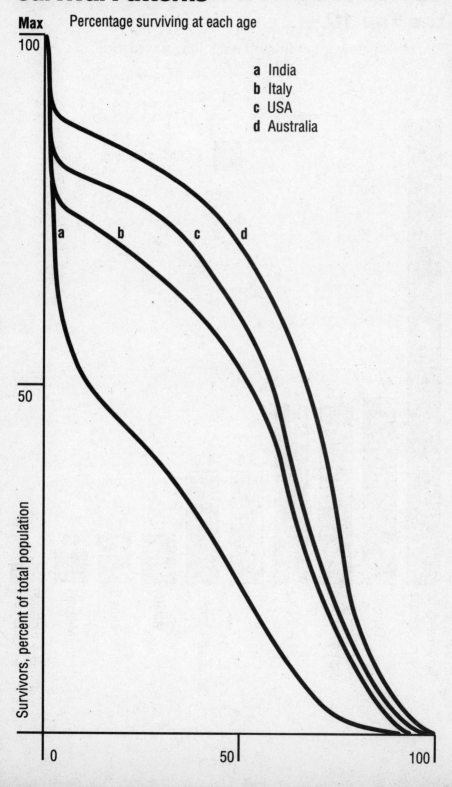

Percentage surviving at each age

Max
100

a India
b Italy
c USA
d Australia

2

50

a b   c   d

Survivors, percent of total population

0   50   100

Causes of Death Worldwide: the Top 10

The table below gives the top ten killers worldwide.

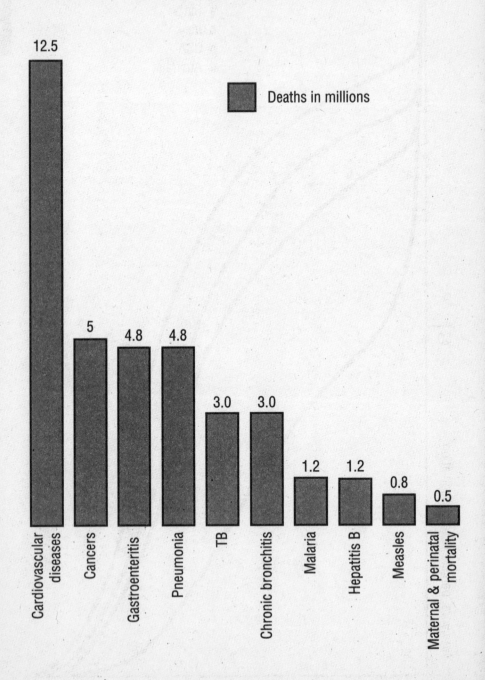

Deaths in millions

Cause	Deaths in millions
Cardiovascular diseases	12.5
Cancers	5
Gastroenteritis	4.8
Pneumonia	4.8
TB	3.0
Chronic bronchitis	3.0
Malaria	1.2
Hepatitis B	1.2
Measles	0.8
Maternal & perinatal mortality	0.5

The table below gives the major causes of death in the United States.

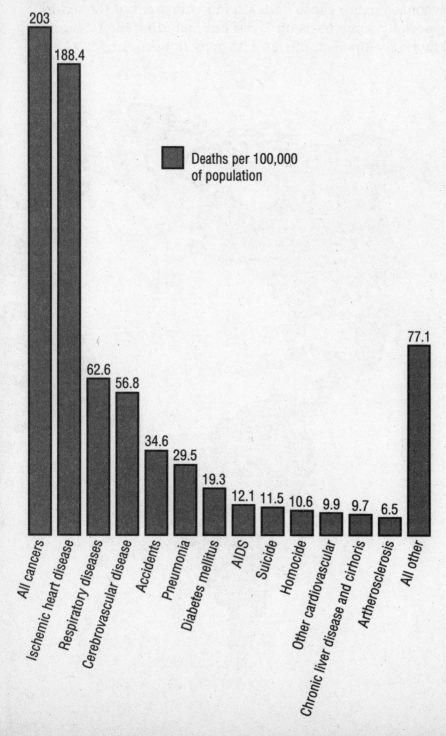

Deaths per 100,000 of population

Cause	Deaths per 100,000
All cancers	203
Ischemic heart disease	188.4
Respiratory diseases	62.6
Cerebrovascular disease	56.8
Accidents	34.6
Pneumonia	29.5
Diabetes mellitus	19.3
AIDS	12.1
Suicide	11.5
Homocide	10.6
Other cardiovascular	9.9
Chronic liver disease and cirrhoris	9.7
Artherosclerosis	6.5
All other	77.1

AIDS and HIV

The Human Immunodeficiency Virus (HIV) and the Aquired
Immune Deficiency Syndrome (AIDS) that it produces have
become a major cause of death in many areas of the world,
especially some parts of Africa but including the USA and
other developed countries. HIV may not produce any

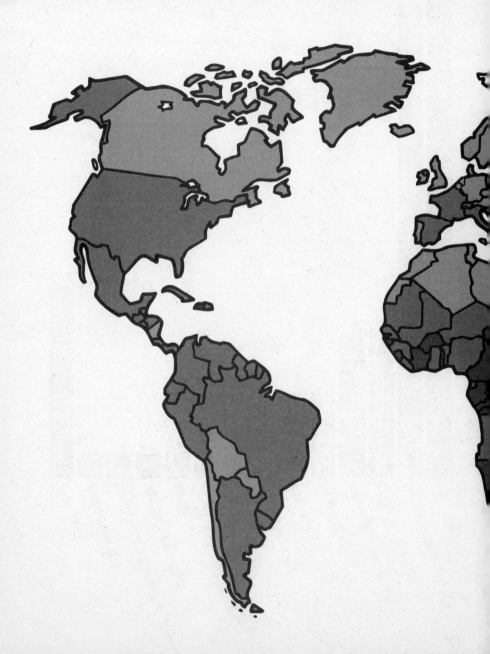

Prevalence of HIV infection (per 10,000 population)

- Less than 1
- 1 - 10
- 10 - 100
- 100 - 1000

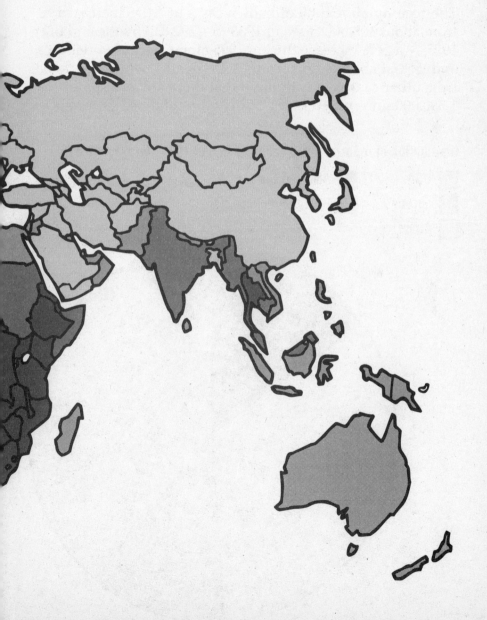

symptoms until long after it has been contracted so that infection may be transmitted by people who do not realise they have the disease.

Figures for people who are HIV+ (who carry the virus) are based on estimates, since so many are unaware that they are infected but in 1994 the World Health Organization estimated that some 17 million people were HIV+. They also estimate that figures will have quadrupled by the end of the millenium.

The accumulative total of known cases of AIDS increased from about 108,000 cases in 1988 to 1,292,810 by the end of 1995 — a 26% increase during 1995 alone. Because prejudice and lack of knowledge lead to AIDS deaths being reported as from other causes, it is thought that there are also some 1,500,000 unreported cases. Many more of those suffering

Distribution of reported AIDS cases up to end 1995 : total 1,291,810

- USA
- Europe
- Africa
- Asia and Oceana
- Rest of Americas

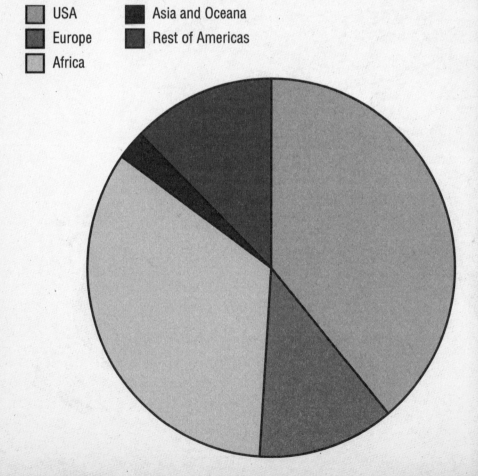

from HIV will go on to develop full blown AIDS.

The 501,310 reported AIDS cases in the US equal almost half the world total and more than those in the whole of Africa, although WHO estimated that of those globally with HIV at the end of 1994 some 11.2 million, 66%, lived in sub-Saharan Africa.

HIV is now the eighth leading cause of death in the US, accounting for 2%, fourth for those under aged 65 at 9% and the leading cause for persons aged 25-44 at 19%. HIV is not passed on through everyday contact but through transmission of body fluids mainly through unprotected sex, sharing equipment for injecting drugs and from infected mother to unborn child. It can be avoided by adopting safe practices to avoid infection (see pp151-2).

Estimated actual AIDS cases up to end of 1995 : total 6,000,000

- USA
- Europe
- Africa
- Asia and Oceana
- Rest of Americas

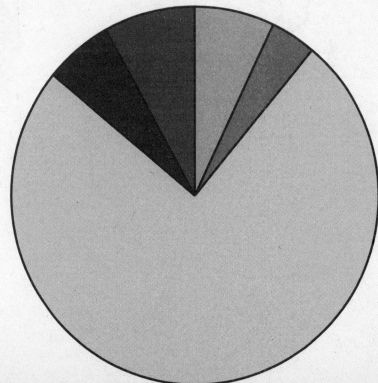

Tuberculosis

Tuberculosis re-emerged in the industrialized world during the early 1990s after a century of improvement and gradual abolition. In the United States the number of cases reported increased by 16% in the first half of the decade.

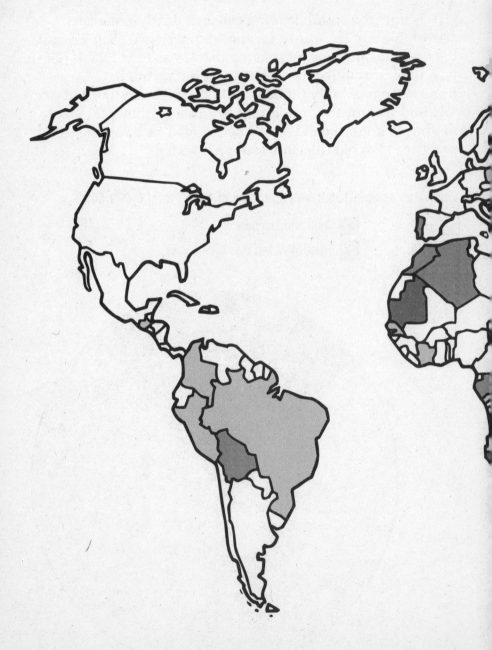

Reported new cases of TB per 100,000 of population 1990-1994

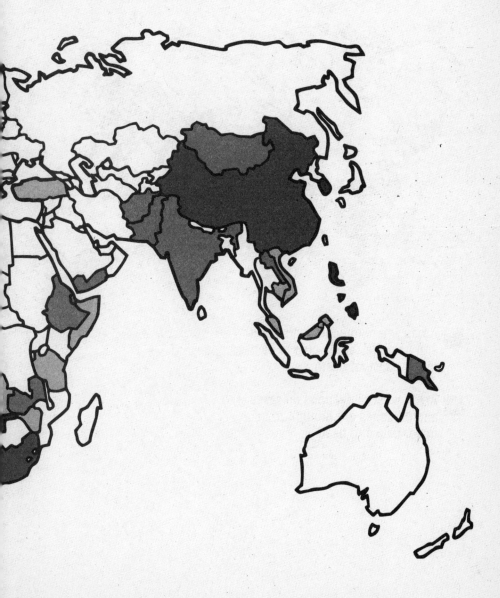

More than 200 new cases

More than 150 new cases

More than 100 new cases

More than 50 new cases

2

Infectious Diseases

These are the killers in the poorer parts of the world: dysentery and diarrhea, malaria, schistosomiasis, filariasis, river blindness, Chagas' disease, Leishmaniasis, leprosy, African sleeping sickness, hepatitis B and measles.

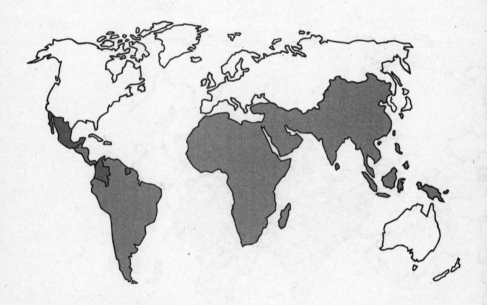

■ Areas where infectious diseases and parasites are known to be a major cause of death

■ Areas where infectious diseases and parasites are thought to be a major cause of death

Respiratory Diseases

Now that habitual smoking has spread to women and is
becoming widespread in the Third World, respiratory diseases
are a scourge of rich and poor countries. In more than 30
countries, more than 50% of men now smoke. Worldwide
annual deaths from pneumonia now total 4.8 million; from
chronic bronchitis 3 million. In the United States about 160,000
die from bronchitis every year.

2

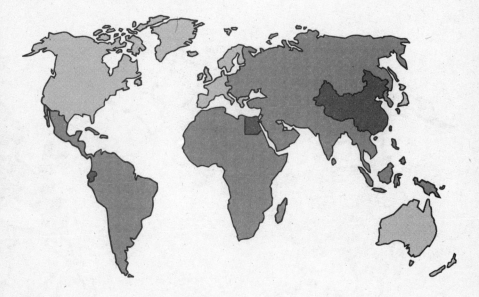

■ Countries where respiratory
diseases are a major cause of
death

▦ Countries where chronic
bronchitis kills 6% of the
population

□ Countries where chronic
bronchitis kills 3% of the
population

Cardiovascular Disorders

The affluent world can deal with infection, but its life-style creates its own problems: degeneration of the blood vessels, thromboses and embolisms, high blood pressure and heart failure.

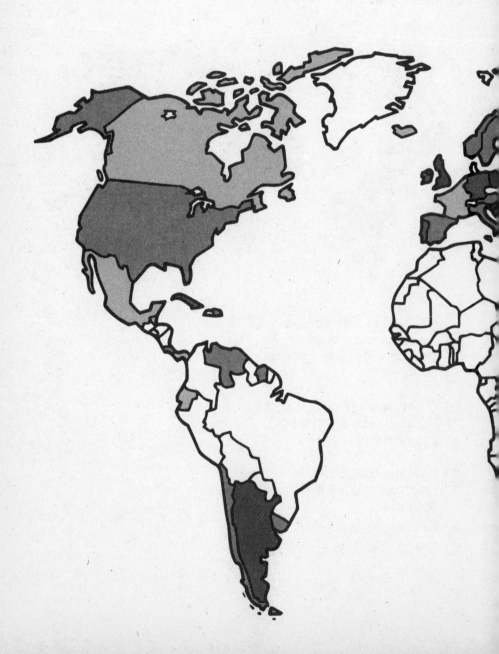

Areas of the world where cardivascular disease is a major cause of death (per 100,000 population).

- More than 500 deaths
- More than 400 deaths
- More than 300 deaths
- More than 200 deaths

2

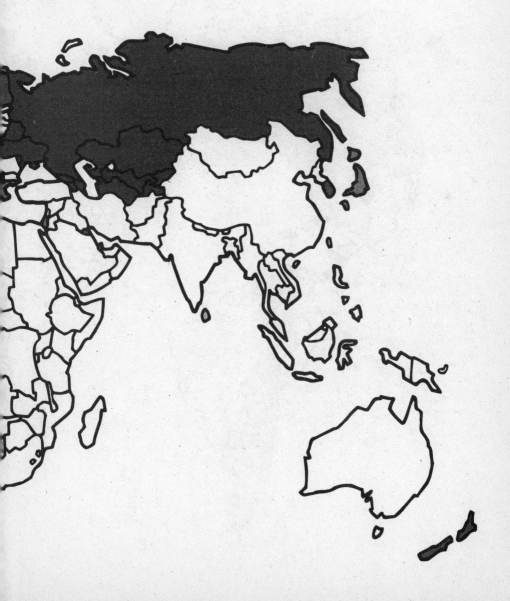

Cancers

One of the main problems of western society: cancers of the lung, intestines, prostate, lymph glands and stomach; cancers of the breast, ovary and uterus in woman; and leukemia.

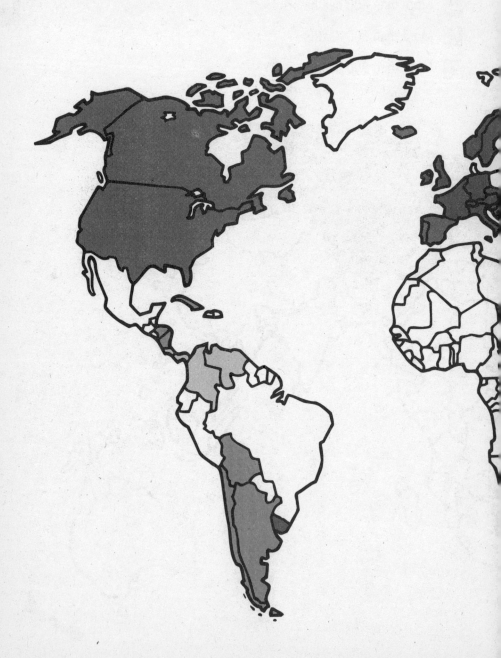

Annual deaths from cancer worldwide per 100,000 people.

More than 200

More than 150

More than 100

More than 50

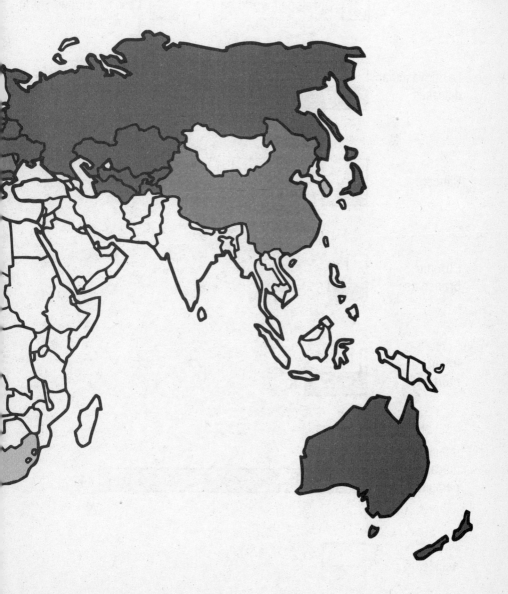

Rich Death and Poor Death

The table below shows the percentage of deaths accounted for by certain major causes in developed and developing countries. The more developed countries have more heart disorders, the less developed more infectious diseases and higher maternal and infant mortality.

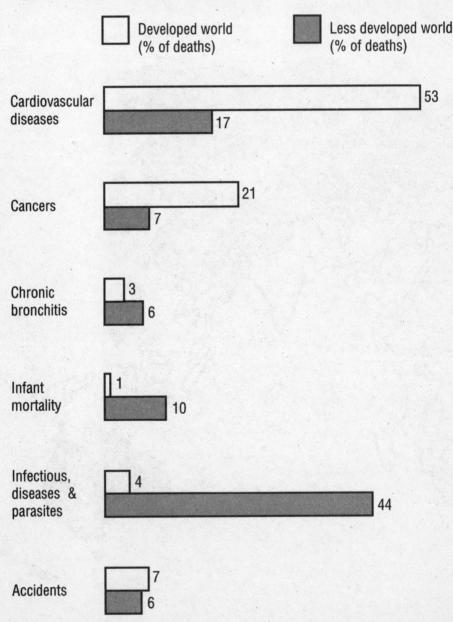

Developed world (% of deaths)

Less developed world (% of deaths)

Cardiovascular diseases
53
17

Cancers
21
7

Chronic bronchitis
3
6

Infant mortality
1
10

Infectious, diseases & parasites
4
44

Accidents
7
6

The Heart

The blood system supplies the cells of the body with oxygen and nutrients, and carries away waste materials.

The heart is the vital center of this, being the pump that drives blood through the body. It weighs under 1 pound (0.45kg), measures on average about 5in (12.5cm) long by 3$\frac{1}{2}$in (8.75cm) wide, and comprises four muscular chambers.

The heart is positioned under the rib cage and in front of the lungs. It lies on the center line of the body, but not symmetrically: one end slants out to a point just to the left of the breastbone (sternum). The heartbeat is most noticeable here, giving the impression that the heart lies on the left side of the body.

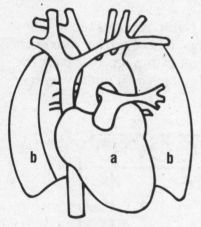

Exterior view

a Heart
b Lungs
c Aorta
d Right atrium
e Left atrium
f Right ventricle
g Left ventricle

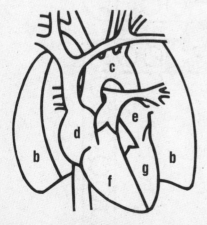

Sectional view

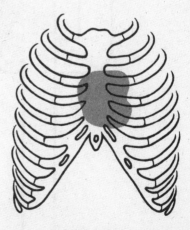

Position of heart

Vital Statistics

The adult heart beats 60-80 times a minute, and about 40 million times a year.

The smaller the heart, the faster it beats. An average male heart is about 10 ounces in weight, and a female heart 8 ounces. So a woman's heart makes about 6 to 8 more beats a minute than a man's.

At each beat the heart takes in and discharges over $1/4$ pint (.14 litre) of blood. It pumps over 2000 gallons (9100 litres) a day, and 50 million gallons (227 million litres) in a lifetime. In a healthy man the heartbeat during exercise may increase to 180 beats a minute, pumping 40 pints (22 litres) a minute.

Heart-lung System

The heart is really two pumps. One pump receives blood from the body and sends it out to the lungs, where carbon dioxide is exchanged for fresh oxygen. The other pump receives back the oxygenated blood from the lungs, and speeds it on its way to the rest of the body.

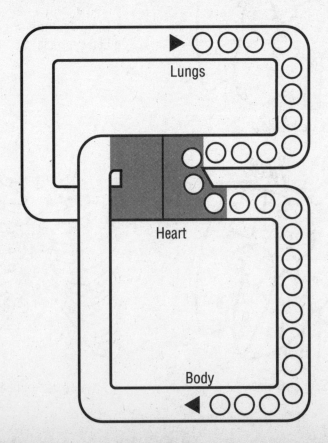

How the Heart Works

The heartbeat is in two stages: contraction and relaxation. As the heart begins to contract, both atria and both ventricles are already full of blood.

The left atrium and ventricle contain deoxygenated blood, the right contains oxygenated blood.

1 The atria contract slightly before the ventricles. This builds up the pressure in the ventricles. **2** Eventually back pressure closes the valves between the atria and the ventricles. **3** The ventricles contract, and pressure forces open the valves between the ventricles and the arteries that lead from them. From the right ventricle, deoxygenated blood is sent to the lungs. From the left, oxygenated blood from the lungs is sent out to the body. **4** When most of the blood has passed, the valves close, because there is no longer enough pressure to keep them open. The heart relaxes, and atria and ventricles begin to fill with blood. After about 0.4 seconds, a nerve impulse triggers off the next contraction.

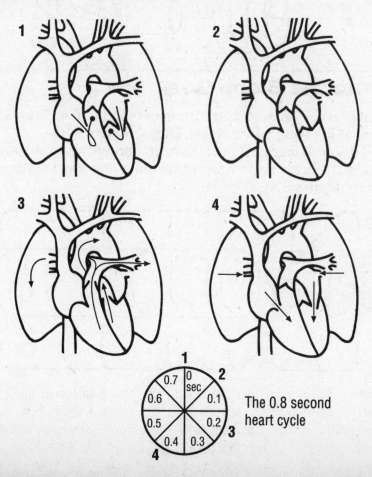

The 0.8 second heart cycle

Blood Vessels

Blood vessels are of three types: arteries, veins and capillaries. Arteries carry oxygenated blood from the heart to all parts of the body. They have strong elastic walls that squeeze the blood along with waves of contraction. After profuse branching the blood passes via the arterioles through the tissues of the body in tiny (thin-walled) capillaries, where nutritive substances and oxygen are exchanged for waste products. The blood is then conveyed back through the venules and to the heart along veins. These have thinner walls than the arteries, and contain valves to prevent a back flow of blood.

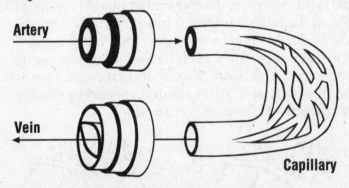

Where the Blood Goes

This shows the relative distribution of blood to the various organs of the body when at rest. During exertion, the distribution changes. At rest, the heart-lung-heart route takes 6 seconds, the heart-brain-heart route 8 sec, and the heart-toe-heart route, 16 sec.

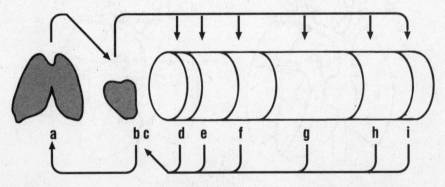

a Lungs
b Heart (right)
c Heart (left)
d Heart blood vessels 5%
e Brain 15%
f Muscles 15%
g Intestines 35%
h Kidneys 20%
i Skin, skeleton, etc 10%

Blood Pressure

Blood pressure is expressed in two figures that indicate the pressures in the aorta: on contraction, called systolic pressure; and on relaxation, called diastolic pressure.

For a healthy young man at rest the systolic pressure is usually between 100 and 120mm Hg, and the diastolic between 70 and 80mm Hg. ('Hg' is the height of a column of mercury measured in millimeters.) Pressure in the right ventrical only rises to about 20mm Hg. This is enough to send blood through the lungs and back to the left ventricle.

Pressure variations in the system

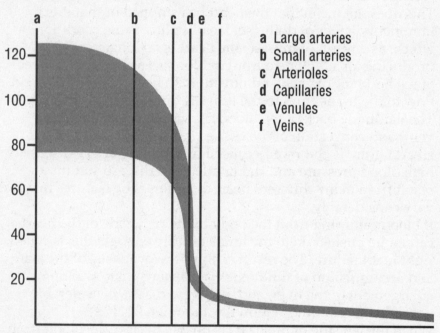

a Large arteries
b Small arteries
c Arterioles
d Capillaries
e Venules
f Veins

Heart Disorders

Angina pectoris

Angina is the Latin word for 'sore throat' and persists in that sense in the name 'Vincent's angina' — a severe infective ulceration on the tonsils. Nowadays, the word is used almost exclusively to refer to the pain or gripping sensation felt in the center of the chest when more work is demanded of the heart muscle than its blood supply, through the coronary arteries, can support. Coronary artery blood carries oxygen and fuel (glucose) to the heart muscle and if this is insufficient, pain-stimulating substances are produced by the muscle.

The symptoms can vary in intensity and may be severe and frightening. The pain often spreads up the neck and down the left arm. It is brought on by physical exertion, emotional tension, a heavy meal or cold weather. The symptom is quickly relieved by resting or by drugs, such as nitroglycerine, which temporarily widen the coronary arteries. Angina is a symptom, not a disease, but it is nearly always an indication of atherosclerosis of the coronary arteries (see pp 76-7). The arterial narrowing that is a feature of this disease is the cause of the inadequacy of coronary blood flow.

Heart failure

This does not mean that the heart has stopped or that it is in imminent danger of doing so. Heart failure is the condition in which, as a result of disease, the heart is no longer capable of producing an adequate output of blood so as to meet the needs of the body for oxygen and nutrition. In heart failure the blood flow to the tissues and to the lungs is diminished and slowed. The damming back of the blood causes engorgement of the veins and congestion of the tissues, leading to symptoms.

Heart failure is commonly caused by coronary artery disease, high blood pressure and rheumatic heart disease, but may result from many different heart disorders. The features may vary considerably.

If blood returning from the body to the right side of the heart cannot be pushed on to the lungs quickly enough, this is called right heart failure. The result is blueness (cyanosis) of the skin and accumulation of fluid (edema) causing ankle swelling, enlargement of the liver, and, in severe cases a considerable accumulation of fluid within the abdomen (ascites).

When the left side of the heart is unable to clear the blood from the lungs quickly enough, there is fluid accumulation in the lungs. This is called left heart failure. The main feature is breathlessness. This may occur on mild exertion or even when the affected person is at rest. There may be attacks of sudden breathlessness during the night. As the condition worsens, the tendency to breathlessness increases. Eventually, the degree of disability becomes extreme and the state pitiful. In both right and left heart failure there is severely restricted activity.

Heart failure can usually be helped, especially if the underlying cause of the heart damage is remediable. The drug digitalis is valuable in increasing the strength and effectiveness of the heart beat (contraction) and its use often greatly improves the condition. Other stimulating drugs, such as norepinephrine, may also be used. Fluid in the lungs and the tissues can be removed by the use of diuretic drugs, which greatly increase the urinary output. Free fluid in the abdomen may sometimes be sucked out through a wide-bore needle.

2

Heart attack

A coronary thrombosis, or heart attack, is usually described by doctors as a 'myocardial infarction'. This is the result of an obstruction to blood flow in one of the branches of the two coronary arteries through which the heart muscle is supplied with blood. Because it must beat (tighten or contract) continuously, the heart has a considerable oxygen and fuel (sugar) requirement. Any substantial diminution in this fuel supply to any part of the muscle interferes, not only with its ability to function, but even with its survival as a living tissue. The arterial obstructive disease, atherosclerosis, is present, to some degree, in most adults in the Western world, and affects particularly the coronary arteries. The disease is much worse in men than in women before the menopause and increases in both sexes with age. This is why coronary thrombosis is responsible for about half of all deaths in Western countries and is generally regarded in medical circles as the major problem in preventive medicine.

Blockage of a main coronary artery branch (coronary thrombosis) occurs when blood is prompted to clot by a roughened plaque of fatty, degenerative, cholesterol-containing material called atheroma (see pp 76-7) in the inner lining of the vessel. Cholesterol (see p 298) has an important role to play in the body but excess in the bloodstream can be deposited on the walls of arteries as part of these atherosclerotic plaques which, prior to the thrombosis, cause no symptoms, nor any other indication of their presence, until they narrow the artery so severely — to less than half its normal bore — that the blood flow is insufficient to permit full exertion. At rest, the person affected may seem normal, but a fixed amount of exertion causes the heart pain of angina pectoris (see pp 67-9).

When total blockage occurs, part of the heart muscle loses its blood supply and dies. Depending on the size of the artery blocked, this dead area may involve the full thickness of the heart wall, or only part. The heart cannot continue to function as a pump if more than a certain proportion of the muscle is destroyed. Blockage of a major branch, with destruction of about half of the muscle in the main, left, pumping chamber, is almost always immediately fatal. Previous smaller attacks make death more likely.

Coronary thrombosis usually causes a severe pain, or sense of pressure, in the center of the chest. The pain often spreads through to the back, up into the neck, or down either arm. There is often extreme restlessness, and a horrifying sense that one is about to die. The pulse is weak, difficult to feel and often irregular. Sometimes it is very slow. Severe pain is not always a feature. In less major cases pain may be absent and there is evidence that up to 20% of mild coronaries are not recognized as such by those affected. This means that there are millions of people who, because of previous unrecognized attacks, are much more vulnerable than average.

Half of those who die from a particular attack do so, from heart stoppage (cardiac arrest), within three or four hours of onset, so there is always great urgency to get a person with a coronary thrombosis to hospital with minimum delay. Many who might have been saved have died because they did not recognize or believe that they had a life-threatening condition. Factors which increase the risk of coronary thrombosis are, or should be, well known. They are:

- smoking
- lack of exercise
- a high fat diet
- a lack of adequate levels of the antioxidant vitamins C and E
- parents who died of arterial disease.

Only the latter factor is beyond individual control and there is now ample evidence that people able to benefit by advice are now reducing the likelihood of having a heart attack by changing their lifestyle. Since these facts have been widely known, the incidence of coronary thrombosis has declined significantly in certain social groups. Regrettably, all have not seen the light. In a study of 7735 middle-aged men, coronary thrombosis was found to be 44% higher in manual workers than in non-manual workers. This was attributed mainly to cigarette smoking, obesity and lack of exercise in leisure time. A strategy for the prevention of coronary artery disease, based on the concordant views of experts from 19 countries, has been published. The main points are directed to the eradication of smoking, reduced cholesterol intake with emphasis on unsaturated fat and high fiber content, and the promotion of exercise. The aim was to reduce obesity, lower blood cholesterol levels and reduce blood pressure. There is particular emphasis on encouraging social pressures against smoking. In recent years, the importance of antioxidant vitamins has become apparent.

Rheumatic heart disease

In spite of the name, rheumatic fever does not seriously affect the joints, and, although arthritis does occur, this is fleeting and does not produce any permanent disability. Rheumatic fever is important because of the frequency with which it affects the heart and because of the severity and permanence of the resulting damage. Happily, rheumatic fever is becoming rare in the US. The Centers for Disease Control reported in 1989 that the incidence of rheumatic fever, nationwide, had dropped to only about 1.3 cases per million.

The cause of the disease is unknown, but rheumatic fever always follows a throat infection with a particular strain of streptococcus – the Group A hemolytic streptococcos. It is not caused by the normal processes of infection and is generally believed to be some form of immune system disorder induced by streptococci. No positive proof of this has yet appeared. It can always be prevented by prompt treatment of the streptococcal throat infection with antibiotics. The avoidance of overcrowding and of other conditions promoting the spread of respiratory infection is also important in prevention.

The heart involvement is often insidious and there may be no symptoms until a late stage. The commonest and most serious effect on the heart is a fibrous thickening and scarring of the valves, with narrowing or leakage. This may seriously interfere with the heart's action and cause severe secondary effects on the health of the affected person, even heart failure (see pp 67-9). Heart valve replacement may be necessary.

Blockage and Tissue Death

Thrombosis

This means clotting of blood within an artery or vein. This is always abnormal and often dangerous as it may restrict or even totally cut off the flow of blood. Thrombosis, when it affects vital arteries, such as the coronary arteries to cause a coronary thrombosis (heart attack), or the arteries supplying the brain with blood to cause a cerebral thrombosis (stroke), is a major cause of death and serious illness. Thrombosis of arteries supplying the limbs leads to pain, disability and, if severe, even gangrene and loss of the limb. The arteries to the intestines sometimes suffer thrombosis, leading to gangrene of a segment of bowel, calling for emergency surgery. Thrombosis seldom occurs in healthy arteries because the smooth inner lining prevents the starting of the sequence of events that leads to blood coagulation. Injury to a vessel, or any disease process affecting the smoothness of the inner lining may, however, initiate thrombosis. By far the commonest cause of thrombosis is the common artery disease atherosclerosis (see pp 76-7). Even when arteries are normal, a clotting tendency may, rarely, occur as a result of hormonal or biochemical changes in the blood. The tendency to thrombosis in arteries may be greater during pregnancy, in women using oral contraceptives, in people with cancer which has affected vessels, and in people whose blood is more viscous than normal (polycythemia). Thrombosis in veins is encouraged by local pressure, inflammation (thrombophlebitis), and stagnation of blood flow, as occurs in varicose veins.

The clot (thrombus) which forms in arteries is called a white thrombus. It is securely fixed and tends to progress in layers until the artery is blocked. Thrombi in deep veins are red, soft, loose, and easily detached, and may break loose to cause embolism. Thrombosis may be prevented by the use of anticoagulant drugs, such as heparin and warfarin, and the risk can be reduced, to some extent, by small daily doses of aspirin. The use of enzymes to break down the thrombus ('fibrinolytic therapy'), as soon as possible after its formation, is an important factor in treatment. There is good evidence that the combination of birinolytic drugs, such as streptokinase, with aspirin, can significantly reduce the death rate from coronary thrombosis.

Embolism

This is the sudden blocking of an artery by solid, semi-solid or gaseous material brought to the site of an obstruction in the bloodstream. The object, or material, causing the embolism is called an embolus (plural emboli). It is always abnormal for any non-fluid material to be present in the circulation, and because blood proceeding through arteries encounters ever smaller branches, such material will inevitably impact and cause blockage, thereby depriving a part of the body of its essential blood supply.

Many different forms of emboli can occur. Embolism is commonly caused by blood clot emboli, often arising in the veins and passing through the right side of the heart to enter the arteries carrying blood to the lungs. It may also be caused by:

- crystals of cholesterol from plaques of atheroma in large arteries
- clumps of infected material in severe injuries
- air or nitrogen in diving accidents
- bone marrow and fat in fractures of large bones
- tumor cells and other substances.

The chief danger in deep vein thrombosis is the formation of long, soft, snaky blood clots which may become very large before breaking loose into the bloodstream. Such clots pass quickly through the right side of the heart and impact in the main branches of the arteries to the lung. This is called pulmonary embolism and is a common cause of sudden, unexpected death. Similar, but smaller, emboli may form on the inner lining of the heart, often on the left side, after a coronary thrombosis. These can be carried upward to cause embolism in vital brain arteries, leading to stroke. Small cholesterol emboli, arising from disease of the carotid arteries, commonly cause 'mini-strokes' (transient ischemic attacks).

A. A thrombosis in the leg (**a**) may become detached and cause an embolism at (**b**).

B. Three pulmonary embolisms showing their areas of effect.

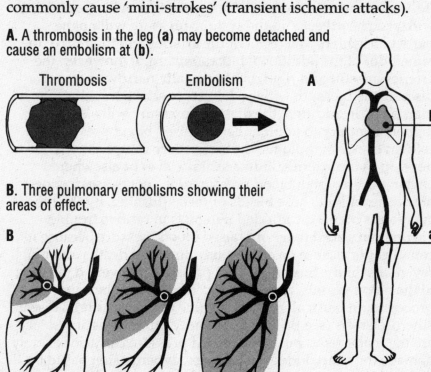

Thrombosis   Embolism   A

B

High Blood Pressure

Abnormally high blood pressure is called hypertension. The circulation is a closed system in which, under the influence of the tightening (contractions) of the chambers of the heart, the pressure varies constantly, rising to a peak (the systolic pressure) soon after the contraction, and falling to a lower level (the diastolic pressure) between heartbeats. Because of this dynamic situation, a person's blood pressure cannot be represented by a single figure, but is given as two numbers, the systolic first and then the diastolic, commonly thus: 120/80. These numbers indicate the pressure in terms of the distance in millimetres which a column of mercury would be forced up a glass tube by the pressure.

Blood pressure also varies constantly with the level of physical exertion, with anxiety, emotional stress and other factors. So a single measurement is not significant and the blood pressure should be checked repeatedly under resting conditions, at different times.

If the main arteries are healthily elastic, they will stretch a little with each heartbeat and the systolic pressure will not be particularly high. The recoil of the arteries will then drive the remainder of the additional blood onward. If, however, the arteries are stiff and rigid, or abnormally narrowed from disease, the pressure with each heart contraction will rise to a high peak. In addition, the diastolic pressure will also be higher. Contrary to popular belief, raised blood pressure seldom causes symptoms until secondary complications develop in the arteries, kidneys, brain, eyes or elsewhere. Uncomplicated high blood pressure does not cause dizziness, headache, fatigue, nose bleeds or facial flushing. By the time symptoms occur, the affected person is in serious trouble.

No one can afford to ignore raised blood pressure because its complications cause an enormous number of deaths and much severe disability. Sustained high pressures are very damaging to the blood vessels, causing an acceleration of the aging processes. In particular, they promote the killer arterial disease atherosclerosis (see pp 76-7). Coronary thrombosis and stroke are the major risks, but raised blood pressure can also severely damage the heart, kidneys and eyes. Hypertension has to be looked for, and every adult should have regular checks. Fortunately, proper and effective treatment can largely eliminate the additional risk of these serious complications. In many cases, the change to a healthy, natural lifestyle with regular exercise, reduced food intake, no smoking and perhaps a reduction in salt intake will be sufficient to get the blood pressure down to normal. Regular visits to a physician for check-ups will give confidence and help to reduce stress levels. The three main classes of drugs used to treat hypertension are:

- diuretics, which act on the kidneys to cause them to pass more water and salt in the urine and reduce the volume of the blood, so bringing down the pressure
- beta blockers, which interfere with the hormone and nervous control of the heart, slowing it and causing it to beat less forcefully, so reducing the pressure
- vasodilators, which act on the arteries to widen them. This group contains drugs acting in different ways. They include the alpha blockers, the calcium antagonists, and the ACE inhibitors.

In some cases the drug treatment of hypertension may cause the patient to feel worse for a time, rather than better. Until readjustment to normal pressures has occurred there may be weakness, lack of energy, depression and a tendency to dizziness or faintness on standing up.

Cholesterol

Cholesterol is a waxy substance produced in the liver, and also acquired from outside in certain foods, especially animal fats, milk products and eggs. It is found throughout the body, but especially in the brain, nervous tissue and adrenal glands. It is important in the repair of ruptured membranes, and in the production of sex hormones and bile acids. Blood cholesterol level varies with age, sex, race, hormone production, climate and occupation, and is thought to depend mainly on the amount manufactured in the body. Surplus adrenalin, due to stress situations, may be one cause of excess cholesterol. However, nutrition does not affect the level to some extent - though in this the cholesterol content of the diet seems less significant than the fat content. A diet rich in 'polyunsaturated fatty acids' (i.e. those of most vegetable oils) can lower the blood cholesterol level if saturated fat consumption is reduced.

High cholesterol level

Cholesterol is a main part of the substance deposited on the arterial walls in atherosclerosis. It has been established that heart disease is more common in those with a high blood level of cholesterol than in those with a low level, though no reason for this has been demonstrated to everyone's satisfaction.

Arterial Degeneration

Atheroma

This means, literally, 'a lump of porridge'. Atheroma is the degenerative, fatty material containing cholesterol and other fats, broken down muscle cells, blood clot, blood-clotting elements (platelets) and fibrous tissue, which forms on the inner surface of arteries and which eventually may lead to obstruction and serious blood deprivation.

Atheroma is deposited. Clots of blood adhere to it. Finally a large thrombus blocks the artery. But blood may find ways through, or take alternative routes.

Atheroma forming inside an artery leading to atherosclerosis

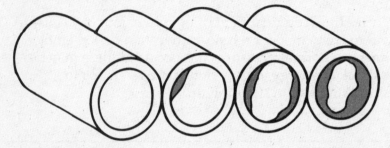

Atherosclerosis

This form of arterial degeneration is the number one killer of the Western world. It is a disorder of arteries in which fatty plaques (atheroma) develop on the inner lining of arteries so that the normal flow of blood is impeded. Atherosclerosis affects almost everyone, the earliest signs being apparent in childhood, and the condition is, in general, steadily progressive with age. Although most arteries are affected, those in which the condition is most dangerous are the coronary arteries supplying the heart muscle with blood, and the carotid and vertebral arteries and their branches, which supply the brain. Atherosclerosis of these two systems leads, respectively, to coronary thrombosis and stroke.

Atherosclerosis is responsible for more deaths than any other single condition and it should be the object of everyone to delay, or halt, the progress of the disorder. This can be achieved by adopting a number of life principles. The informed and responsible person will:

- eat little more than is required to maintain normal body weight
- avoid saturated fats (from dairy products and meat)
- take exercise to the point of breathlessness, once a day
- never smoke cigarettes

• drink alcohol in moderation
• have regular blood pressure checks
• take adequate antioxidant vitamins C and E.

Arteriosclerosis

This word, once widely used, has become so imprecise that it is now seldom heard in medical circles. Literally, it means 'hardening of the arteries' (see above under **Atherosclerosis**) which more accurately describes the common degenerative disease of arteries.

Aneurysm

Aneurysm is a bulge in the wall of a vein or artery at a weak point. Under pressure of blood, the aneurysm may balloon out, and finally break, spilling out blood.

Heart Surgery

Before the development of the heart-lung medicine, sugeons could only carry out heart operations that did not interfere with the heart's pumping action. For if the flow of oxygenated blood to the body stops, brain damage and death follow within 4 minutes due to lack of oxygen. Nowadays, the heart-lung machine take-over the functions of the heart and respiratory system, while the heart is being operated on. Usually, the two large veins that lead into the right atrium are connected to the machine instead. Deoxygenated blood flows into the machine, where it is mixed with oxygen, in a way similar to the lungs' processes, and the blood flows back into the body through a connection to one of the branches of the aorta. This allows sufficient time for certain procedures, especially
• closure of actual or ventricular septal defects (see p 80) or
• replacement of diseased valves, such as the aortic or mitral. (The mitral valve is that between the left atrium and left ventricle, and is often damaged in cases of rheumatic fever). Difficulties that can arise afterwards, especially when the machine is used for longer than normal, include: kidney damage and psychological psychosis (from which recovery usually occurs). Both are possibly due to the pressure output of the machine being too low for pumped blood to reach some tissues.
Other surgical techniques include:
• replacement of segments of coronary artery or aorta;
• artificial pumping aids for the left ventricle; and
• use of artificial,'pacemakers' to stimulate the heartbeat.

Brain Disorders

Arteriosclerosis Psychosis

Atherosclerosis can impair the blood supply to the brain. It is a condition usually associated with old age, but may occur earlier. An affected person feels restless and emotional, is inclined to wander at night, and complains of headaches, giddiness and momentary blackouts. Memory may fail and strong personality traits become exaggerated. These symptoms fluctuate.

As the physical change is permanent, treatment concentrates mainly on creating a relaxing environment. Drugs may be used when the person is overactive or worried (sedative), or depressed (anti-depressant); also to try to increase cerebral circulation (but this usually has little effect).

'Stroke'

Technically known as a cerebrovascular accident (CVA), a stroke results from failure of the blood supply to a part of the brain. This may be due to a thrombosis or embolism, or to a hemorrhage in the brain from a ruptured blood vessel. Infarction (death) of part of the brain may occur. A stroke is more common in men than women. It can vary in severity from a minor disturbance, forgotten in a few minutes, to a major attack causing unconsciousness and death. The severity depends on the position and extent of the damage. In a severe attack, the patient loses consciousness almost immediately. Death may then follow in a matter of hours; alternatively, consciousness is regained, but there is usually lasting damage. An attack may also show itself in sudden paralysis of one side or part of the body, without loss of consciousness. Or, again, it may develop over several hours, with persistent throbbing headache, vomiting, dizziness and numbness of the limbs. Recovery depends on age, general health, and the site and size of damage. Even if recovery is possible, it may take years. In some cases, control of the body has suffered permanent damage, with muscles paralyzed or very weak. The effects occur in the opposite side to the side of the brain affected (because one side of the body is controlled by the opposite side of the brain). A stroke in the side of the brain that is 'dominant' may also affect speech. Mentally, concentration may be impaired, but judgment and basic personality need not be. Treatment consists mainly of rest and prolonged convalescence, with careful nursing, physiotherapy and (if needed) speech therapy.

Drugs are sometimes used to lower the blood pressure, if it is high, and so help prevent further damage.

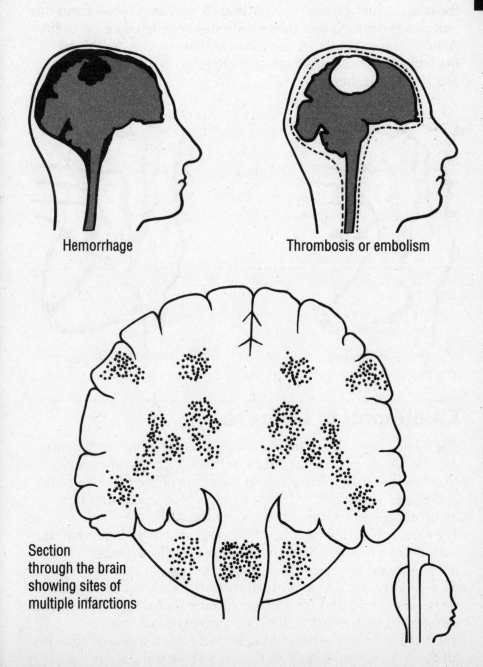

Hemorrhage

Thrombosis or embolism

Section through the brain showing sites of multiple infarctions

Congenital Heart Defects

Two common types of congenital heart defect are shown here: atrial septal defect (**a**) which is the presence at birth of a large hole between right and left atria; and ventricular septal defect (**b**) which similarly is the presence of a hole between right and left ventricles. In each case, because pressure in the left side of the heart is higher, the result is that oxygenated blood from the left passes through and mixes with deoxygenated blood in the right.the heart is higher, the result is that oxygenated blood from the left passes through and mixes with deoxygenated blood in the right.

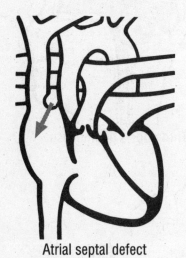

Atrial septal defect

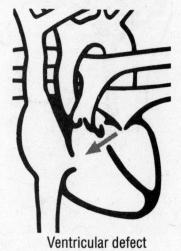

Ventricular defect

Likelihood of Disease

These diagrams show the likelihood of a person getting heart disease (i.e. angina, heart attack or death). They compare the likelihood at different ages, and the effect of the three biggest and most measurable risk factors: high blood pressure, high blood cholesterol level and cigarette smoking.

They show how the likelihood changes with age. For example, with no risk factor, a 35-year-old man is in little danger – but his likelihood has risen considerably by age 50, and again by 65. Similarly, for a man with all three risk factors, likelihood rises between 35 and 50. But then it falls slightly by 65, because so many of the easiest victims are by then dead.

The final bar shows that the likelihood for a woman of 65, with all the risk factors, is only 2/3 that of a 65-year-old man.

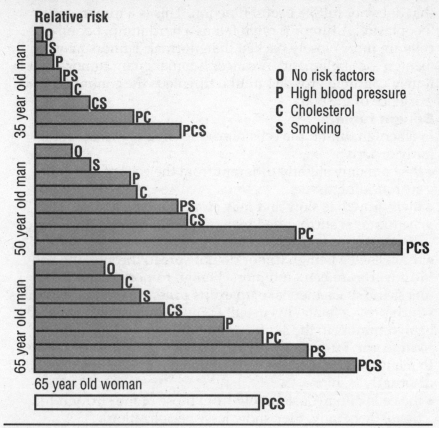

Relative risk

35 year old man
- O
- S
- P
- PS
- C
- CS
- PC
- PCS

50 year old man
- O
- S
- P
- C
- PS
- CS
- PC
- PCS

65 year old man
- O
- C
- S
- CS
- P
- PC
- PS
- PCS

65 year old woman
- PCS

O No risk factors
P High blood pressure
C Cholesterol
S Smoking

2

What is Cancer?

Cancer is one of several disorders which can result when the process of cell division in a person's body gets out of control. Such disorders produce tissue growths called 'tumors'. A cancer is a certain kind of tumor. Cancer attacks one in every four people.

Normal Cell Division

The body is constantly producing new cells for the purpose of growth and repair – about 500,000 million daily. It does this by cell division – one parent cell divides to form two new cells. When this process is going correctly, the new cells show the same characteristics as the tissue in which they originate. They are capable of carrying out the functions that the body requires that tissue to perform. They do not migrate to parts of the body where they do not belong; and if they were placed in such a part artificially they might not survive.

Tumors

In a tumor, the process of cell division has gone wrong. Cells multiply in an uncoordinated way, independent of the normal control mechanisms. They produce a new growth in the body, that does not fulfil a useful function. This is a tumor, or 'neoplasm'. A tumor is often felt as a hard lump, because its cells are more closely packed than normal. Tumors may be 'benign' or 'malignant'. A cancer is a malignant tumor. That is, it may continue growing until it threatens the continued existence of the body.

Benign tumors

In a benign tumor, the cells reproduce in a way that is still fairly orderly;

- they are only slightly different from the cells of the surrounding tissue;
- their growth is slow and may stop spontaneously;
- the tumor is surrounded by a capsule of fibrous tissue, and does not invade the normal tissue; and
- the cells of a benign tumor do not spread through the body.

Most warts are benign tumors. Benign tumors are not fatal unless the space they take up exerts pressure on nearby organs which proves fatal. This usually only happens with some benign tumors in the skull.

Malignant Tumors

In malignant tumors, the cells reproduce in a completely disorderly fashion;

- the cells differ considerably from those of the surrounding tissue (generally, they show less specialization);
- the tumor's growth is rapid, compared with the surrounding tissue;
- the tumor has no surrounding capsule, and can therefore invade and destroy adjacent tissue;
- the original tumor is able to spread to other parts of the body by metastasis and produce secondary growths there; and
- a malignant tumor is usually fatal if untreated, because of its destructive action on normal tissue.

Biopsy

A biopsy is the most certain way of distinguishing between benign and malignant tumors. A piece of the tumor is surgically removed, and then studied under a microscope.

Cancer Growth

Cell division

Cancerous cells cannot divide faster than normal cells. But normal cell division reaches its maximum rate only in times of injury and repair. Cancerous growths are continually producing cells at this maximum rate without check. They are

Cell structure of healthy and unhealthy tissue growth

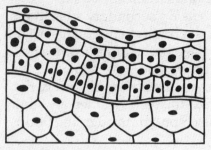

Normal body tissue

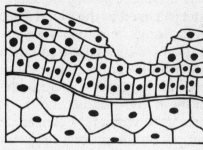

Damaged body tissue

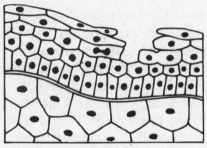

Normal cell replacement

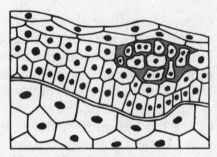

Abnormal malignant growth

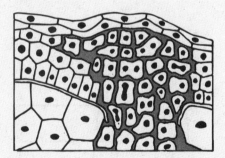

Loss of basement membrane integrity

less successful than normal tissue could be, because many of the faulty cancerous cells die. Nevertheless, the result is that cancerous growths grow faster than normal tissue.

Metastasis

Metastasis is the process by which cancerous cells travel from the original (primary) cancer site to other parts of the body. It occurs when cancerous cells get caught up in the flow of blood or lymph. The cells are carried along in the vessels, until they lodge in another part of the body. If they succeed in establishing themselves there, this becomes a new (secondary) cancer site. If a secondary site gets large enough, it can also metastasize in turn.

Cancer that has metastasized along the lymph vessels normally sets up its secondary sites in the glands. Cancer that has metastasized in the blood stream sets up secondary sites in the bone, lungs, and liver. Cancers in the brain do not metastasize, but cancers elsewhere can metastasize to the brain. Some sites are more receptive than others. Common locations for secondary growths include the lungs, the bones, the brain, the kidneys, the bladder and the larynx, the testes in men and the breasts in women. A cancer can also spread through the body simply by the process of growth.

Sites of Cancer

Cancers can grow almost anywhere in the body, but the most common sites are shown here. Cancers are classified by the kind of tissue in which the primary growth occurred. Tumors originating in the 'epithelial' cells (e.g. skin, mucous membrane and glands) are called carcinomas; those in connective tissue (e.g. muscle and bone), sarcomas. Secondary sites are classified by the kind of primary tumor that they came from. This is possible because metastasized growths still show some of the characteristics of the tissue from which they originally came.

**The most common
cancers: USA**
a Lung
b Prostate
c Digestive
d Colon/rectum
e Urinary
f Pancreas
g Stomach
h Esophagus
i Lymph glands (not shown)
j Leukemia (not shown)

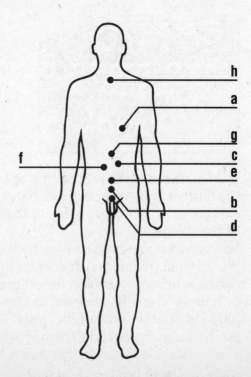

Common Cancers

Lung cancer

This is one of the most deadly forms of cancer if the tumor is malignant, for it is not usually diagnosed until too late. The tumor begins in the walls of the bronchial passages or sometimes in the body of the lung, and usually produces no symptoms until it has become firmly entrenched in the lung tissue and has even metastasized. Only one in twenty cases lives for more than two years after lung cancer has been diagnosed. Lung cancer is very much associated with cigarette smoking. Over 95% of all lung cancer patients are smokers or victims of secondary smoking.

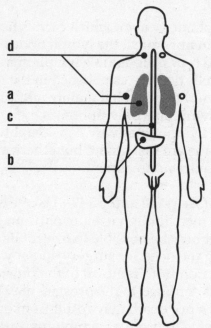

Lung cancer metastasis
Primary site:
a lung

Secondary site:
b liver
c spine
d lymph nodes

Leukemia

The leukemias are a form of cancer that affect the blood cells, causing them to reproduce without control. If untreated, they increase very fast and eventually replace the platelets, red blood cells and other blood components. Death occurs from infection or from a lack of red blood cells.

The different types of leukemia affect different blood cells. Leukemia can be caused by radiation, by viruses, by some cytotoxic (anti-cancer) drugs and by some industrial chemicals. In many cases, however, the cause is not known.

Leukemia may be acute (appearing suddenly) or chronic (developing over time). This type of leukemia tends to affect the young and people from middle age on. Chronic leukemia, which is more common in men, develops gradually over up to 20 years. It tends to affect the over-50s.

Symptoms of leukemia include lack of color, tiredness and paleness. Infections are common since there is shortage of normal white blood corpuscles. The legs and feet may swell, and there may be diarrhea.

Advances in treatment in recent years has resulted in a higher cure rate for certain leukemias, especially if they are diagnosed in the early stages. Treatment is usually by chemotherapy. Blood or white cell transfusions, antibiotics, surgical removal of the spleen, and bone marrow removal, or transfusion after total body radiation are other types of treatment, some are still at an experimental stage.

Lymphomas

These are cancers of the lymphatic system, which carries tissue fluid to the body cells. They mainly affect the lymph nodes and the spleen. There are two types: Hodgkin's lymphoma, in which very large abnormal cells become established in the body; and non-Hodgkin's lymphoma, which mainly affect the body's B-lymphocytes. The symptoms of lymphomas are similar to those of leukemia. Lymphomas vary considerably in their degree of immunity. Some are malignant, but others may take years to develop and require no treatment.

Male specific cancers

Cancer of the prostate gland (see p 142 and p 147-8) is one of the most common cancers in men, though usually only among older men. In younger men it may be possible to control its growth, avoiding or delaying the need for surgery and any interference with sexual function from removal of the prostate. In elderly men small growths confined to the prostate may be monitored but left untreated since death may result from other causes before the tumour begins to produce symptoms.

Cancer of the penis is rare and found most usually in uncircumcised men who do not keep their penis clean. A wart-like lump or ulcer appears on the foreskin or the head of the penis and if untreated slowly develops into a cauliflower-like growth. Early radiation treatment usually makes surgery unnecessary.

Cancer of the testicles is rare, especially before puperty or in old age, tending to occur mainly in men between 15 and 40. It usually appears as a firm, painless swelling of one testis, though in some cases there may be pain and inflammation. The risk is higher in men with only one testes or who as young boys had undescended testis.

Causes of Cancer

Chromosome damage
The characteristics of a cell are inherited from its parent cell.
They are passed on in the DNA (deoxyribonucleic acid), which
is a very long molecule with a skeleton in the form of a double
helix. It contains the complete instructions for the development
and functioning of the human body and it controls the cell's
structure and function. In cancerous cells, the characteristics of
malignant growth are passed on from one generation to
another. This means that the genetic code must have been
damaged. This, in fact, is seen if the chromosomes of cancerous
cells are examined. Normal cells have 46 chromosomes
arranged in 23 pairs. Almost all cancer cells are abnormal in
the number and/or the structure of these chromosomes.

Normal deviancy
Cells with genetic defects appear in the body every day: so
many millions of cells are being made that some mistakes are
inevitable. Most faulty cells die almost immediately because
they are too faulty to survive, or because they are recognized
as abnormal and are destroyed by white blood corpuscles.
Others are only slightly defective, and non-malignant. Only
very rarely do malignant cells survive and reproduce
successfully. Appearance of cancer in a person may simply be
due to this unlucky change. Alternatively, it may be that the
body has an 'immunity' to such malignant cells, and that this
sometimes breaks down. This would explain why cancer can
remain dormant in a person for many years.

Special factors
A few factors have been recognized that make genetic damage
in cells more likely. But they can only explain a tiny proportion
of cancers that occur.
- Certain chemicals can cause cancer to form, if they are
  repeatedly in contact with the body over a period of time.
  Such chemicals are called carcinogens, and they include
  some hydrocarbons. Apart from tobacco smoke, these
  carcinogens usually only affect workers whose job brings
  them into regular contact with them. (However,
  atmospheric pollution may also be carcinogenic.)
- Certain viruses can pass malignant tumors from one animal
  to another, and the same may occur in man. But so far only
  one rare form of cancer is thought to be caused this way.
  Apart from this, human cancer seems not to be virus
  induced – and therefore not infectious.
- Ionizing radiation. Without correct protection, X-rays can

cause skin cancer, and radiation can cause leukemia. Also ultraviolet rays (as in sunlight) may cause skin cancer, especially in regions where the ozone layer has broken down.

● Continued physical irritation. Repeated physical disturbance of the skin or a mucus membrane can cause cancer. For example, the white patches called leukoplakia, which are a symptom of cancer of the mouth, are caused by repeated irritation by cigarette smoke. Such irritation can also accelerate an existing cancerous growth.

Correlative Factors

Some individuals are more likely to develop cancer than others for the following reasons:

Heredity. Cancerous growths are not inherited. But a predisposition for cancer can be passed on. It may be that some inherited characteristics make a person's cells more likely to become malignant.

Age. Most cancers occur in the 65+ age group. However, children and adolescents are susceptible to leukemia, brain tumors, and sarcomas of the bone.

Sex. In almost all countries, cancer occurs more frequently in men than in women.

Geographical location. Gastric cancer is most frequent in coastal countries with cold climates.

Cultural habits. Cancer of the penis is less common in societies where circumcision is usual.

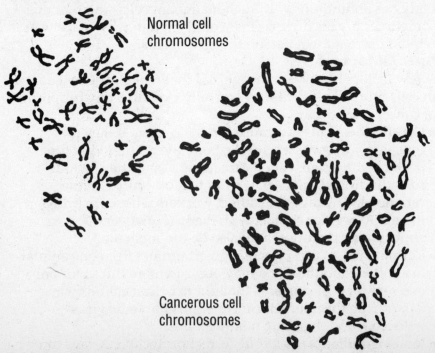

Normal cell chromosomes

Cancerous cell chromosomes

Changing Death Rates

Cancer is not a modern disease – it has been found in dinosaur fossils and in the remains of Java man who lived about 500,000 years ago. But in the present century it has become vastly more prevalent. In 1900 it was the seventh main cause of death in the USA. Today it is the biggest. Some experts believe this is simply because people are living longer – for likelihood of cancerous growth increases with age. However, some types of cancer have shown a dramatic fall in recent years, eg stomach cancer. (This particular example may be linked with changes in techniques of food preservation.)

Symptoms of Cancer

- Any unusual bleeding or discharge from the mouth, the genitals or the anus.
- Any lump, thickening or swelling on the body surface, or any swelling of one limb.
- Any increase in size or change in color or appearance in a mole or wart.
- A sore that will not heal normally.
- Persistent constipation, diarrhea or indigestion that is unusual for the person.
- Hoarseness or a dry cough that lasts more than three weeks.
- Difficulty in swallowing or urinating.
- Sudden unexplained loss in weight.

If you develop any of these symptoms, you should see a physician. Nearly always, the cause will be something else, not cancer. But do not delay. If it is cancer, quick diagnosis is essential.

Treatment

Treatments for cancer have a good chance of success only if the tumor is still localized. Early diagnosis is vital. Once a tumor has metastasized, successful treatment is almost impossible.

Surgical

Surgical removal of localized malignant tumors at an early stage is still the only completely successful form of treatment for some types of cancer. In the later stages, surgery may be attempted in conjunction with other techniques to reduce symptoms.

Radiotherapy

Cancer cells are killed by radiation more easily than normal cells. Radiotherapy seeks to destroy cancerous tissue by focusing a stream of radiation on it. This is most successful if the cancer is still localized, and can be destroyed without causing radiation damage to the rest of the body. The rays used are either X-rays or those of radioactive materials such as radium or cobalt.

Chemotherapy

This is treatment by the administration of chemicals. Again, the major difficulty is finding drugs that will destroy cancer cells without harming normal cells. Three main types of chemical are used: those that interfere with the cancer cells' reproductive processes; those that interfere with the cells' metabolic process; those that increase the natural resistance of the body to the tumor cells.

These chemicals can affect the whole of the body, specific regions, or the tumors themselves, depending on how they are applied.

Hormone therapy

Used mainly for tumors of the endocrine glands and related organs and in treatment for prostate cancer in its early stages. it is also useful in the treatment of metastases originating from these areas. Success depends on whether the cancerous cells still have the specialized relationship with the hormone that the original tissue had.

Immunotherapy

This form of treatment is based on the supposition that a person who has cancer has a malfunctioning immune system: phagocyte cells are failing to respond to the presence of alien cells by destroying them. Treatment aims to strengthen the patient's immune system. Several different approaches are used. The general approach seeks to improve the patient's general health and uses preventive methods, such as immunization with, for example, BCG (tuberculosis) vaccine. Specific approaches attempt to find antigens or substances that act like antigens and attack the tumor, such as killed cancer cells or a chemical extracted from the cancer cells. In another approach, healthy lymphocyte cells, or even RNA are transferred from one patient to another in an attempt to stimulate the immune system. These treatments are still at an experimental stage, and their degree of success is not yet known.

Much publicized 'natural' approaches to the treatment of
cancer by learning relaxation techniques to minimize stress and
following a very strict vegetarian diet have not gained wide
support in the medical profession. Physicians believe that
stress does not play an important role in the development of
disease; and they believe that following a very limited
vegetarian diet might further harm patients who are already
terminally ill. However, such methods and the practice of
mental disciplines to give 'mind-over-body' control have in
numerous instances been claimed as the cause of remissions or
the retarding of cancer growth.

Lungs and Breathing

The two lungs lie in the chest (pleural) cavity, bounded by the
ribs and the chest muscles and back muscles, and beneath by a
muscular wall called the diaphragm. Breathing occurs because
muscular effort enlarges the chest cavity: the diaphragm
moves down, and the cavity skeleton forward and outward.
This threatens to create a vacuum in the cavity, so air rushes
into the lungs under atmospheric pressure, and the lungs
enlarge and fill out the cavity. Breathing out also occurs
through muscular effort: the chest cavity contracts, forcing air
out of the lungs.

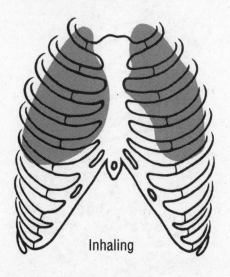
Inhaling

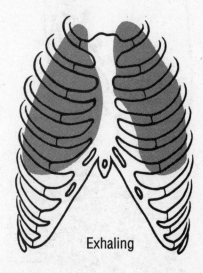
Exhaling

The Respiratory System

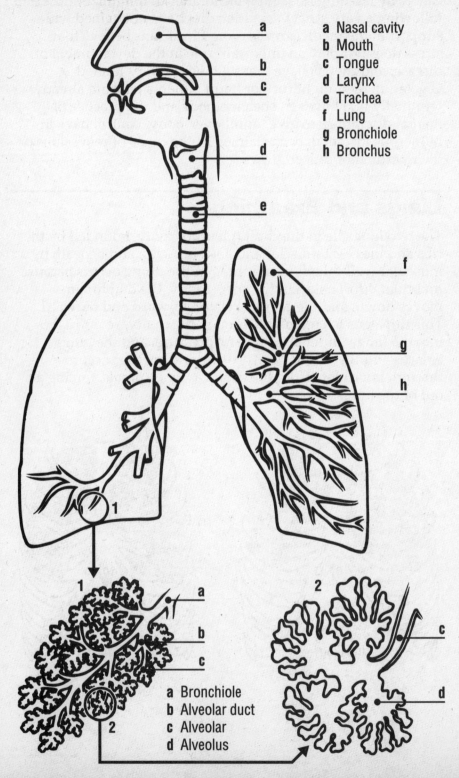

a Nasal cavity
b Mouth
c Tongue
d Larynx
e Trachea
f Lung
g Bronchiole
h Bronchus

a Bronchiole
b Alveolar duct
c Alveolar
d Alveolus

Pneumothorax

This is air in the chest cavity. It may have come form outside through a wound, or from inside through a hole in the lung. The lung on that side collapses as a result, causing sudden severe pain and breathing difficulties. But it expands again in a short time, because air in the chest cavity is quickly absorbed. Pneumothorax may be induced surgically, in cases of tuberculosis for example, to allow the collapsed lung to rest and heal.

2

Sounds of Disorders

As all passes in and out of the lungs, it makes sounds that can be heard through a stethoscope. In a healthy person, these have a sighing or rustling character. But in an unhealthy person, unusual sounds and their location can tell of lung disorders. Tubes that are constricted but dry cause whistling and 'snoring'; those narrowed by mucus, sibilant sounds; those filled with fluid, bubbling noises. In each case the coarseness and loudness of the sound suggests the size of the tube involved.

Bronchitis

Bronchitis is an inflammation of the bronchi – though the bronchioles and small passages are often involved too. Its severity varies. Mild cases may seem like a severe chest cold. Severe cases lead to pneumonia and death. Bronchitis is most prevalent in the UK, where it kills more than 30,000 people a year. The high level of air pollution is thought to be a factor contributing to this statistic. However, cigarette-smoking is the major cause of bronchitis. Cigarette smoke irritates the lungs, and deposits tar in the alveolar tubes, preventing the cilia (tiny hairs in the lungs) from helping to clear the lungs of mucus. There are two main types of bronchitis:

Acute bronchitis

This results from: viral and bacterial infection following colds and flu; inhaling cigarette smoke and other irritating dust or vapors; exposure to damp cold air; or from combinations of these. The attack begins with a short, dry, painful cough and a general feeling of acute illness. There may also be slight fever. After two or three days the cough begins to bring up sputum (mucus from the lungs) in increasing quantities. The symptoms may begin to subside at this point. The cough may last for three or four weeks, but the more distressing symptoms pass off in about ten days. The condition is most dangerous in the old, especially if emphysema is also present. Treatment consists of antibiotics, bedrest, warmth, hot drinks, inhalation of steam preparations and abstention from smoking.

Chronic bronchitis

Chronic bronchitis mainly affects the middle aged and the old. It can lead to emphysema and heart failure. It usually develops after repeated respiratory infections. There are several major contributing factors: excessive cigarette smoking; exposure to a cold, damp climate; damp living conditions; exposure to irritating environmental dust and fumes (e.g. from industrial pollution); obesity; and, probably, constitutional predisposition. The disease produces a constant cough which is worse during the night and in the mornings. The mucous membranes of the bronchial tubes become thickened, and the nutritional blood supply to the lungs may be impaired. Emphysema and other complications may lead to constant breathlessness. Treatment depends on the patient's age, the severity of the illness and whether there are complications. It may include: expectorants to loosen the mucus in the air passages, steam inhalations, and antibiotics if there is any bacterial or viral infection. To prevent recurrence, a sufferer should avoid cold, dusty or polluted air, and must never smoke. Care must be taken to prevent colds from developing into bronchitis.

Bronchitis and emphysema
a Duct blocked with sputum
b Mucous membrane swollen
c Alveolus swollen

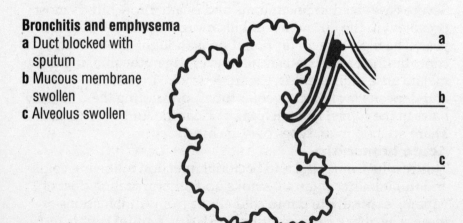

Emphysema

Emphysema is linked with bronchitis and cigarette smoking. It also sometimes results from constant overstraining of the lungs (as with glass-blowers). Due to infection, inflammation and obstruction of the air passages, the lungs lose their elasticity. The small alveolar air spaces become enlarged: the dividing walls are stretched thin and break down, and large air sacs are formed. This greatly reduces the surface area available for gas exchange; the blood and body get less and less oxygen for each breath. Breathing becomes increasingly labored, as more breaths are needed to take in the necessary oxygen. The lung's deterioration often also hinders the passage of blood through the arterioles. This puts a strain on the right side of the heart. It becomes weakened and dilated, and death from heart failure can result. The chest becomes barrel-shaped. Emphysema is most common in older people.

Asthma

Asthma is a disease in which inflammation narrows the bronchioles, the small airways in the lungs, causing attacks of breathlessness. The inflammation leads to increased sputum production, adding to the blockage. The number of asthmatics seems to be growing in the US and the developed world and blame has often been laid on traffic exhaust and other air pollution but, those these may trigger an attack, there is no evidence that they are the initial cause of the disease. Children are ten times more likely to be affected than adults, the first attack usually occuring before age five, though it can develop at any age. Fortunately in most cases attacks become less severe with age; more than half the children affected do not suffer at all as adults and treatment enables others to lead a normal life. There are two main forms:

● Extrinsic asthma, triggered by an allergy such pollen, house-dust mites, animals fur or feathers, a particular food or drug, tobacco smoke and other air pollution, a respiratory infection or even by exercise (especially in cold air).

● Intrinsic asthma, which often first appears after a respiratory infection, usually develops later in life. Attacks are often triggered by stress.

Symptoms

Attacks, which tend to be most frequent in early morning, vary greatly in severity ranging from slight breathlessness through wheezing, a dry cough and a tight feeling across the chest to such loss of breath that there is sweating, a racing pulse and such lack of oxygen that the skin becomes pale and clammy with a purplish discoloration, especially of the lips, a condition which is life threatening.

Similar symptoms are produced by cardiac asthma, but this is caused by fluid collecting in the lungs and usually The result of inefficient pumping of the heart.

Treatment

There is no known cure, although if particular allergens can be identified it may be possible to avoid them, for example by sealing matresses in airtight covers, strictly controlling household dust or staying indoors when there is a heavy pollen count. A drug to relax and widen the airways, administered through an inhaler, is used to treat the symptoms.

Pneumonia

Pneumonia is a disease in which large parts of the lungs become inflamed and filled with fluid. It is often caused by infection by bacteria. When one or more lobes of one lung are infected, it is called lobar pneumonia. If both lungs are involved it is called bilateral pneumonia. Broncho-pneumonia occurs in patches of the lung tissue, not in whole lobes. It often comes about as a complication of bronchitis and other illnesses. Hypostatic pneumonia occurs in bed-ridden people, especially the elderly. Fluid collects in the lungs because of lack of movement. Primary atypical pneumonia is caused by viral infection. Predisposing factors for pneumonia include the common cold, chronic alcoholism, malnutrition and bodily weakness.

Symptoms

In lobar pneumonia the illness begins with chest pains, vomiting and shivering, closely followed by a rapid rise in temperature as high as 104°F (39.6°C). Breathing is difficult. A harsh, dry cough brings up rust-colored sputum which may contain blood in untreated cases. The temperature stays high for about a week. It then falls within 24 hours to normal, and pulse and breathing become regular. The patient recovers quickly (but may be fatigued for many weeks). Broncho-pneumonia and other forms have similar symptoms, but do not end suddenly. The temperature tends to fall and rise, gradually returning to normal over a number of weeks.

Treatment

Treatment includes antibiotics and measures similar to those for severe bronchitis. An oxygen tent is used in extreme cases. Convalescence should last for a month or two. Pneumonia can be fatal in weak or aged people, in cases where the extent of inflammation prevents respiration; and in those whose resistance is low for other reasons (e.g. because of other illness, or alcoholism). Because of this it is often quoted as a cause of death for old people who could not withstand the illness or the accompanying fever and fatigue. But apart from these and other extreme cases, it is not normally fatal.

Pleurisy and Empyema

Pleurisy is inflammation of the pleura – the membrane which lines the chest cavity and covers the lungs. It nearly always accompanies pneumonia and other lung inflammation. In dry pleurisy, the inflamed membranes rub against each other as the patient breathes, causing acute pain. In wet pleurisy, the pleural cavity fills with fluid – there is no pain, but breathing is impaired. Pleurisy is seldom fatal in itself, but may increase the risk of fatality in the diseases it accompanies. Empyema is any condition in which there is pus in the pleural cavity. It usually results from pneumonia, tuberculosis or cancer of the lung. It causes the lung to collapse and restricts breathing. Treatment involves removing the pus.

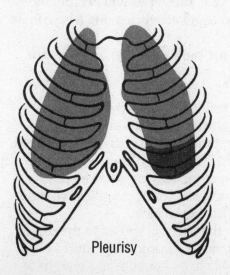

Pleurisy

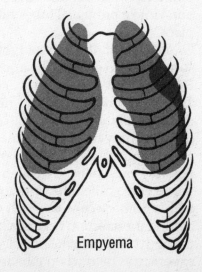

Empyema

Tuberculosis

Tuberculosis (TB) is not just a respiratory disorder. It is a general term for diseases caused by the bacterium *myobacterium tuberculosis.*These are contagious: the bacteria are carried in the sputum of the patient, and are spread when he sneezes or coughs. They enter other bodies by being breathed in or swallowed. Since the bacteria are also very hardy and can survive for a long time in dried sputum and dust, everything within the vicinity of a patient soon becomes infected. The most common form of tuberculosis is pulmonary tuberculosis, because the lungs, in adults, are the most common point of entry of the bacteria into the body. But tuberculosis can also affect bones, joints, skin, lymph nodes, larynx, intestines, kidneys, testes, prostate gland and nervous system.

Systemic tuberculosis is transmitted in milk from cows that have bovine tuberculosis. It causes tissue breakdown in the affected areas.

Process of the disease

The bacteria enter the body through the lungs or through the intestines (most common in children). They are carried in the lymph or blood vessels, settle in an organ, multiply, and produce small grayish nodules or ('tubercles') around themselves big enough to almost visible to the naked eye. When adjacent tubercles touch they fuse, forming a larger, yellow tubercle. This has a soft, yellow, cheesy substance inside.

As fusion spreads, the healthy tissue is broken down, to be replaced by the disease substance of the yellow tubercles. In pulmonary tuberculosis, this infected substance will eventually burst into a bronchial tube and be coughed up, leaving a hole in its place.

Often areas of fibrous scar tissue are built up as the body tries to surround and contain the infection.

Symptoms

These depend on the organ attacked. In all cases the bacteria disrupt and then destroy the organ and its functions.

In pulmonary tuberculosis the first infection is often unrecognized, and thought of as a bad cold or flu. There is a cough, fever and possibly chest pain. This often clears up, leaving a hardened, scarred area called the primary complex. Many people have signs of this primary complex with no further trouble.

Secondary infection occurs when the bacteria spread to the rest of the body. The patient spits blood, has a chronic cough and experiences pain when inhaling. He loses appetite and weight, is constantly tired and sweats profusely.

Treatment

Tuberculosis is treated with the antibiotic streptomycin, and a range of other drugs, for up to 1 year. Surgical treatment is now seldom needed, though fresh air, a healthy diet and plenty of rest are still essential to full recovery.

BCG vaccine is recommended for anyone who does not have a natural immunity and who may be exposed to the disease, such as social and health care workers. Anyone who is HIV positive should be immunized.

Control

After the 1950s, when immunization programs were introduced in the USA and many European countries, the incidence of TB fell dramatically. By 1990, the number of new cases notified in the UK had fallen to fewer than 1 in 100,000 people. In the late 1980s, a sudden resurgence of cases in the large cities of the US and Europe has been attributed to several factors:

● homelessness
● drug abuse
● increased immigration from countries with a high TB incidence
● overcrowding in shelters, homes for the poor, and prisons.

However, a major underlying cause of the resurgence is now known to be reduced resistance in the large numbers of people who are HIV positive. Up to 40% of people with AIDS, or who are HIV positive, become ill with TB; normally only 10% of people who are exposed to TB infection become ill.

Accidents

Accidents are a leading cause of death in all modern societies. In the USA they claim more than 90,000 fatalities every year, ranking beneath heart disease, cancer, strokes, and respiratory diseases in the number of their victims. And in the under-24 age group accidents are the second major cause of death, outnumbered only by AIDS.

Men are far more likely to suffer accidental death than women. One-third of all accidental deaths are male, for all causes and all ages. Among young people aged 15 to 24, there are more than four male deaths to every female death. In the over-75 age group there are twice as many male accidental deaths, despite the fact that women considerably outnumber men in this category.

The countries shaded in which more than 150 people per 1,000,000 are killed each year in accidents are:

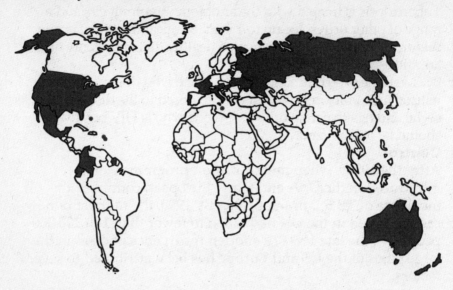

Causes

Motor vehicle accidents are the major cause of accidental death. Although the numbers of deaths caused by motor vehicle accidents has fallen over the last 25 years, they still account for more than half of all accidental deaths in many of the countries for which figures are available.

Americas		**Europe**		**Asia/Australasia**
Bahamas	Martinique	Austria	Luxembourg	South Korea
Barbados	Mexico	Belgium	Malta	Australia
Colombia	Surinam	France	Portugal	New Zealand
Ecuador	USA	Hungary	Russia	
		Italy	Ukraine	
		Lithuania		

Accidental Death Rate

The table gives a late-1980s breakdown of deaths per year from different types of accidents in the US:

2

Cause of death	No. of deaths	% of all deaths
Motor-vehicle accidents (total)	47,865	19.9
Traffic (**1**)	46,867	19.4
Nontraffic (**11**)	998	.4
Water transport accidents (**9**)	1,102	.5
Air and aerospace accidents (**8**)	1,148	.5
Railroad accidents (**13**)	556	.2
Accidental falls (**2**)	11,444	4.7
Accidental drowning (**5**)	4,777	2.0
Fire (**3**)	4,835	2.0
Firearms (**4**)	4,835	2.0
Electrocution (**12**)	854	.4
Accidental poisoning by:		
Drugs and medicines (**6**)	4,187	1.7
Other solids and liquids (**14**)	479	.2
Gases and vapors (**10**)	1,009	.4
Inhalation and ingestion of objects (**7**)	3,692	1.5
Other	8,743	3.6
Total	**95,277**	**39.5**

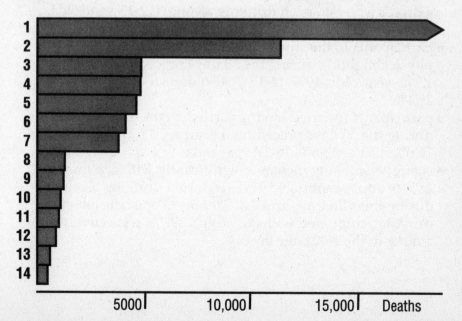

Age and Sex

Although the total number of accidental deaths have fallen since 1970, men in all age groups are more than twice as likely to die from accidents as women. The table gives a breakdown of male accidental deaths by age for the late-1980s:

Age group	Male deaths per 100,000 population
15-24	118.8
25-34	102.5
35-44	80.6
45-54	78.6
55-64	82.1
65-74	105.7
75-84	204.3
85+	428.8
Total (including under-15s)	**33.2**

A survey carried out in 1992-4 as part of the US Youth Risk Behavior Survey looked at health-risk behavior among people aged 12-21 discovered that:

- people aged 12-13 are less likely to use safety belts when riding as a passenger in a motor vehicle
- people in the age group studied reported having ridden with a driver who had been drinking alcohol (12-13-year-olds, 11.3%; 14-17-year-olds, 21.7%; 18-21-year-olds, 34.5%).
- participants in the study reported having taken part in physical fighting during the 30 days preceding the survey: 12-13-year-olds, 49%; 14-17-year-olds 43.8%; 18-21-year-olds, 29.4%.
- participants reported having carried a gun, knife or club during the 30 days preceding the survey:12-17-year-olds, 12.6%; 17.1%; 13.6%, 14-17-year-olds.
- cigarette-smoking increases significantly with age group.
- 28% of adolescents aged 12-13 reported drinking alcohol during their lifetime, and 4.3% reported episodic heavy drinking, compared with 86.7% and 39.7% respectively among in the 18-21 age group.

Motor Accidents

The main types of fatal motor vehicle accidents are, beginning with the most common: collisions with other motor vehicles (42%); overturning or going off the road (28%), hitting a pedestrian (17%); collisions with fixed objects (7%); collisions with trains (2½%); and collisions with bicycles (1½%). Most causes distribute over the age groups to coincide with the general age pattern of motor vehicle fatalities, i.e. they are much more common in those of working age (15 to 65). However, pedestrian deaths are spread much more evenly over all age groups – with the result that almost half of those killed under 14 are pedestrians. Also over a third of those 75 and over are pedestrian deaths but even more, in this age group, are deaths in motor vehicle collisions.

Percentage of death and injured, by action

Drivers

Killed

Action	a	b	c	d	e	f
Percent	41	16	15	13	10	5

Injured

Percent	42	7	19	19	7	6
Action	a	b	c	d	e	f

a Exceeding speed limit
b Driving on wrong side of the road
c Reckless driving
d No right of way
e Driving off highway
f Others

Pedestrians

Killed

Action	a	b	c	d	e	f	g	h	i
Percent	41	16	9	8	7	5	5	5	4

Injured

Percent	32	8	10	8	17	6	9	4	6
Action	a	b	c	d	e	f	g	h	i

a Crossing intersection with signal
b Walking or rural highway
c Crossing intersection against signal
d Crossing intersection no signal
e Crossing from behind parked car
f Others
g Crossing between intersections
h Not on roadways
i Children playing in street

Home Accidents

Home accidents claim over 25,000 victims every year in the USA. About a third of these are 75 or over, and almost a quarter of the remainder are in the 0 to 4 age group. The main types of accident in the home are, beginning with the most common: falls (36%); deaths associated with fire (21%); poisoning by solids and liquids (9½%), choking (8½%), firearms and poisoning by gas (each 4½%); and 'mechanical' suffocation (4%).

Falls are most prevalent in the old; suffocation in the under-5s; and poisoning with solids and liquids in the 25 to 44 age group, as well as in the under-5s. Also, among other unspecified causes of fatal home accidents, one-third of the victims are children under five. Other causes distribute comparatively evenly over the age groups.

Suicide

Suicide is the act of killing yourself. There are as many as 365,000 suicides in the world every year, and some 3 to 4 million attempts. In the US there is 1 suicide approximately every 20 minutes, and about 28,000 suicides a year, or about 11 or 12 people per 100,000 people of all ages. Suicide is the seventh major cause of death.

Suicide has occurred in many societies in the past. In some eras it was more frequent than in others. Today it occurs in most societies, but is more common in some than in others. The suicide rate appears to rise as a society increases in prosperity. Suicide seems to be rare in poor countries. It is common in cities and in prosperous regions and neighbourhoods.

In many societies past and present, suicide has been and still is rare because it is proscribed by religious beliefs. When the restraining influence of religious belief and moral principles breaks down, the suicide rate rises. However, in Imperial Rome and in feudal Japan, the suicide rate was high because suicide was valued as an act of personal pride.

Age

In modern industrial societies, suicide is more common in certain age groups. As societies change from a form of organization based on extended families to a nuclear family-based organization, the suicide rate often increases among old people, whose traditional roles within the family cease to be seen as important. Suicide among children is rare, but in recent years, there has been a rapid rise in suicides among the under-25 age group.

Gender

Men have always been more likely to commit suicide than women. Today they are more than three times more likely to commit suicide than women.

Skin color

US statistics show that white-skinned people are twice as likely to commit suicide as black people.

Suicide compared with other causes of death in the USA

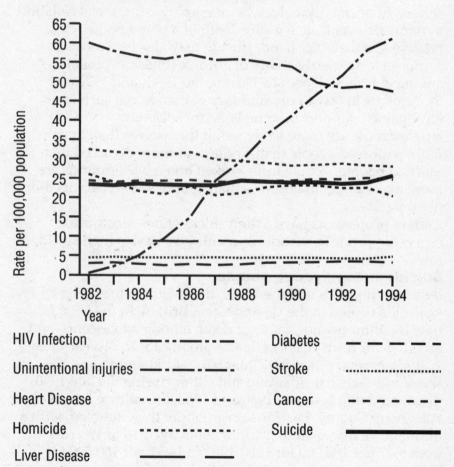

HIV Infection	— ·· — ·· —	Diabetes	— — — —
Unintentional injuries	— · — · — ·	Stroke	·················
Heart Disease	···············	Cancer	– – – – –
Homicide	··············	Suicide	▬▬▬▬▬
Liver Disease	— — —		

Reasons for Suicide

In Western industrialized societies, more than 90% of suicides are thought to be the result of mental illness or disturbance:

Suicides by people with mental illnesses

Disorder	%
Clinical depression	15
Schizophrenia	10
Alcoholic dependence	7
Neuroses and personality disorders	5

Suicide may be a reaction to a perceived problem, such as serious financial difficulties, or unemployment, social isolation, a traumatic event, such as the death of a wife or other close relative. On the other hand, suicide may also be a rational response to severe disability or chronic illness, especially among elderly sick people. During the 1980s and 1990s, movements in favour of voluntary euthanasia in such cases have gained support in some Western societies.

Single people are more likely to kill themselves than married; more widowed people than single; and more divorced than married people. People from broken home backgrounds are more likely to kill themselves than people whose parents did not separate.

Certain professions have a high suicide rate – doctors are especially prone to suicide. Students also have a high suicide rate.

Suicide among young people

Between the 1970s and the 1990s, the suicide rate among 15-19-year-olds tripled in the US and Great Britain. In the US it is now the third leading cause of death among adolescents, and accounts for nearly 12% of deaths among 15- to 24-year-olds.

A study carried out at the University of Pittsburgh and the Western Psychiatric Institute and Clinic during the late 1980s discovered that between 1960 and 1983, the suicide rate in Allegheny County, Pa. (Pittsburgh) more than doubled, with a dramatic increases among white males aged 15 to 19 years from 6.47 per 100,000 for 1960-1962 to 14.37 per 100,000 for 1978-1983. During the period studied, the use of firearms as a suicide method increased by 2.5 times, whereas other suicide methods increased only 1.7 times. An increase in domestic firearm sales took place during the same period.

The study also found an increase of more than three-and-a-half-fold of blood alcohol levels in suicides over the same period, from 12.9% in 1968-1972 to 46% in 1978-83. The researchers also reported that suicide victims who used firearms were also five times more likely to have been drinking than those who used other means of suicide. A national increase in alcohol abuse among adolescents of epidemic proportions in the same period was noted by the researchers.

2

Attempted Suicide

There are ten times more attempted suicides than successful ones. Of every four men who try suicide, three kill themselves. Many who genuinely think of suicide are deterred by the thought of the pain and grief they would leave behind. Attempted suicide can be a way of trying to call on those emotional ties: it can be an appeal for help.

People who talk of suicide must not be ignored. Two-thirds of people who kill themselves have told someone beforehand that they intend to take their lives. Contrary to common belief, talking about suicide is not a sign that the talker is not serious. It is also important to bear in mind that people who try once often try again and succeed.

Suicide Method

US suicides by method used 1986

Method	Total male	Percent
Firearms (a)	15,518	65
Poisoning (b)	3,516	15
Hanging and strangulation (c)	3,478	14.5
Other (d)	1,431	5.5

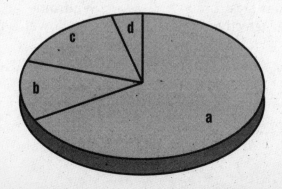

ILLNESS

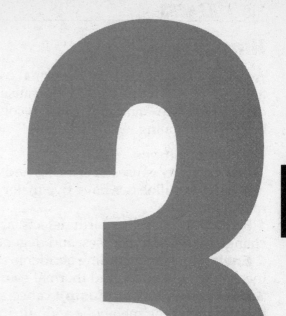

Illness

A sickness or disease is an abnormal condition of the body or any part of it. All diseases have a cause – though this is often difficult to trace – and they cause recognizable changes in the body's functioning.

Causes of illness

There are many causes of sickness and disease, including accidents, but illnesses have five major causes, all of which may interact:

1 Heredity: including birth defects, abnormal developmental changes, inherited diseases, and degenerative processes

2 Environment: including accidents and irritation by mechanical, chemical, and thermal sources, and from radiation

3 New growths(neoplasia): cancers

4 Diet: including metabolic and nutritional disorders, and poisons

5 Infections

Signs and symptoms

A symptom is an outward manifestation of an illness – a signal, such as a pain, which indicates to the sick person that something is wrong. But not everyone with an illness notices any symptoms, especially in the early stages. There are, however, indications – abnormal patches on the tongue, for example – that are obvious to the trained eye of a doctor. Doctors call these indications 'signs', not 'symptoms'.

Acute illnesses

Acute illnesses are short-term illnesses, which tend to start abruptly. They may clear up quickly – e.g. a cold or chicken pox; or become persistent and long-lasting – e.g. malaria or asthma; or cause rapid death if not treated by drugs or surgery – e.g. pneumonia or acute appendicitis.

Chronic illnesses

Chronic illnesses may be mild (e.g. varicose veins) or severe, (e.g. osteoarthritis) but they are always persistent and long-lasting.

Incidence of Illness

The frequency of different sicknesses varies considerably from country to country – even region to region – due to differences in climate, diet, standard of living, health care availability and lifestyle.

The occurence of illness also changes over time as medical

advances and social customs change. Over the 25 years up to the 1980s in the US and Europe, once-prevalent diseases, such as measles, whooping cough and poliomyelitis, were declining as a result of mass immunization programs. More effective drugs and careful control also brought syphilis and tuberculosis (TB) in check.

Between 1986-1992, however, statistics showed:

- **re-emergence of TB:** partly because of increased poverty, homelessness, overcrowding and poor nutrition; and partly because of the spread of the HIV virus, which causes AIDS.

- **re-emergence of syphilis:** partly because of the spread of the HIV virus.

- **emergence of AIDS:** a new disease, the spread of which has been facilitated by increased sexual freedom.

- **an increase in salmonella poisoning and listeriosis:** the result of intensive farming, and carry-out cooked food.

3

Chronic Health Conditions in the USA 1991-1993

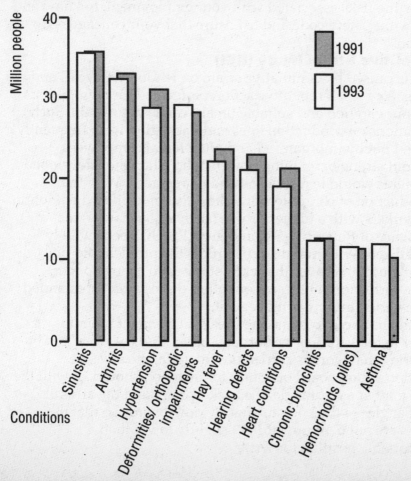

Workplace Illness

Some jobs have a high risk of accident and injury if safety measures are not strictly observed and there are many others that involve the risk of exposure to dangerous substances, from the coal dust which can produce pneumoconiosis in miners to the hazards of radiation in the nuclear industry. Mineral oils, for instance, can create skin problems and may be carcinogenic, oil-soaked overalls of a man straddling a machine may increase the risk of testicular cancer. Many processes involve the use of poisonous or corrosive chemicals and they are not confined to heavy industry: some pigments used by artists and the solvents used in glues can be dangerous when inhaled or ingested. Photocopiers and printers can emit harmful radiation and hydrocarbons — toner dust is suspected of being carcinogenic. Noisy machinery can produce hearing loss and vibrating tools can damage tendons and lead to other disorders, as can excessive vehicle vibration. It is important to know the risks associated with your employment, to know and follow the safety code and to ensure that your colleagues do so, too.

Repetitive Strain Injury (RSI)

This is caused by cumulative strain on tendons, muscles and joints. Any small repetitive action performed for long periods without varation and suitable breaks can lead to strain. Such operations on production lines and packaging were frequently carried out by unorganised and often female employees without strong bargaining powers who when they developed problems would leave the job and be replaced. With the introduction of computers and the effect of keyboard operation on workers with a higher profile (such as journalists) the incidence of Repetitive Strain Injury (RSI) has been widely recognized. With manual typewriters the problem did not usually occur because the typist stopped to change paper, make corrections and carry out other duties which demanded more varied muscular movement.

RSI can be avoided by taking breaks at frequent intervals, either in recreation or performing other kinds of work and by ensuring that work is carried out in ergonomically safe positions: a keyboard operator, for instance, should sit with the knee joint at a rightangle, the back upright and the arms at right angles to the body or slightly downwards so that the wrists are not bent upwards — slightly lower than a comfortable position for writing.

Sick building syndrome

Workers in and users of some buildings suffer from a high incidence of illness for no identifiable reason. Symptoms may include irritation of the eyes, nose and throat, headaches, recurrent gastric upsets, rashes, itching, coughs and colds and mental tiredness.

Poor ventilation and lighting, an even warm temperature with no variation, low humidity, pollution from chemicals used in or with equipment and furnishings and poor hygiene in kitchens or refreshment dispensers have all been suggested as possible causes. Germs can be spread by ventilation systems and some forms of humidifier.

Humidifier fever is an influenza-like illness caused by the inhalation of contaminated water droplets from the tanks of humidifier systems. Symptoms range from mild headaches and muscle aches to coughing, breathlessness and acute fever, most noticeable four or more hours after starting work, especially after a holiday or weekend break. In most cases the body overcomes them after 12-16 hours but they recurr on return to work. Diagnosis can be confirmed by tests on the sludge in the tanks of the system. Steam humidifiers or others which do not produce water droplets avoid the problem.

Legionnaire's disease is a fortunately rare but potentially lethal bacterial illness also caught by breathing contaminated water droplets. Symptoms include high fever, chills, headache and muscle pain, developing into a dry cough and pneumonia. Smokers, diabetics and those with respiratory and kidney problems appear to be more at risk and men more than women. In the case of an outbreak anyone who is likely to have been exposed to infection is in danger.

Infectious Illnesses

The infectious illnesses are those with which non-medical people are most familiar, and expect to have to deal with in everyday life. During the 20th century, antibiotics have given doctors in industrialized countries a form of control over infectious diseases, but in the developing countries they are still a major cause of death. Immunisation against disease by vaccination or innoculation can give protection by stimulating the body to produce its own defences (see pp 122-4).

Agents of Infections

Infectious illnesses occur when certain microscopic living organisms gain access to the body. The symptoms of illness arise from their effect on the body, and from the body's attempts to deal with them. The disease-causing organisms are usually single-celled, normally bacteria or viruses. However,

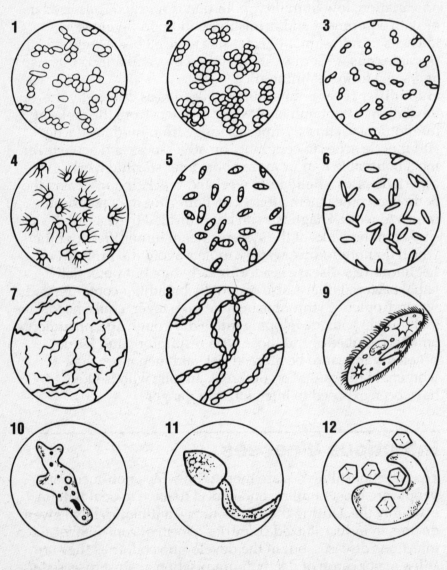

Agents of attack
1 Streptococci
2 Staphylococci
3 Diplococci
4 Typhoid bacilli

5 Tetanus bacilli
6 Tuberculosis bacilli
7 Spirillum
8 Anthrax bacilli
9 Protozoa

10 Amoeba
11 Fluke
12 Viruses
   (surrounding a
   macrophage cell)

infection is also caused by protozoa, amoebae, fungi and multi-celled organisms, such as flukes and worms. Protozoa and amoebae cause toxoplasmosis, as well as malaria, sleeping sickness, amoebic dysentery, and other tropical diseases. Microscopic fungi cause infections such as thrush (see p 163). These days, however, bacterial infection is the source of most infectious illness in the industrialized countries.

Bacteria

These are a form of tiny single-celled plant life, round or rod shaped and each from one to 20 thousandths of a millimeter in diameter. They consist simply of an outer wall inside which there is protoplasm and DNA. Most are incapable of any independent movement. They almost always reproduce simply by dividing in two; and many can form themselves into spores – a seed-like inactive state, in which they can survive adverse conditions. The conditions they prefer vary greatly between the different types, but mostly they do not like too great heat or cold, and like moisture which is not too acidic.

Bacteria commonly occur in vast numbers in almost every corner of life – including on and in man's body. Most are utterly harmless and some no life forms could exist without. Bacteria, for example, play a vital part in the body (e.g. in digestion, vitamin manufacture and destruction of dangerous substances), while all life depends on bacteria in the air and soil without which dead matter would not decay and return into the cycle of existence.

Illnesses from bacteria arise in two ways. Firstly, because bacteria that normally exist on, or in, the body – and may be very useful – get into the wrong part of the body. Examples of this include acne, pimples, and boils; some meningitis; and many urinary infections (especially in women). The first group are caused by normal skin surface bacteria gaining entry into a sweat duct or skin wound; the second by throat bacteria gaining access to the brain; and the third by bacteria from the rectum finding their way into the urinary tract.

Secondly, illnesses can occur because bacteria that are always harmful gain access to the body. Examples of illnesses that are always carried by one specific organism include scarlet fever, tuberculosis, whooping cough, typhoid, syphilis and gonorrhea. Examples that can be caused by a range of bacteria include tonsilitis, dysentery, most pneumonia and 'food poisoning'. In fact, certain types of bacteria have so far evolved from being free living, that they are dependent on other living cells for their very existence. Some of these are useful or harmless – but others are among the most dangerous to man. Outside the living cell, they either die immediately (e.g. syphilis bacteria) or have to form spores (e.g. tetanus).

Viruses

Bacteria are giants compared with viruses, the most primitive form of life. They consist of minute quantities of nucleic acid – DNA or RNA – wrapped in a protein sheath. They can survive in varying conditions, but become active and reproduce only inside another living cell. Having gained entry to a cell (sometimes by a syringe-like injection process), a virus takes over the cell's chemical processes and reproduces inside it until the cell breaks open and dies, freeing the new viruses to enter other cells.

The cells attacked are sometimes easily replaced – as in the nose lining, for example, during a cold. But a virus attack usually interferes with physiological processes and may cause irreparable damage – if nerve cells are destroyed, for example. Illnesses caused by viruses fall into two groups: those that attack specific organs (the influenza virus attacks the respiratory system; the mumps virus the salivary gland; the polio virus attacks the nervous system); and those that cause generalized symptoms, often including a skin rash (measles, rubella, chicken pox, yellow fever).

Retroviruses

These are viruses with a genome (complement of genetic material) consisting of a single strand of RNA. The action of an enzyme called reverse transcriptase enables the cell to synthesize DNA from this. This is unusual: normally RNA is synthesized from DNA. HIV (the AIDS virus) is a retrovirus.

Rickettsiae

These are intermediate between viruses and bacteria. Most live in the intestines of insects, and can infect a human being if the insect is a parasitic blood-sucker. Typhus fever and Rocky Mountain spotted fever are both caused in this way.

Toxins

Toxins are not organisms in themselves – they are immensely powerful chemical poisons, produced by certain bacteria when active in the human body. For example, it has been estimated that one-6000th of an ounce of pure botulin (the cause of botulism food poisoning) would be enough to kill the entire population of the world. Other toxic infections include tetanus and diphtheria. In many toxic illnesses, the bacteria themselves are not harmful to the body – only the substance they produce, if it is not neutralized.

How Infections Occur

Routes into the body

Infective agencies have four main routes into the body:

- through breaks in the skin, or in the mucous membrane that lines the mouth, nose, etc (the breaks may be wounds, which infection happens to enter, or bites made by the same insect that brings the infection, or, in the case of hepatitis B and AIDS, often through punctures made by drug abusers using infected needles).
- down the respiratory tract into the lungs;
- down the digestive tract, into the stomach and bowels; and
- up the reproductive and urinary systems, via the genitals.

In all cases, the infectious agent may remain localized at its point of entry, or may enter the blood or lymph system and be distributed through the body. For example, infection of a wound may result in an abscess filled with pus; and/or may burst onto the surface, possibly infecting other flaws in the skin; and/or may travel up the lymph canals to the regional lymph nodes – perhaps being trapped there and causing a further abscess. Serious blood-borne infections are rare, but blood-borne bacteria do often attack already damaged heart valves. HIV, the AIDS virus, is carried in the bodily fluids and may be transmitted in the saliva, the seminal fluid, or the blood.

The Body's Defenses

The skin, especially if it is kept clean and healthy, offers excellent resistance to infective organisms. Most organisms that are swallowed are destroyed by the stomach acid, but some, such as those in the *Salmonella* genus, can pass through

Agents of defence
White blood corpuscles:
1 Neutrophil
2 Basophil
3 Eosinophil
4 Monocyte
  Lymphocyte
5 T - Lymphocyte
6 B - Lymphocyte

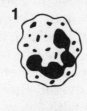

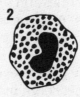

Stages in the phagocytic digestion of a bacterium

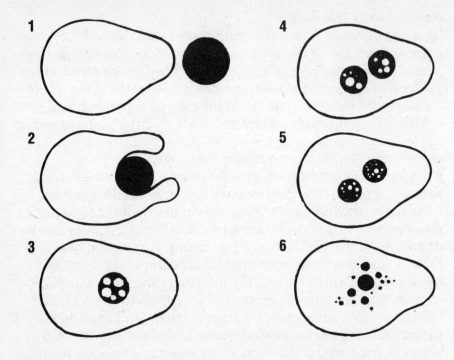

the stomach unharmed. Many of the germs that penetrate the skin and intestinal barriers are killed by scavenging cells called phagocytes that are present everywhere in the tissues.

The term 'immunity' is rather loosely applied to the body's ability to resist infection by means of antibodies and a complex defense mechanism involving the cells of the immune system. Absolute immunity to infection does not exist. To many organisms, our immunity is almost absolute, but to many others it is relative only. Whether or not an infection becomes established so that germs are able to form colonies in the body is, essentially, a question of the relative strength of the opposing forces. A minor assault by a small dose of organisms of fairly low virulence is easily repulsed. But a large dose of highly virulent organisms might be overwhelming. Organisms mutate and vary in the severity of their effects. The immune system also varies, both in its overall efficiency, and in its specific ability to deal quickly with a new invader.

Defense Cells in Action

All infective organisms or foreign biological materials carry surface markers (antigens) identifying them as dangerous.

Certain cells of the immune system, large phagocytes called macrophages actively engulf foreign organisms or tissue and display these surface markers on their own surfaces. Other cells, called helper T lymphocytes (helper T cells) identify these markers on the macrophages and carry the information to cells of another class of lymphocytes, the B cells.

There are thousands of different kinds of B cell, each capable of producing a specific antibody to deal best with a particular invader. The helper T cells seek out the B cell that best fits with the marker information they carry. This selected B cell now starts to reproduce itself and produces a large number of identical copies of itself (a clone). The cloned B cells then produce millions of protein molecules called antibodies. These latch on to the invading organisms and immobilize them so that they can easily be destroyed by phagocytes.

Some of the cloned B cells become 'memory cells', which remain available almost indefinitely. If another infection by the same organism occurs later, the memory cells can clone to produce antibodies more quickly than on the first infection. This is why we have resistance to many diseases after a first attack. It is also the basis of artificial immunization (see below).

Antibodies are not the only way in which the immune system guards the body. Some T-cells — the natural killer T cells — can attack foreign organisms directly. Others take part in a remarkable process of surveillance of our body cells to check whether they are likely to cause danger to the whole body. When normal body cells are attacked by viruses or begin to develop the DNA abnormality that leads to cancer, they always put out surface markers indicating that something is wrong. These markers are identified by helper T cells, and antibodies or killer T cells are called up to destroy the affected cells. Without this constant process of surveillance, most of us would already have died from cancer or virus infection.

Immunodeficiency Disorders

This is an important class of diseases in which the body's immunological system of defense against infection, foreign material generally, and some forms of cancer, is in some way defective. The best known example of this group of disorders is the acquired immunodeficiency syndrome, AIDS (see below), but immunodeficiency disorders were well known in medical circles long before AIDS appeared. They may be congenital (i.e. of genetic origin and present at birth) or they may be acquired later. The immunological mechanisms are so important for survival that major congenital defects are seldom seen.

Some deficiency in the production of immunoglobulins is normal in the early years of life and it is not until adult life that full production occurs. This is why children are so susceptible to infections. Children depend on antibodies supplied by the mother before birth and provided in the early breast milk — the colostrum — after birth. Premature babies may not, because of early birth, have received the full quota from the mother.

Antibodies are soluble globulin proteins known as immunoglobulins. Immunoglobulin deficiency (agammaglobulinemia) is the most important genetic immunodeficiency disorder. People with this condition have a variable degree of B-cell deficiency, and may survive for many years, although very susceptible to bacterial and other infection and requiring constant treatment.

Another form of immunodeficiency disorder is a selective deficiency of the T cell group of lymphocytes. When this is present from birth the outlook is poor, but in some cases treatment by human fetal thymus gland transplantation has been effective.

Acquired immune deficiency may be caused by necessary medical treatment to prevent the rejection of transplanted organs, or it may be caused by disease. Diseases causing immune deficiency include AIDS, many types of cancer, and severe dietary deficiency states, especially when the protein necessary to form antibodies is absent. Old age features a relative immune deficiency, as a consequence of a gradual using up of the total stock of both kinds of lymphocytes. So conditions such as shingles and certain cancers, which have been kept in check by the immune system, become more common. People with immunodeficiency disorders suffer recurrent infection, not only by the common organisms, but also by those which do not normally cause disease. These infections are known as 'opportunistic', and include such conditions as *Pneumocystis carinii* pneumonia, cytomegalovirus infections and extensive herpes simplex and thrush infections (see p 163), involving not only the skin but also the intestinal and respiratory systems.

AIDS

AIDS was first reported in June 1981, when the Centers for Disease Control, Atlanta, Georgia, were informed of a strange outbreak among homosexual men in Los Angeles of two very uncommon diseases — a form of pneumonia caused by an organism called *Pneumocystis carinii*, and a rare cancer called *Kaposi's sarcoma*.

As further similar reports came in, CDC set up a task force to investigate and soon found that the numbers of such cases were doubling every six months. In addition to *Pneumocystis* pneumonia and Kaposi's sarcoma, these men were developing widespread herpes and thrush infections, tuberculosis, and a variety of infections with organisms normally hardly able to attack humans. It was not long before it became clear that the men were suffering from immune deficiency. They were developing these rare infections and cancers because they had lost their resistance to them. The term 'acquired immune deficiency syndrome', soon abbreviated to 'AIDS', was coined. In 1983, scientists in Paris and Maryland were able to establish that AIDS was caused by a virus of a type related to other known viruses. It is now known as the human immunodeficiency virus (HIV), and is spread mainly by sexual contact. HIV is an RNA virus that carries an enzyme called reverse transcriptase that enables it to make DNA copies of itself in the helper T cells it invades. The virus binds to the surface of the T cell and injects its genetic material. This replicates rapidly in the T cell to form thousands of copies of the virus, which then burst out of the cell and spread to other helper cells. The result is a profound deficiency of helper T cells. B cells are not affected and some antibody production occurs, although the only value of this appears to be to enable tests for HIV infection to be performed. Unfortunately, in the absence of helper T cells, the antibodies do not have any significant effect on the virus. HIV also invades the brain and can cause destruction of brain cells and dementia.

See p 151 for information about safe sex practices; for HIV infection, treatment and the progress of AIDS, see p p152-3.

Medicine and Infection

Artificial immunization

Immunization, either by the introduction of a live agent of a disease (innoculation) or of a dead or attenuated form (vaccination) into the body has been highly successful against infectious diseases. In areas where there has been a good acceptance rate, it has led to a large reduction in the incidence of diseases such as diphtheria, measles, rubella (German measles), poliomyelitis and whooping cough (pertussis). Smallpox has been eradicated, largely due to immunization. The effect of these successes is a major improvement in the health of the communities concerned and a substantial reduction in the tragedy of early death and of congenital and acquired defects. But there is concern among public health authorities that parents who have never known diseases such as diphtheria or polio will not have the necessary motivation to see that their children are immunized. The danger is the greater because, after a generation of freedom from such diseases, there is little or no natural immunity in the population, and the reintroduction of the disease might lead to major epidemics. In the USA, legislation ensures compliance by prohibiting entry to schools of unimmunized children. Germs carry surface markers called 'antigens', which prompt the immune system to manufacture antibodies against them (see above). Fortunately, infective organisms can be modified so that, although no longer causing danger to the infected person, they retain their antigens. If such modified organisms are introduced into the body, the immune system reacts to them exactly as it would to the normal virulent strains and produces defensive antibodies.

Immunity can also be achieved in a passive way. Antibodies produced in another person, or in an animal, as a result of infection, can be injected into someone suffering from the same infection. The antibodies are protein molecules and are not cellular organisms, so do not carry antigens. Human immunoglobulin (gamma globulin) is derived from pooled donated blood and contains a considerable collection of antibodies to the diseases common in the general population, including measles, mumps, hepatitis A, rubella and chickenpox. Immunoglobulins can also be taken specifically from donors who have had particular diseases. In this way, immunoglobulins are available for rarer diseases, such as tetanus, rabies and hepatitis B.

Active immunization is always to be preferred but, since it takes time for the necessary levels of antibodies to build up, passive immunization is often necessary in the treatment of serious illness. The two are often combined, passive immunization giving immediate cover while the active production of the patient's own antibodies is getting under way. Everyone should receive routine immunization, starting in infancy, against diphtheria, whooping cough, tetanus, poliomyelitis and measles, and against other diseases as appropriate. Vaccination against smallpox is no longer required and should not be done. HIV-positive people, whether they have symptoms or not, should be immunized against measles, mumps, rubella, polio, whooping cough, tetanus, diphtheria, typhoid, cholera and hepatitis B.

3

Antibiotics

The benefits conferred on humanity by the antibiotics are beyond computation. Most people alive today have no concept of the terrors of a world without antibiotics. These drugs were originally derived from cultures of living organisms, such as fungi or bacteria, but today, many can be chemically synthesized. These drugs are able to kill germs (micro-organisms) in the body, or to prevent their growth or reproduction, without harming the recipient. As a result, almost all diseases caused by infecting bacteria can now be cured by antibiotics. These drugs have no effect on viruses, however.

Ideally, antibiotics should be used only for serious, or potentially serious infections, or to prevent dangerous conditions in specially susceptible people. When a course is prescribed, it should be taken completely and the dosage should be regular.

Antibiotics are often unnecessarily prescribed. Sometimes, this misuse stems from pressure from patients, and sometimes it occurs because busy doctors feel they cannot take chances with possibly potentially serious infections but do not have time to investigate the cases as thoroughly as they might. Hospital doctors are understandably often more concerned with the immediate pressing needs of their patients than with the possible future hazards to society as a whole, and sometimes prescribe powerful new drugs when safer, established remedies would suffice.

Such misuse results in two problems: the development of

strains of bacteria resistant to antibiotics; and the risk of undesirable side-effects. If antibiotics are used casually and in inadequate dosage, the bacteria that are sensitive to them will be killed but those which, by chance, have a natural genetic resistance may survive. When these reproduce, clones of resistant organisms result. This process of natural selection is accelerated by the short bacterial reproduction time – only about 20 minutes. As a result, many organisms are now resistant. This has put a heavy demand on research workers to produce new and better antibiotics, so as to keep ahead. A race is now on between the development of resistance in bacteria and the development of new antibiotics.

The many antibiotics fall into two groups, the members of each of which are related chemically, or by derivation, to each other.

Main Antibiotic Groups

Penicillins penicillin G, penicillin V, cloxacillin, flucloxacillin, etc.

Cephalosporins cephaloridin, cephalothin, cefuroxime, etc.

Aminoglycosides gentamicin, streptomycin, tobramycin, netilmicin, amikacin, neomycin, framycetin

Tetracyclines tetracycline, chlortetracycline, methacycline, oxytetracycline, etc.

Imidazoles metronidazole, ketoconazolew, miconazole, nimorazole, mebendazole, thiabendazole

Individual antibiotics

These include: chlorampbenicol, erythromycin, lincomycin, clindamycin, spectinomycin.

Side-effects

Powerful antibiotics often produce undesirable side-effects:

- **Allergies** to some, especially **penicillin**, are common and may be serious or even fatal.
- **The aminoglycosides** can cause deafness, permanent singing in the ears (tinnitus), kidney damage, or interference with normal blood production if used in large dosage, or in people who cannot excrete them normally.
- **The tetracyclines** can cause permanent staining of teeth if given to young children.
- **Wide-spectrum antibiotics** can destroy normal, health-giving body bacteria and allow overgrowth of undesirable organisms, such as the *Candida* fungus that causes thrush. If used for long periods, they can interfere with the functioning of the immune system.

- **Most antibiotic drugs** can cause nausea and intestinal upset, diarrhea, and skin rashes.

Contagious Diseases

The known contagious diseases can be divided into four main groups, as set out below. There are many contagious diseases - we list only the most common. Several new diseases have been discovered over the last two decades – Legionnaire's disease, AIDS, Ebola fever. No doubt others will be discovered in coming years. In addition, mutant strains of infectious organisms evolve, resistant to known antibiotics, causing virulent strains of formerly mild illnesses. Recently, strains of the salmonella bacterium that cause food poisoning have evolved which are resistant to known antibiotics.

1. Children's diseases
These include chickenpox, measles and rubella (German measles) (all caused by a virus), scarlet fever and whooping cough (bacterial infections), and roseola infantum (cause unknown). Anyone who has had theses diseases is immune - but adults with no natural immunity can be infected with all but roseola. Vaccines are available against all but roseola, but the whooping cough vaccine may cause side-effects and is controversial. Vaccination against Hib type hepatitis is available and vaccination against the rarer meningococcal strains of bacterial meningitis may be introduced to control a local epidemic, but does not work in small children who are most at risk.

2. Common diseases affecting adults
Vaccines are available to prevent all of these diseases, and anyone who was not vaccinated as a child should be protected. Men are more often affected than women by viral hepatitis. In the US about 40% of young adults have been exposed to hepatitis A. Both forms of hepatitis are more prevalent in places with poor hygiene. See holiday diseases, below.

3. Holiday diseases
Before travelling abroad, check with your physician or a vaccination clinic and arrange to have the necessary vaccinations against the diseases prevalent in the region you will be visiting. Bear in mind that the prevalence changes from year to year, so you should check regularly.
The most widespread, or commonly occurring diseases for

which vaccines are available, are listed below. Others are
tetanus and polio, listed above, cholera, rabies, sleeping
sickness and typhoid. For malaria a course of drugs must be
started some days before entering a malarial area and
continued for four weeks after leaving it. Vaccines are not
available for all diseases, so in some areas you may need to
take special precautions:

Lyme disease is a bacterial infection, which is transmitted by
tick bites. It occurs throughout the temperate climatic zones: in
the US, Europe, Australia, the former USSR and China. In the
US and Europe, the disease is prevalent among hunters. The
disease begins with heachache, fever, and aches in the joints,
and progresses to damaged joints and disorders of

CONTAGIOUS DISEASES CHART

	Incubation	When contagious
Glandular fever (virus)	4–7 weeks	Usually a few weeks
Diphtheria (bacterial)	2–5 days	While symptoms persist
Legionnaire's disease (bacterial)	2–10 days	About 3 weeks
Polio (virus)	3–35 days	Up to 6 weeks
Mumps (virus)	14–24 days	From 6 days before glands swell till 9 days after swelling.
Tetanus (bacterial)	2–50 days	Not transmissable under normal conditions
Tuberculosis (bacterial)	infection is immediate	While the disease is active

the nervous system, including inflammation of the brain coverings (encephalitis) and paralysis of certain nerves. Treatment is with antibiotics. Covering the legs and arms when outdoors, and using insect repellents can help to reduce the likelihood of tick bites.

Lassa fever is a viral disease occurring only in West Africa. Its sources are food contaminated by rats, and contact with the body fluids of infected people. The disease begins with a sore throat and tiredness, but the symptoms become rapidly more acute, eventually leading to death from kidney and heart damage. Treatment is with intensive care. The disease can be prevented by scrupulous attention to hygiene and avoiding contact with infectious people.

3

Symptoms	Treatment
Headache, muscle pains, fever, sore throat, swollen lymph nodes. Loss of appetite.	For symptoms: rest, throat wash, aspirin, Also for complicationss if any.
Raised temperature, rapid pulse, swollen neck glands, sore throat, hoarseness. A greyish membrane covers the throat and may obstruct breathing.	Emergency opening into the windpipe to restore breathing; antibiotics and antitoxins.
Mild flu-like symptoms worsening to high fever, cough, chest pains, labored breathing, diarrhea, vomiting.	Antibiotics. Bedrest.
Initially mild headache with fever; in serious cases neck stiffness, raised temperature, rapid pulse, progressive muscle weakness, paralysis of part of the body.	None. Symptoms alleviated by bedrest and painkillers.
Chill and fever, headache, temperature, swollen salivary glands (pain on chewing). Other glands may be swollen. In men, painful swelling of the testicles.	For symptoms: rest, soft diet, aspirin, perhaps sedatives. Also for complications if any.
Fever, sore throat, headache, spasm of the chewing muscles, difficulty in opening the jaw; risus sardonicus (snarling smile, rigid, backward-arching smile).	Tetanus antitoxin, antibiotics, and antispasmodics.
Fever, fatigue, loss of appetite and weight, night sweats, persistent cough and blood-streaked sputum.	A range of drugs.

Disease	Occurrence	Transmission	Symptoms
Hepatitis A (viral)	Central and South America, Africa, the Middle East, South, East, and SE Asia.	Contaminated food and water	Inflammation of the liver, fever, jaundice
Hepatitis B	Central and South America, Africa, the Middle East, South, East, and SE Asia.	Contact with body fluids of infected people; shared infected needles	Inflammation of the liver, fever, jaundice
Malaria (protozoal)	Central and South America, especially Brazil, Africa south of the Sahara, South, East and SE Asia	Bite from an *Anopheles* mosquito	Recurrent, severe fevers, dizziness, delirium
Meningococcal meningitis (bacterial)	Parts of Central Africa and Asia	Droplets spread by an infected person	Fever, stiff neck, vomiting, coma
Yellow fever* (virus)	Tropical Africa and America	Bite from an *Aedes Aegypti* mosquito	Fever, headache, jaundice, vomiting blood, coma

*You need an official certificate of protection against yellow fever for entry to Benin, Burkina Faso, Cameroon, Central African Republic, Chad, Congo, French Guiana, Gabon, Ghana, Ivory Coast, Liberia, Mali, Mauritania, Niger, Panama, Rwanda, Senegal, Togo and Zaire.

4. Sexually transmitted diseases

These include: AIDS, syphilis, gonorrhoea, chlamydial infections, herpes, Gardnerella infection, genital warts, thrush, trichomoniasis, and others. They are covered in detail in pp 155-64.

Inherited Disorders

A few disorders exist that usually occur only in men, but that are always inherited through their mother. These include hemophilia, red-green color blindness, and two forms of muscular dystrophy.

Of course, many defects can be inherited. Each chromosome inherited from a parent carries many thousands of 'genes' or units of genetic information. If any one of these genes is faulty, it will not pass on the correct instructions and a defect can occur. However, these few disorders such as hemophilia are passed on in the odd way described because they are linked with the X chromosome. This is one of the chromosomes that determine sex; but other genes on the same chromosome have other jobs – including helping to ensure normal color vision, blood clotting; and so on.

Both men and women have X chromosomes, and both men and women can have X chromosomes in which one of these genes is faulty. But whenever the defective chromosome is matched by another, normal X chromosome, the defect will not appear: the correct function (e.g. color vision) is guaranteed by the normal chromosome (i.e. the normal gene is 'dominant').

So in any woman the defective chromosome is normally masked by a healthy one from the other parent. And a father with the defective gene cannot pass it on to his son at all, because to them he contributes only his Y chromosome. But a mother can pass it on to her sons, because to them she contributes their X chromosome which may be defective and their other Y chromosome will not 'mask' it, because it does not have a gene responsible for the defective function.

The only way in which a woman can show the signs of one of these defects is if she has inherited defective X chromosomes from both sides of the family. This is very unlikely, but does happen rather more often in the case of color blindness.

A woman who does not herself show signs of the disorder, but can pass it on, is called a 'carrier'. Only chance decides whether or not any one of her children inherits the defective X chromosome: the child can equally inherit the healthy one. So if a carrier becomes pregnant, there is a one in four chance of her having a normal son; the same chance of her having a normal daughter; the same of her having an affected son; and the same of her having a carrier daughter.

If a woman is found to be a carrier, there is risk not only to her own subsequent children, but also to those of her female relatives on the maternal side – because they may also have inherited the defective gene. If no previous family history is discovered after careful check, it is likely to be an isolated mutation in either mother or child. If in the mother, she can still pass it on to subsequent children.

Hemophilia

This disorder is characterized by uncontrollable bleeding, even after slight wounds. It is caused by a deficiency of one of the elements needed to make the blood clot. There are about 8 cases per 10,000 of the population and about 3 to 4 severe cases per 100,000.

Symptoms

In mild cases, the disorder may remain undiscovered until revealed by some incident (e.g. loss of a tooth). In severe cases, it will be obvious soon after birth. There is persistent blood flow from any cut, or in any bruise. Without special treatment this may continue for hours or even days, despite normal attempts to stop it. Even when the flow does finally stop, it may recur soon after. The real danger, however, is from internal bleeding. Superficial cuts and scratches are not threatening unless the mucous membrane is involved, and deep cuts do not kill unless a major vein or artery is involved. But bleeding in soft tissues, such as the kidney, is serious, and bleeding in large joints can eventually cripple them. Both conditions can occur spontaneously in severe cases. The symptoms may decline with age, and at any age there may be periods free from trouble. Laboratory tests are necessary for diagnosis.

Treatment

The hemophiliac has to take special care in all he does and in

Hemophilia carriers and sufferers

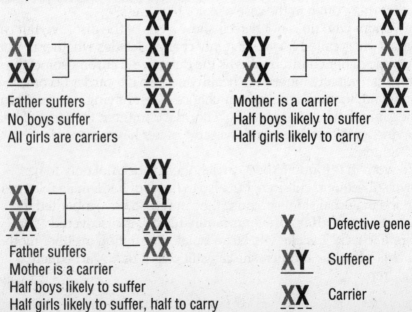

XY
XX
Father suffers
No boys suffer
All girls are carriers

XY
XY
XX
XX

XY
XX
Mother is a carrier
Half boys likely to suffer
Half girls likely to carry

XY
XY
XX
XX

XY
XX
Father suffers
Mother is a carrier
Half boys likely to suffer
Half girls likely to suffer, half to carry

XY
XY
XX
XX

X   Defective gene

XY   Sufferer

XX   Carrier

severe cases his sphere of activity is drastically curtailed. Any sports involving bodily contact or danger of injury must be avoided. Hemophiliacs often wear warning tags, in case they are involved in an accident or need an emergency operation. If bleeding occurs, the missing blood factor is injected intravenously to promote clotting. Since the appearance of AIDS, this need has exposed hemophiliacs to infection by the HIV virus as a result of being injected with infected blood products. Since this tragic situation first came to light, most health authorities have instigated rigorous screening procedures at blood banks. However, that does not protect hemophiliacs who need blood products when travelling abroad, and there is no answer to this difficulty. Carrying emergency blood supplies is not a practical proposition, since they need to be kept in controlled conditions.

3

Muscular Dystrophy

This is a disease in which the muscles waste away. Muscle tissue does not replace itself, and slowly gives way to fibrous tissue and fat. It may be due to absence or excess of protein, or the presence of abnormal protein. There are several forms of the disease. All are usually inherited, but two are sex linked – inherited almost only by men, and through female carriers. The carriers themselves may have slight muscle weakness, but are usually apparently normal.

Duchenne Type

This is the most common and most severe form. Half of those with muscular dystrophy are boys with the Duchenne type. The disease is usually fatal by the age of 25. The first symptoms develop between the age of 2 and 5. Walking is clumsy, running poor, falls frequent. Later, climbing stairs and getting up after falls becomes difficult. Weakness begins with certain muscles of the shoulders, upper arms, and thighs. Diagnosis is by measuring enzymes in the blood serum, and examining small muscle samples under a microscope. (If muscular dystrophy is suspected in a family, these tests can also diagnose it within a few days of a child's birth.) There is at present no cure or effective drug treatment. Exercise and muscle stretching can slightly slow the progress of the disease, but eventually (usually between 8 and 11) the child has to take to a wheelchair. The spine curves, muscle weakness spreads, eventually affecting even eating and drinking, and muscle contraction distorts limb positions. Finally respiratory and heart muscles are involved, and death occurs, usually between

16 and 25. There are tests that prove a woman is a carrier
(though none can prove she is not).
Becker Type
This is similar in the muscles affected and pattern of
inheritance, but rarer, later, slower, and milder. Patients can
usually still walk in their thirties and often into middle age.

Color Defective Vision

Color defective vision may be caused by poisoning and by
certain diseases, but it is most commonly inherited. Women
are usually carriers and men inherit the defect. The condition is
due to a reduced number of cone cells in the retina of the eye,
which are responsible for color vision. There are three types,
sensitive to blue, green and yellow light respectively. The
nature and degree of an individual's defect depends upon
which groups of cells are affected. Difficulty in distinguishing
gray from purple is the most common defect, but many men
have difficulty in distinguishing shades of red and orange
from shades of yellow and green. The ability to read red and
green signals is essential in many areas of work. The condition
may be diagnosed by a number of color tests, but there is no
cure for color defective vision.

Hernias

A hernia has occurred if a body organ protrudes through the
wall of the body cavity in which it is sited. This happens most
often in the abdomen: part of the stomach or intestine is
pushed through the abdominal wall.
Hernias occur where the cavity wall is weak, either because of
a natural gap where a blood vessel or digestive tube passes, or
because of scar tissue. They are often called 'ruptures', but this
really means any tearing or breaking of tissue (e.g. ruptured
blood vessels).

Types of Hernias

Inguinal Hernias are by far the most common. In men, the
inguinal canal is the pathway down which the testes descend just
before birth. In later life it contains the spermatic cord and blood
vessels. In an inguinal hernia, part of the intestine protrudes down

this canal, into the scrotum. Since the inguinal canal is much smaller in women (containing only a fibrous cord), inguinal hernias are much more common in men.

Femoral Hernias are more often found in women. The femoral canal is the route through which the main blood vessels to the leg pass from the abdomen. In a femoral hernia, part of the intestine passes down the canal and protrudes at the top of the thigh.

Umbilical Hernias occur where the abdominal wall has been weakened at the navel by the umbilical cord. They are found mostly in young children.

Ventral Hernias occur where the abdominal wall has been weakened by the scar of a wound. (When the scar is due to an operation, it is called an incisional hernia.)

Epigastric Hernias are protrusions of fat and sometimes intestine through the abdominal wall between the navel and the breastbone.

Obturator Hernias occur when part of the intestine passes through a gap between the bones of the front of the pelvis.

Hiatus Hernia occurs when the upper part of the stomach protrudes upwards through the hole in the diaphragm occupied by the esophagus.

Hernias can also be classified in other ways.

Congenital or Acquired Congenital hernias exist at birth. All others are acquired. The only congenital hernias are umbilical or inguinal but congenital weakness in the abdominal wall may give rise to hernias.

Reducible or Irreducible Reducible hernias can be pushed back into place in the abdomen. Irreducible hernias cannot – the opening is too small.

Inguinal and femoral hernias

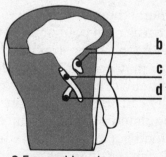

1 Inguinal hernia

2 Femoral hernia

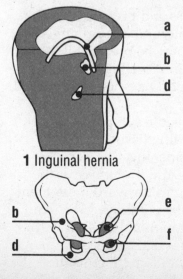

a Spermatic cord	e Site of inguinal
b Pubic bone	hernia
c Femoral canal	f Site of femoral
d Ischium	hernia

Strangulated or Unstrangulated Strangulated hernias are those in which the tightness of the opening has cut off the blood supply. This is a very serious condition, leading rapidly to tissue death, gangrene and death. In unstrangulated hernias, the protruding tissue still has its blood supply.

Hernias: Causes, Symptoms, Treatment

Causes

Congenital hernias are caused by the failure of some channels to close properly during fetal development. The intestine is either displaced at birth or easily becomes so. Acquired hernias are caused by any form of straining or exertion that increases pressure in the abdomen, and forces it through a weak spot in the abdominal wall (e.g. physical work, straining at the bowels, violent coughing, etc). Strain and exertion equally act as predisposing factors (i.e. they weaken the abdominal wall) as also does any large, sudden gain or loss in weight (including pregnancy). Men who do heavy manual work are much more likely to suffer from hernias.

Symptoms

These depend on the type and condition of the hernia, the size and tightness of the opening, and the amount of the organ involved. Also the onset of the hernia may be gradual, with the symptoms increasing till they become noticeable; or sudden (perhaps while lifting a heavy weight), in which case the person is often aware of something having 'given way', perhaps with varying degrees of pain.

In general there is a feeling of weakness and pressure in the area, occasional pain or a continual ache, and a gurgling feeling in the organ under strain. A swelling may be present all the time or may appear only under pressure. Swellings that are continually present may increase in size. Digestion is disrupted, usually causing constipation.

Strangulated hernias produce special acute symptoms. When the blood supply is cut off, the protruding tissue dies and swells, increasing the pressure in the opening. The hernia becomes inflamed and acutely painful and the skin over the area may redden. (With intestinal hernias, forward movement in the intestine ceases, and there may be vomiting.) The dead tissue in the hernia quickly becomes gangrenous, often within five or six hours, and this in turn causes peritonitis – inflammation of the abdominal lining and its contents. If untreated, death occurs within a few days.

Treatment

Reducible hernias are sometimes held in place by a truss – a belt with a pad which is fitted over the hernia. But as long as the hernia exists, the risk of future strangulation remains. Most hernias are therefore treated surgically. Any damaged tissue is removed, the protruding organ replaced in the abdomen, and the opening stitched up again. Strangulated hernias require immediate operation.

3

Trusses

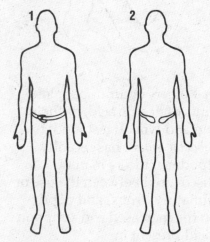

1 Truss for right inguinal hernia
2 Double truss

A truss is a belt that presses against the hernia so that the gut cannot protrude through it. Surgery, however, is a more effective treatment.

Peptic Ulcer

An ulcer is a breach in the surface of the skin or in the membranes inside the body. The breach does not heal, and it spreads across, and through, the tissue. Peptic ulcers are small breaks in the mucous lining of any part of the gastrointestinal tract. There are two main types: ulcers of the stomach, called gastric ulcers; and ulcers of the duodenum (the first part of the small intestine). They occur if the lining of the stomach or duodenum becomes eroded by the stomach acids and digestive enzymes (i.e. the stomach and intestine begin to digest themselves). Peptic ulcers can also occur in the lower part of the oesophagus, but these are very rare.

Causes

Important advances have been made during the 1980s and 1990s in the understanding of the causes of peptic ulcers. It is now known that gastric ulcers are more common in people who take large amounts of aspirin and other salicylate drugs, in smokers, and in people who drink excessive amounts of

Sites of peptic ulcers

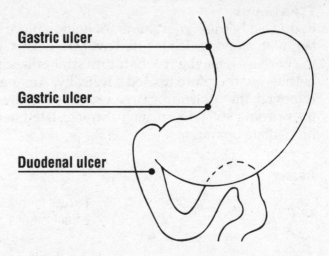

Gastric ulcer

Gastric ulcer

Duodenal ulcer

coffee or alcoholic drinks. Duodenal ulcers occur in people who secrete unusually large amounts of gastric acid, or their stomach acids are unusually strong, and who digest food rapidly. An organism called *Helicobacter pylori* has recently been discovered to be a cause of duodenal ulcers in many people. A link has recently been discovered between the use of NSAIDs (non-steroidal anti-inflammatory drugs) and peptic ulcers. A link is suspected between the increased consumption of lineolic acid (an essential fatty acid present in polyunsaturated fats), which has been found to decrease the production of gastric acids, and a fall in the occurrence of peptic ulcers, but this link has not been proved.

Associated Factors

Some things are known to increase the likelihood of developing a peptic ulcer: living under considerable stress; drinking large amounts of alcohol; eating rich food; having excess acidity of the stomach; suffering from frequent stomach or intestinal infection; being of blood group 'O' having a family history of ulcers, and being of 'personality type A'.

Symptoms

Peptic ulcers may be acute or chronic. Recurring indigestion is a common first symptom, followed by heartburn, pain and nausea. Untreated ulcers may lead to an intensification of the pain, bleeding from the ulcer, and perforation - the ulcer eventually eats through the wall of the digestive tract, causing a serious and often fatal inflammation of the abdominal cavity, called peritonitis.

Gastric ulcers: pain in the upper abdomen after eating, usually slightly to the left-hand side of the body, and is not relieved by eating. Indigestion, nausea and vomiting are common.

Duodenal ulcers: pain in the centre of the upper abdomen may occur before meals and in the early hours of the morning, and can be relieved by eating. The abdomen may feel tender around the site of the ulcer.

	Duodenal	Gastric
When does pain occur?	Before meals or 2 to 2½ hours after	½ to 2 hours after meals
Is it made better by food?	Yes	Somtimes
Vomiting?	Rare	Common
Appetite?	Good	Fair

3

Treatment

Modern treatment for peptic ulcers concentrates on medication to eliminate the *Helicobacter pylori* organism and to reduce the acid secretions of the digestive system, especially overnight. These measures, continued for 6 to 8 weeks, will heal most ulcers. Combinations of antibiotics have been found effective in eliminating *Helicobacter pylori*; Zantac (ranitidine) has been found effective in reducing stomach acid.

Peptic ulcers have a high recurrence rate. To prevent recurrence, foods that increase the production of stomach acids, such as highly seasoned and gas-forming foods, and foods high in roughage, should be reduced in the diet, and alcoholic drinks should also be reduced. But frequent bland meals are no longer recommended, since they are thought to increase gastric acid production. It is believed that the role of stress as a cause of peptic ulcers has been overestimated, so long periods of bedrest are no longer recommended. Smoking and drinking alcohol are discouraged. Antacids are not thought to be effective in treating peptic ulcers. People with resistant ulcers may be offered a 'maintenance' treatment to prevent recurrence of the conditions that produced the ulcer. Acute ulcer disease, with bleeding, vomiting blood and perforation, may need to be treated by surgery to remove the affected part of the stomach, or to sever the nerve that stimulates the stomach to produce acid.

Gout

Gout is a form of arthritis, an acute – and extremely painful – inflammation of joints, tendons and other tissues. It is caused by an excess of uric acid in the blood – a condition that may be hereditary. Uric acid is produced during the breakdown of proteins, and is normally excreted from the body in the urine. The excess uric acid cannot be excreted by the kidneys, and it collects, in the form of monosodium urate monohydrate crystals, around the joints and tendons.

People with a family history of gout are thought to have a predisposition to the condition. Men constitute over 90% of all sufferers; some post-menopausal women develop gout, so they may be protected from developing the disease by the female sex hormones. However, gout rarely occurs before the age of 45.

Acute gout

Attacks of gout are usually sudden, often beginning at night, with acute pain in the big toe or thumb. The joint becomes red, inflamed and excruciatingly painful. The sufferer is feverish and passes less, more intensely coloured urine than normal. If untreated, an attack can last for four to ten days.

Chronic gout

Gout tends to recur, initially on the site of the first attack, but later involving more joints. In chronic gout, acute attacks occur more frequently, but with less intensity. The affected joints become arthritic as the crystal deposits gradually form stones called 'tophi'. Eventually, crystals may be deposited in the kidneys, beneath the skin, in the eyes and in the cartilage of the ear. In the long-term, the kidneys, liver, arteries and heart may degenerate.

Treatment

Gout is easily treated these days with non-steroidal anti-inflammatory drugs (NSAIDs), which reduce the inflammation and relieve the pain; and uricosuric drugs, which increase the excretion of uric acid, or inhibit the formation of uric acid salts. Eating plain foods, cutting down on alcohol, drinking plenty of fresh water – at least five pints per day – and regular exercise also help.

The intestines

The intestines are the long tube by which food leaves the
stomach and is eventually excreted from the body. The tube is
made up of sheaths of muscle, coated on the inside with
mucous membrane. The small intestine leads directly from the
stomach. It is about 22ft (6.6m) long, and up to 1½in (3.75cm)
wide. It continues the process, begun in the stomach, of
absorbing nutrients from the food.

The large intestine (the 'colon') follows on from this. It is about
6ft (1.8m) long and up to 2½in (6.25cm) wide. Its main function
is the absorption of water from the waste products ('feces').
Many physiological disorders may affect the small intestine

3

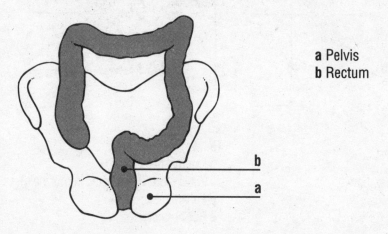

a Pelvis
b Rectum

(e.g. bacterial infection or fever). It can also be a site for ulcers
and cancer. However, the term 'bowels' refers mainly to the
large intestine – and often simply to the last 6 to
8in (15–20cm) (the 'rectum') and the surface opening (the
'anus') through which the waste products are excreted, usually
in a fairly solid form known as 'stools'. This is another
potential cancer site. But it is also affected by certain well-
known disorders, linked with the physical process of waste
evacuation, and dealt with on the following pages.

Normal and Diseased Bowels

Normal bowels

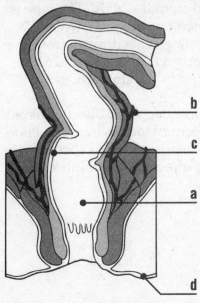

Diseased bowels

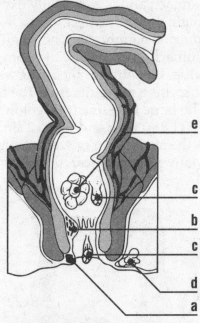

a Rectum
b Veins
c Mucus membrane
d Skin

a Internal hemorrhoid
b External hemorrhoid
c Polyp (fibrous elongated hemorrhoid)
d Perianal abscess
e Rectal carcinoma

Diarrhea and Constipation

These common complaints are both usually caused by the
failure of the colon to carry out its job of controlling the level of
water in the feces. This may be due to any one of many causes:
a change of eating habits; gastritis (inflammation of the
stomach); gastro-enteritis (inflammation of stomach and
intestine); or bacterial or viral infection of the intestine.

Diarrhea

Diarrhea is the excessive discharge of watery feces. The
primary danger in serious cases is body dehydration, and this
can be combated by an increased intake of fluid.

Constipation

Constipation is infrequent or absent defecation. It is usually
caused by a poor diet, especially one lacking in roughage. But
it may follow diarrhea in the course of an infection – and is
also sometimes caused by intestinal obstruction. However,

much imagined constipation is only the consequence of judging bowel habits by an excessive norm of 'regularity'. In fact, 'normal' bowel motions may occur as often as three times a day, or as infrequently as once every three or four days, depending on the individual. Constipation can be both relieved and prevented by a healthy lifestyle: a largely vegetarian diet with a high fibre content; regular exercise, especially walking; and drinking plenty of fresh water — at least five pints per day is recommended.

Hemorrhoids (Piles)

Hemorrhoids (piles) come about through the enlargement of veins in the wall of the rectum or in the anus.

This may be due to acute constipation, or overstraining during excretion. It can also result from tumors.

The swellings cause the mucus membrane to press against passing feces, causing discomfort, pain and sometimes bleeding.

Internal hemorrhoids occur at or before the rectum's junction with the anus. If they protrude beyond the anal opening the pressure of the anal muscle (the 'sphincter') often causes great and constant pain – this is known as 'strangulation'.

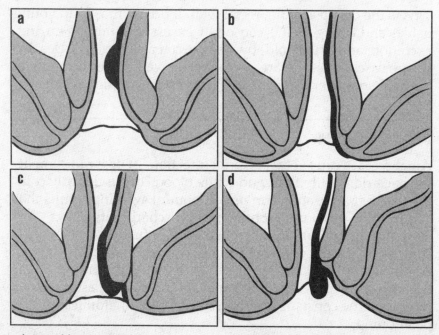

a Internal hemorrhoid
b External hemorrhoid
c Enlarged hemorrhoid
d Strangulated hemorrhoid

External hemorrhoids occur under the skin just outside the anus. In addition to the usual causes, they can also result from a ruptured vein leading to a hemorrhage. Internal hemorrhoids may eventually develop 'polyps'. This is a condition in which the hemorrhoidal protrusion becomes fibrous and elongated.

Colitis

Colitis is inflammation of the colon – often with an associated ulcer. The symptoms are abdominal discomfort, diarrhea, blood in the feces and fever. Anemia and even emaciation result. The first (acute) phase can be fatal if untreated. More usually, a prolonged (chronic) phase develops.
The causes are unknown, but may be linked in different individuals with: infection; allergy; deficiency of vitamin B and certain proteins; or simply nervous stress. Sometimes several causes occur together. Treatment involves bedrest until the fever has passed; and also careful dietary control using highly nutritious foods, high in protein. Steroids may be used. Relapses are frequent. In extreme cases surgery is needed.

Rectal Prolapse

This is the collapse of the rectal wall. It occurs mostly in young babies and the aged. It is caused by excessive straining during excretion, and (in the old) by weak rectal and anal muscles. In severe cases, an entire area of the rectal wall passes through the anal sphincter. Extreme pain from strangulation results.

Abscesses

An abscess is caused by bacterial infection. In order to combat the bacteria, bodily fluid and white blood corpuscles collect in the tissue spaces, and form pus. A painful swelling results that continues to grow until it bursts and discharges its fluid.
To avoid discomfort and the possibility of further complications abscesses are usually drained surgically. Anorectal and perianal abscesses are extremely painful, because of the pressure of the anal sphincter, the passage of feces, and the constant irritation due to their anatomical positioning.

Fissure-in-ano

This is splitting of the walls of the anus. It is usually due to the passing of an exceptionally large stool. An 'acute' fissure involves only the outer surface of the wall (the mucous membrane). If it does not disappear after a few days, it develops into a 'chronic' fissure, which is deeper. This causes great pain and needs intensive treatment.

3

Irritable Bowel Syndrome

Recurrent pain, tummy rumbling, excessive gas production, and frequent diarrhoea alternating with constipation. It is more common in women than men, and in people aged between 20 and 40. The condition is believed to be common among people who are excessively anxious, and can be worsened by stress. Psychotherapy may help to reduce the symptoms, but food intolerance is also thought to be a cause. Treatment may therefore consist of an elimination diet, in which fresh meat, fish, vegetables, rice, and any milk are eliminated from the diet for a period of three weeks, then one food is reintroduced each day or two to identify the food that causes the symptoms. This treatment is thought to be effective in up to 50 percent of cases. A decrease in overall food consumption may also help.

Gay Bowel Syndrome

A condition affecting mainly those homosexual men who practice "fisting" (inserting a fist into the lower part of the rectum), or inserting other objects into the rectum during sex. The practices damage the margin of the anus and the rectum, and results in anal abscesses, causing anal fistulas (a persistent discharge from the anus) and anal fissures (see above).

The Urinary System

In the male body, the urinary and reproductive systems are interconnected. This complexity makes the urinary system a likely and troublesome site for infection. The system consists of those organs that produce and excrete urine: a pair of kidneys; a pair of tubes called ureters; a muscular bag called the bladder; and another single tube called the urethra.

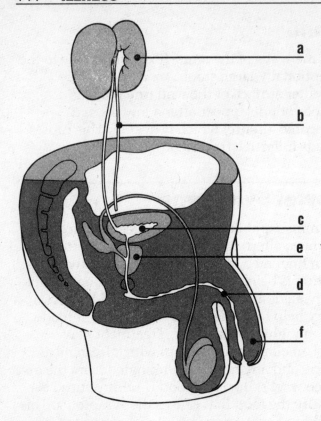

a	**a** Kidneys
	b Ureters
	c Bladder
b	**d** Urethra
	e Prostate
	f Penis
c	
e	
d	
f	

The kidneys

The kidneys are located on either side of the spine, in the region of the middle back. The right kidney lies slightly lower than the left. Each kidney is bean-shaped, and about 4in long, 2½in (6.5cm) wide, and 1½in (4cm) thick. Each weighs about 5 ounces (142g). The kidneys are chemical processing works. In them, waste matter in the blood – crystalline particles and fluids – is filtered off under pressure, through more than 2 million glomerules – tiny filtering units. Some glucose, amino acids, electrolytes and water are reabsorbed into the bloodstream. The waste matter is excreted as a fluid called urine.

The Ureters

The ureters are muscular tubes, each one about 10in (25cm) long. One tube leads from each kidney, and down them the urine passes to the bladder, at the rate of a drop every 30 seconds.

The Bladder

The bladder is a balloon-like, muscular bag that acts as a reservoir for the urine. When full it holds about 1.2pt (US) (0.6 litres) of urine – though the desire to urinate is usually felt

when about half that amount is present. A muscular ring
(sphincter) surrounds the exit from the bladder into the
urethra. When this is contracted, it prevents leakage of urine
out of the bladder. Upon urination the sphincter is relaxed, and
the urine passes into the urethra. During sexual excitement, the
internal part of the sphincter closes, preventing urine from
passing into the urethra during ejaculation.

The urethra

The urethra is an S-shaped muscular tube about 8in (52cm)
long in a man. It leads from the bladder, along the penis, to the
external opening. In men it has two functions: to transport
urine from the bladder during urination (called 'micturition');
and to carry semen from the prostate during ejaculation (see p
361).

The prostate

The prostate is a gland lying just under the bladder and
surrounding the urethra at its upper end. Its secretions keep
the lining of the urethra moist, and during sexual excitement,
form part of the seminal fluid (see p 373).

Urine

Urine consists of 96% water and 4% dissolved solids. Only 60%
of the water taken into the body is normally eliminated as
urine. The rest passes out in sweat and feces, and through the
lungs. Urine is normally straw-colored or amber. In 24 hours
an adult usually passes about 2.2pt (US) (1 litre), spread over 4
to 6 occasions (and most do not find it necessary to get up to
pass urine at night). However, all these characteristics vary
normally with: the amount of fluid drunk, and when; the
amount lost in sweat; the size of the bladder; etc.

Urinary Disorders

Urethritis

Urethritis is inflammation of the urethra. The most common
cause is a sexually transmitted disease (STD), but any irritation
of the urethra can cause an attack. Sources of irritation can
include alcohol consumption, ingredients in the diet and the
passage of instruments along the urethra during surgical
examination. The symptoms are discharge of pus from the
penis, pain on urinating, tenderness of the urethra and
possibly inflammation of other organs such as testes, bladder
and even kidneys. If an obstruction, such as an enlarged
prostate, prevents the flow along the urethra, an infection in
the urethra can lead to cystitis, an inflammation of the bladder

lining. Treatment for urethritis depends on the cause. Drinking large quantities of fluid usually helps.

Retention

Retention refers to the involuntary holding back of urine in the bladder, due to some obstruction of the urethra. The bladder enlarges behind the obstruction as the quantity of urine increases, and may be stretched and weakened. Eventually the ureters and kidneys also dilate, and kidney infection may occur. Rapid surgical treatment is needed, before the kidneys suffer permanent damage.

Retention is most common in elderly men, due to enlargement of the prostate gland. Strictures are another cause.

Strictures

A stricture is an abrupt narrowing of the ureters or urethra. In the ureters, it may be congenital, or caused by physical irritation such as the passage of kidney stones or surgical instruments. Treatment is difficult, and surgery is usually necessary.

Strictures of the urethra are more common. They may also be congenital, but are usually 'spasmodic' or 'organic'. Spasmodic strictures are temporary, and due to irritation by cold, excess alcohol or physical objects. They last only a few hours or days, and cause no permanent discomfort. Organic strictures follow prolonged inflammation or laceration, and if untreated may cause distension and inflammation of the bladder and kidneys. Both forms are treated by stretching the urethra with special instruments. In organic strictures this must be repeated regularly.

Kidney Disorders

These mainly result from infection or kidney stones. Bacterial infection can reach the kidney through the blood stream, or pass back along the urinary system from a site of stagnant urine or sexually transmitted disease. If kidney damage results, waste products left in the blood can cause poisoning, while rising blood pressure can lead to heart failure or brain hemorrhage. The same may occur if back pressure from retention damages the kidneys. Kidney stones (which generally have unknown causes) may stay in the kidney or pass out without trouble, but they can also cover the entrance to the ureter, or get stuck in ureter or urethra. This can be violently painful, and surgery may be needed.

Incontinence

Incontinence is inability to control the bladder: urination occurs when the person does not want it to. Causes include psychological stress (e.g. severe fright), disorders of the bladder, and, especially, impairment of the controlling nerves due to injury or disease. Incontinence due to old age is also common.

Bladder Tumors

Tumors of the lining of the bladder cause about 4% of all cancers diagnosed in the United States, and affect about three times more men than women. Most are benign wart-like growths called papillomas. They are painless, but as they develop they may cause bleeding, or retention (stagnation of urine in the bladder). They are caused by smoking.

3

Preventing Urinary Disorders

• drink plenty of fluids, especially clean water, daily
• pay careful attention to personal hygiene: shower or bathe daily, cleaning the genital and anal regions; wear clean underpants daily
• use a condom during sex with another person
• exercise regularly to keep the pelvic muscles in tone
• do not smoke; avoid areas where you may be subjected to secondary smoking.

Prostatics Disorders

Prostatitis

This is inflammation of the prostate, usually caused by infection in the urinary tract – most commonly the urethra – which has spread to the prostate. It may be due to a sexually transmitted infection, such as gonorrhea (see p 157). Prostatitis is most common in men aged between 30 and 50.
Symptoms are pain when urinating, more frequent urination than usual, a discharge from the penis, blood in the urine, and pains in the lower back or abdomen or around the rectum. The disorder is diagnosed by internal examination and urine test, and treated with antibiotics. However, prostatitis tends to recur and can become chronic. An abscess may develop, and need to be drained.

Enlarged prostate

In adult men the prostate (see p 145 is normally about 1in by ¾in by 1½in (2.5cm by 1.9cm by 3.75cm). In later life, however, for reasons not yet understood, it enlarges. Enlargement of the prostate affects about 43 percent of men aged over 60.

Symptoms

In the early stages, there are rarely any symptoms, and no treatment is necessary. Eventually, however, the enlarging gland compresses the urethra. If untreated it may eventually cause retention- it blocks the passage of urine. Early diagnosis and treatment are essential, as retention carries a risk of serious damage to the kidneys. Noticeable symptoms are:

- urination is slow to begin, lacks force, and is often interrupted by pauses
- the desire to urinate occurs with increasing frequency especially at night
- there are further dribbles of urine after the main flow has stopped
- urethritis or prostatitis may occur if the urine retained in the bladder sets up infection
- there may be a desire to urinate, but urination is difficult or impossible.

Treatment

Severe symptoms usually necessitate urgent drainage of the bladder by inserting a catheter into the urethra. Removal of part of all of the prostate – a prostatectomy – is still the most common treatment, but major advances in the treatment of prostate enlargement have taken place over recent years. As we write, experiments are taking place in the widening of the compressed urethra by balloon dilatation (similar to the treatment used to unblock arteries, see p 76); and in the insertion of a tube, called a prosthetic stent, into the urethra, to give permanent support. A drug called Proscar has been found to be effective in shrinking an enlarging prostate, and is now in general use. Microwaving of the prostate is also used.

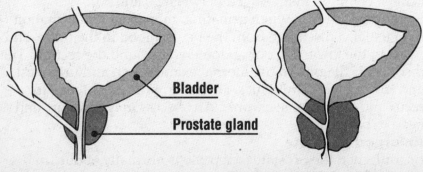

Bladder

Prostate gland

Enlarged prostate constricts urethra, causing retention

Radical Prostatectomy

Removal of the prostate is now nearly always done through the urethra instead of through an incision made in the abdomen. In trans-urethral prostatectomy (TURPS), a resectoscope is passed through the urethra and heated wire or laser beams are used to cut away the prostate tissue. This operation is safer, minimizes bleeding, and preserves nerves and blood vessels, so that 50% of patients retain their potency and fertility after the operation.

3

Transurethral Prostatectomy

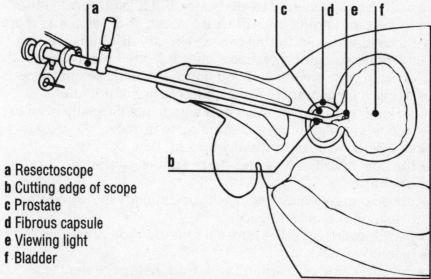

a Resectoscope
b Cutting edge of scope
c Prostate
d Fibrous capsule
e Viewing light
f Bladder

Prostate Tumors

This is the second most common cancer affecting men. It occurs as early as 50, but is most common in men aged over 60. Early diagnosis is vital: 32,000 American men die every year from malignant cancer of the prostate, but if diagnosed in its early stages, this cancer is curable.

Cancer of the prostate has a genetic link: if your father or brother had it, you are twice as likely to develop the disease as someone with no family links. If two of your first-degree relatives had it, you are four times as likely to develop it.

Diagnosis

Diagnosis is by rectal examination and biopsy. Difficulties in distinguishing between benign and malignant enlargement have been reduced by the PSA blood test carried out over a period of 1 year. The PSA (prostatic specific antigen) rises rapidly if the enlargement is caused by a malignant tumor.

Treatment

Prostate cancer is hormone dependent - the male hormones affect its development. In its early stages it may be made to shrink and its further development brought under control, by treatment with female hormones, or by surgical castration.

Monitoring Symptoms

Changes in urination and in the composition of urine are early-warning signs of a disorder, but men tend to be slow to report such changes to their physicians. Minor urinary problems can usually be cleared up if treated early, but if left untreated they may become chronic and difficult to treat, or develop into more serious illnesses, including cancer. Urinary disorders are also sometimes symptoms of illness affecting other parts of the body. Report to your physician if you notice any of these symptoms:
- changes in quantity of urine, or frequency of urination
- waking up to urinate at night if you do not normally need to
- difficult in beginning or continuing to urinate
- slow and weak, or unusually forceful flow
- the flow of urine stops and starts; sudden stopping
- dribbling
- unusual urgent needs to urinate or difficulty in restraining urination (i.e. incontinence)
- pain, burning, or other unusual sensations on urination
- inability to urinate
- unusual color, odor, cloudiness, frothiness or content (e.g. blood or pus in the urine)
- itching, redness or stickiness on the tip of the penis
- discharge from the tip of the penis
- pain or swelling in the back or the ribs around the area of the kidneys
- shivering, temperature or fever combined with any of the above symptoms.

Sexually transmitted diseases (STDs)

The term 'sexually transmitted disease' is used to describe infections that are almost always passed on by sexual contact. They are also known as 'venereal diseases' (VD). They spread because:
- The micro-organisms that cause them usually live in the

infected person's genitals or in some other place (such as mouth or anus) where they have been introduced during sexual activity;
- to infect another person, they usually have to enter the body through an orifice (such as the genital opening, anus or mouth), and sexual activity gives them this chance.

The first symptoms of disorder appear on the part of the body that has been in contact with the infected part of the infected person.

Otherwise, these disorders have little in common. Some are caused by bacteria, some by viruses, some by other micro-organisms. Some are rare in our society, others epidemic. Some may be merely painful or troublesome; others, if untreated, crippling or fatal. Some, such as syphilis, once the most dangerous STD, have been studied for centuries; others, such as AIDS (see pp 154-7), have been discovered only recently. Several other infections, such as genital herpes, are not classed as STD but are typically passed on by, or associated with, sexual activity.

Safer Sex

There is no immunity to or vaccine against any STD, but 'safe sex' practices to prevent the spread of AIDS (see pp 151-2) will protect you from other sexual infections. They are:
- Always wear a condom for vaginal, anal and oral sex (see p 406). As an anti-STD measure, a condom must be put on before any sex play begins. It then guards fairly effectively against all STDs except syphilis.
- Cut down on the number of partners with whom you have sex.
- Before beginning a sexual relationship, you and your partner should be checked for infection at a clinic that specializes in STDs.
- If you are infected with any STD, stop having sex until a doctor confirms that you are clear. If in doubt, ask your doctor.

Other preventive measures
The following practices can help protect against some STDs:
- urinating immediately after sex
- washing the genitals thoroughly before and after sex
- use by the female partner of some contraceptive foams (Delfen, Emko), creams (Cooper, Ortho) and jellies (Cortane, Ortho-Gynol, Milex Crescent, Koromex AII)

- use by the female partner of some noncontraceptive vaginal products (Lorophyn suppositories, Progonaryl antiseptic)
- a 'morning after' antiseptic dose (obtained from a physician or a clinic – but many doctors are reluctant to prescribe these)

AIDS (Acquired Immune Deficiency Syndrome)

Today, the number of cases of AIDS worldwide is estimated to exceed one million. This is probably about one-tenth of the total number of people infected, nearly all of whom will develop the syndrome. More than one million people in the USA are believed now to carry the HIV virus, and about 40,000 more become infected each year. Recent data suggests that in some parts of Africa, AIDS has become the leading cause of death in adults.

The features of AIDS

The initial infection is usually symptomless and the interval between infection and the first appearance of symptoms is from 1 to 10 years. The effects vary. Some 50% of infected people develop the full disorder with serious opportunistic infections and sometimes Kaposi's sarcoma. About 30% develop the AIDS-related complex (ARC), featuring weight loss, thrush, diarrhea and fever. This commonly proceeds to the full syndrome. In over 50% of cases the brain is affected, either directly by the virus to cause dementia, or by opportunistic organisms, such as toxoplasmosis, cytomegalovirus, herpes, fungi or tuberculosis. Once a person becomes infected, that person is probably infectious for life. On current knowledge, 54% of HIV-positive people will develop AIDS within 10 years of infection and almost all will develop the disease if they live long enough. Eighty percent of people who develop the full AIDS disease die within 2 years. Unhappily, although all the various manifestations of AIDS can be treated and life prolonged, no specific treatment for HIV infection has appeared and no effective vaccine has been developed. The research effort to find a cure has been unprecedented, but, so far, unsuccessful.

The disease AIDS first came to public attention as a 'plague' afflicting San Francisco's homosexual community during the late 1970s. But the virus that causes AIDS, though only identified and named in 1983, may have existed as long ago as 1959. It will infect anyone, whatever their sexual orientation. The virus is present in the body fluids (blood, saliva, semen and vaginal secretions) of an infected person. It is transmitted by: sexual activity; by mother to baby; by blood transfusion;

and by carrying out injections using infected needles.

The human immunodeficiency virus (HIV) attacks the body's immune system, but AIDS does not develop immediately after initial infection. Some individuals who are HIV-positive do not show any symptoms for years and may never show any. They are, however, still capable of infecting others. There are several recognized stages. New infections may cause the disease to progress.

There is no vaccine or cure for AIDS yet. Drugs that slow down the growth rate of the virus are effective in dealing with some of the symptoms, and may delay further progression, but they have serious side-effects.

3

Risk groups

There are well-defined, high-risk groups for infections with HIV. These include male homosexuals, drug users, prostitutes, and hemophiliacs who may have received transfusions of infected blood. Once established, the virus can be passed on through heterosexual relationships to people who appear to be outside any high-risk group. Promiscuity and anal intercourse encourage the spread of the virus. The virus in semen passes easily through inflamed or torn membranes. Drug users may pick up and spread the virus through shared needles. Those financing their habit with prostitution spread infection more widely. Hemophiliacs have become infected because of contaminated Factor VIII (a blood derivative) used in the treatment of hemophilia. In most countries, donated blood is now tested for HIV.

The spread of AIDS is hard to measure: an infected person may not feel ill and may unwittingly continue passing the virus on. Everyone who participates in sexual activity with anyone who has had a previous partner is at risk. The only absolute protection is celibacy. Condoms, manufactured to high standards, used correctly, can prevent transmission of the virus.

HIV-positive

Blood tests to detect infection with HIV are available. By about 12 weeks after contact it is usually possible to say whether or not someone has contracted the virus. There may be flu-like symptoms lasting for up to 14 days, but there are frequently no symptoms. Being diagnosed as HIV-positive can be a frightening experience; apart from worries that AIDS may develop, patients are likely to suffer discrimination in employment and life insurance, and possible loss of social and economic status. It is therefore important for patients to seek counseling, and for their families and friends to offer love and support. To be diagnosed as HIV-positive is not an immediate death sentence. In one survey, 75% of HIV-positive men were well and symptom-free two years after diagnosis.

Persistent Generalized Lymophadenopathy (PGL)

About 30% of people with HIV develop persistent swelling of the lymph glands. This is often accompanied by tiredness and malaise. Patients with PGL may be advised to avoid stress as much as possible and to keep to a healthy diet in order to prevent the condition from worsening.

AIDS-related complex (ARC)

A proportion of patients infected with HIV go on to develop definite symptoms of immune system damage: thrush (see p 163); skin disorders; fever; diarrhea; weight loss and constant tiredness.

AIDS

The development of AIDS is the last stage of the HIV infection. The immune system is destroyed, making sufferers vulnerable to a variety of infections, normally trivial, now potentially fatal. In about one-third of patients there are symptoms caused by infection of the brain. An otherwise rare tumor of the blood vessels appears as nodules on the skin called *Kaposi's sarcoma*, it is a common symptom of AIDS; it is sometimes the first symptom. Certain symptoms and infections can be treated, but the underlying damage to the immune system cannot be repaired. AIDS is a terminal illness.

Pregnancy and AIDS

Pregnancy in a woman with HIV can be a two-fold tragedy: the baby may be born infected; the mother runs an increased risk of developing ARC or AIDS. Many of the babies born to HIV-positive mothers are infected at birth; the virus can also be transmitted in breast milk. Babies reach the late stages more rapidly because their immune systems are immature.

Syphilis

Syphilis, nicknamed 'the pox' or 'scab' was, from its sudden unexplained appearance in the 1400s until the discovery of antibiotics that could treat it in the late 20th century, the most serious sexual infection. A decade ago its incidence was declining, but studies in 1988 showed a steady increase among prostitutes, drug users, their sexual partners and newborn babies, and studies during the 1990s have shown a high incidence of syphilis among HIV-infected people. The male homosexual population is an especially high-risk group.

Causation

Syphilis is caused by tiny bacteria shaped like corkscrews: 'spirochetes'. These thrive in the warm, moist linings of the genital passages, rectum and mouth, but die almost immediately outside the human body. So the infection almost always spreads by sexual contact. Whether the probing organ is penis, tongue or (perhaps) finger, and whether the receiving organ is mouth, genitals or rectum, a syphilitic site on either one can infect the other. Very occasionally syphilis does occur from close non-sexual contact (and cases have occurred in doctors and dentists from their professional work); but it cannot be spread by physical objects such as lavatory seats, towels or cups. It can, however, be inherited from an infected mother, resulting sometimes in stillbirth or deformity, and in other cases in hidden infection that causes trouble later.

Incubation

There is an 'incubation period' between catching syphilis and showing the first signs – always between 9 days and 3 months, and usually 3 weeks or more. About 1000 germs are typically picked up on infection. After 3 weeks these have multiplied to 100 to 200 million. If the disorder is untreated, they can invade the whole body, eventually causing death. Syphilis has four stages. Each has typical symptoms, but these can vary or be absent.

Primary stage

The first symptom is in the part that has been in contact with the infected person: genitals, rectum or mouth. A spot appears and grows into a sore that oozes a colorless fluid (but no blood). The sore feels like a button: round or oval, firm and just under ½in (1.25 cm) across. A week or so later, the glands in the groin may swell – but they do not usually become tender, so it may not be noticed. There is no feeling of illness, and the sore heals in a few weeks without treatment.

Secondary stage

This occurs when the bacteria have spread through the body. It can follow the primary stage straight away, but usually there is a gap of several weeks. The person feels generally unwell. There may be headaches, loss of appetite, general aches and pains, sickness and perhaps fever. Also there are breaks in the skin, and sometimes a dark red rash, lasting for weeks or even months. The rash appears on the back of the legs and front of the arms, and often too on the body, face, hands and feet. It may be flat or raised, does not itch and looks like many other skin complaints. Other symptoms can include: hair falling out in patches; sores in the mouth, nose, throat or genitals, or in soft folds of skin; and swollen glands throughout the body. All these symptoms eventually disappear without treatment after anything from 3 weeks to 9 months.

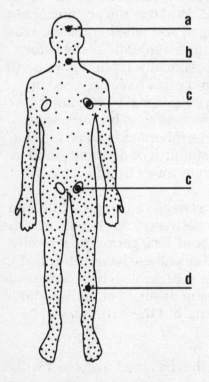

Secondary stage syphilis

a Loose hair
b Mucus patches
c Swollen lymph nodes
d Skin rash

Latent stage

This may last for anything from a few months to 50 years. There are no symptoms. After about two years, the person ceases to be infectious (though a woman can still sometimes give the disease to a baby she bears). But presence of syphilis can still be shown by blood tests.

Tertiary stage
This occurs in about $^1/_3$ of those who have not been treated earlier. The disease now shows itself in concentrated and often permanent damage in one part of the body. Common are ulcers in the skin and lesions on ligaments, joints, or on bones. These are painful, but tertiary syphilis is more serious if it attacks heart, blood vessels or nervous system. It can then kill, blind, paralyze, cripple or render insane.

Tests
Syphilis is not easy to diagnose. Its symptoms are often mild or indistinctive. Testing sores for bacteria or blood for antibodies is necessary. Neither always work, so repeat tests are important.

Treatment
This involves antibiotics – usually penicillin. Given in primary or secondary stages, it completely cures most cases. Tests and examination often last more than two years afterwards, to make sure the cure is complete.

In the latent and even tertiary stages, syphilis can still be eradicated and further damage halted; but existing tertiary stage damage often cannot be repaired.

3

Gonorrhea

Gonorrhea (sometimes nicknamed 'the clap') has spread very rapidly among young people in recent years – partly because it is so easy for a woman to have it without knowing it. There are over 900,000 reported cases in the USA every year, and the true figure is probably many times that number. Several infections in one person in a single year are not too uncommon. Worldwide, there are about 150 million cases.

Causation
Like syphilis, gonorrhea:
- is caused by a bacterium that thrives in the warm moist lining of urethra, vagina, rectum or mouth;
- is normally only passed on by sexual contact, but sometimes may be by close body contact or by inheritance from an infected mother;
- cannot be picked up from objects (though it has been suggested that gonorrhea can be carried by pubic lice, and these can be picked up from objects such as lavatory seats).

Unlike syphilis, the form of sexual contact involved is normally only genital or anal intercourse. Oral contact does not often pass on gonorrhea; if it does, it is usually fellatio rather than cunnilingus, that is responsible. (But some doctors even warn of the possibility of infection through kissing.)

Symptoms in men

After incubation (usually under a week, but sometimes up to a month), gonorrhea in a man shows itself in marked symptoms:
- discomfort inside the penis;
- a thick discharge, usually yellow-green, from the tip of the penis; and
- pain or a burning sensation on urinating.

Later it may spread to near points, such as glands leading off the urethra (e.g. the prostate, seminal vesicles and testes) and the bladder. A resulting abscess may obstruct the urethra, causing difficulty in urinating. Infection of the testes can also cause hard tender swelling: each may become as large as a baseball. If both are involved, and the infection is untreated, sterility may result. Homosexual men can be infected in the rectum during anal intercourse. This may result in soreness, itching, and/or anal discharge, and sometimes severe pain, especially when defecating. But often there are no symptoms, or only a feeling of moistness in the rectum. In either case, though, the infection can be passed on again during subsequent anal intercourse.

If oral contact results in infection, it is mainly as a throat disorder that is often not recognized as gonorrhea. It is also unlikely to infect others, because the lymph tissue where the bacteria can survive are deep in the tonsil area. Unlike syphilis, gonorrhea usually remains fairly localized, but if untreated can finally spread to the blood stream and infect bone joints, causing arthritis.

Symptoms in women

In women the incubation period is longer, and the eventual symptoms, if any, much less severe or identifiable. There may be discomfort on urinating, more frequent urination and a vaginal discharge. The discharge is distinctively yellow, and unpleasant in smell – but this may be unnoticed due to the typically small quantities involved. Seventy to 90% of cases in women occur without the woman being aware of the disease; but she is still just as infectious, even where there are no symptoms.

If untreated, the infection may spread to:
- glands around the vaginal entrance, making them swell, sometimes as large as a golf-ball;
- the rectum (because of the closeness of the two openings), causing inflammation and perhaps a discharge; and or

• the cervix, uterus and Fallopian tubes. Fallopian infection can result in fever, abdominal pain, backache, sickness, painful or excessive periods and pain during intercourse. If not treated quickly, sterility can result. It can also kill mother and fetus, by causing any pregnancy to be ectopic (the embryo implants in a Fallopian tube).

Even where gonorrhea does not affect the Fallopian tubes, it can result in premature birth, umbilical cord inflammation, maternal fever and blindness in the child.

Test and Treatment

Gonorrhea is diagnosed by laboratory analysis of any discharge or of a smear from the affected part. Treatment is with antibiotics – usually penicillin, though many forms of gonorrhea are becoming more resistant to it. Apart from avoiding infecting others through intercourse, the person being treated should also avoid masturbation and alcohol, since both can irritate the urethra and can perhaps delay a cure.

3

The Penis and Sexual Infections

Most sexual infections produce typical symptoms in the penis area, if contracted genitally.

• Primary syphilis: a single, hard, painless sore; glands often swollen.
• Gonorrhea: discharge from tip.
• Chancroid: small painful pimples, breaking down to soft painful ragged ulcers that bleed easily; widely swollen glands.
• Granuloma: red pimple growing into painless raised area, bright beefy red in color.
• Bluish-gray dots about the size of a pinhead or black specks attached to the pubic hair may also appear following sexual contact. They are not symptoms of a disease but an infestation of lice (see p 183).

Chlamydia

A bacterium, *Chlamydia trachomatis*, is the cause of several serious diseases. *Chlamydia* causes what is still often called 'non-specific urethritis' or NSU, the most common sexual infection in men. In women it is responsible for cervicitis — infection of the neck of the womb, and pelvic inflammatory disease, which causes infertility. Babies of infected mothers can be born blind or with eye, ear or chest infections.

More than 3 million new cases of *Chlamydia trachomatis*
infection occur in the United States every year. High-risk
groups are heterosexual blacks, lower socioeconomic groups,
women who have not had babies, teenagers who become
sexually active at an early age, and anyone who is
promiscuous. The sexual transmission of the disease can be
prevented by safe sex practices (see p 151). If untreated, it can
cause infection of the epididymes in men (see pp 360-2, leading
to reduced fertility, arthritis, and infertility in women of
childbearing age. Newborn babies of infected mothers can get
conjunctivitis (infection of the eyelid) and ear infections during
birth.

Symptoms

In men, chlamydia causes symptoms like those of gonorrhea
(pp 159-60), and is often called 'nongonococcal urethritis'. Most
women and about 50% of men develop no symptoms, but the
following symptoms may develop within 4 weeks of initial
infection:

- a greenish-yellow discharge from the penis (most commonly
  in the morning)
- blockage of the penis tip with dry pus
- pain on urinating
- increasing frequency of urination

Treatment

Chlamydia infections are treated with antibiotics.

Lymphogranuloma venereum (LGV)

Certain strains of *Chlamydia trachomatis* cause this illness,
which can become very serious if left untreated. It may initially
cause no symptoms, but about 30 days after the initial
infection, red pimples, sores or blisters may appear on the
penis, scrotum, fingers or tongue; the urethra may become
inflamed; or the penis may swell so that the foreskin cannot be
pushed back.

Stages

Left untreated, the disease causes the lymph nodes in the
grointo swell and become painful. Symptoms during this
secondary stage include pain in the groin, fever, headache, and
a general feeling of malaise. In the tertiary stage, the groin and
legs may swell because of blocked lymph vessels. The disease
may cause permanent damage due to complications affecting
the lungs, liver or heart, so treatment with antibiotics must
begin early to prevent permanent damage.

Herpes Viruses

Altogether, five herpes viruses affect unestimated millions of people annually. They range from HSV-1, which causes cold sores, to the varicella-zoster virus, which causes chicken pox. HSV-2 causes genital herpes, but all five viruses can cause sexual infections.

Genital herpes

This occurs worldwide and is usually sexually transmitted. It affects men and women, and may be transmitted to babies during birth whether or not the mother shows symptoms. Infection may cause death or nerve damage in newborn babies. Within a week of the initial infection, the genitals may itch or be sore, and the groin tender. Symptoms may also include fever and headaches. Red spots or blisters then develop on the penis, scrotum, thigh, and buttocks. In homosexual men they may develop on or around the anus and in the rectum. The sores crust over and heal, usually within two weeks, but they tend to recur.

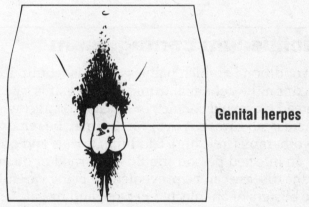

Genital herpes

Treatment

Herpes infections cannot be cured, but drugs can reduce the symptoms. Wearing condoms during sex and washing the genital area afterwards help to prevent the spread of genital herpes

Genital Warts

These occur in clusters in the genital area and area caused by a virus, the human papilloma virus, entering scratches in the skin. They affect men and women and can be passed to babies during birth. In men they may occur as single or multiple growths around the genitals or the anus. There are rarely other symptoms. The warts are generally harmless, but recent research has established a link between them and certain types of cancer affecting the genitals, such as cancer of the penis. The warts can be removed by techniques including cryotherapy, electrosurgery, laser treatment or medication. The spread of genital warts can be prevented by safe sex practices. If not removed surgically, they disappear in time.

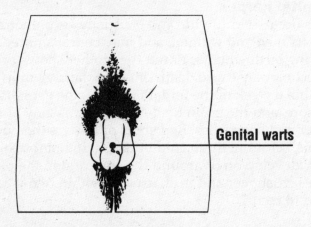

Genital warts

Molluscum contagiosum

A condition in which painless, whitish, button-like growths occur on the genitalia, trunk, and face. It is caused by a virus spread by sexual contact, or by close contact with the blisters. There is no cure, but the growths may be removed by cryotherapy (freezing). Clothing, towels and other articles used by an infected person should be burned or disinfected. Spread of the disease can be prevented by being careful not to touch the blisters of an infected person, and by safe sex practices.

Chancroid

Also called 'soft chancre' or 'soft sore', this disease is caused by bacteria. It is most common in tropical areas, and among uncirumcised men. The main symptom is the formation of one or more painful, irregularly shaped sores on the genitals and sometimes around the anus, which later ooze a foul-smelling pus. Treatment is with antibiotics. Spread of the sores can be prevented by safe sex practices.

Granuloma Inguile

This disease, which is found mainly in the tropics and sub-tropics, affects mainly men in their 20s and 30s. Its main symptom appears after an incubation period that may vary from a few days to several months; it consists of a hard red pimple on the genitals or anus. Similar pimples soon appear and break out into sores. The sores worsen and spread, and begin to destroy the surrounding tissues. In extreme cases, untreated sores have eaten into the tissue of the penis so far as to destroy it. The infection may also spread to the other parts of the body. The infection can be cured by antibiotics, and its spread can be controlled by safe sex practices.

3

Gardnerella

Men can become infected by the organism *Gardnerella vaginalis* after sex with an infected woman. The organism can infect newborn babies as they pass through the birth canal. In men it causes an inflamed foreskin and a slight, thick discharge from the penis. Symptoms are usually mild. Treatment is with a drug called metronidazole.

Candidiasis

Infection by a yeast, *Candida albicans*, is most common in women but can affect men. It can occur in the mouth and throat, anywhere on the skin, and on the genitals. When it is transmitted sexually, it causes itching, burning, and a characteristic white growth on the penis. The condition is treated with anti-fungal creams, such as Canestan. Men usually suffer only mildly from the symptoms, but should be treated in order not to pass on the infection.

Trichomoniasis

A sexually transmitted illness caused by a protozoa, *Trichomonas vaginalis*. It is usually, but not always, sexually transmitted and most commonly affects the 16-35 age group. Symptoms appear within a month of the initial infection. Men rarely show symptoms, although there may be a slight, clear discharge or itching after urination. Men should be treated to avoid passing on the infection.

Infestations

Infestations are passed on by sexual or sometimes other close body contact, and are not especially common. Scabies, or 'the itch', is caused by a tiny mite, which mainly lives on and around the genitals. The female mite burrows beneath the skin to lay her eggs. The symptoms – itchy lumps and tracks – become noticeable after 4 or 6 weeks' incubation. They can occur between the fingers, on buttocks and wrists, and in the armpits, as well as on the genitals. The itching is worse in warm conditions (e.g. in bed). Pubic lice, or 'crabs', are genital versions of the lice that can also occur in other hairy parts of the body. They feed on blood, and cause itching that can be severe. Treatment of both parasites involves painting the entire body with appropriate chemicals.

Symptoms

The following are possible signs of sexually transmitted disease (or NSU):
• sore, ulcer or rash on or around the genitals, anus or mouth;
• an unusual discharge from penis or vagina;
• pain or a burning feeling on urinating;
• increased frequency of urination;
• swollen glands in the groin; and
• itching or soreness of the penis, anus or vagina.
All these usually have some other cause – not sexually transmitted disease. But do not delay in getting proper medical advice. The disappearance of symptoms may not mean the disease has disappeared. It may just mean that the infection has progressed naturally to its next stage. You may still have a sexually transmitted disease; and you may still be able to infect others.

Incidence of Sexually Transmitted Disease

Statistics from state, county, and municipal public health agencies show marked changes in the pattern of sexually transmitted disease in the United States over the last few years. Increased public awareness of the dangers of STD, resulting from publicity about AIDS, may account for some changes. For example, the trend for gonorrhea has been downward, and among the reasons for this have been cited improved public awareness, increased use of condoms, and a decrease in promiscuity among American women – all due, it is believed, to higher awareness of AIDS. Gonorrhea is most prevalent in the south (with some of the poorest and least educated populations), and the east (with large urban centres).

The incidence of syphilis rose through the 1980s, but began to fall at the beginning of the 1990s. The rise was national, but the heaviest concentration of cases is in the South – again, the population most affected has the least education, the poorest living conditions, and the lowest level of access to care. Accompanying the rise in primary and secondary syphilis has been a rise in congenital syphilis babies infected in the womb with syphilis. This can be prevented, but it requires good prenatal care and follow-up by health care providers. During the 1990s, syphilis has become a major problem among HIV-infected patients.

Reported cases of AIDS across the United States rose steadily through the 1980s to more than 45,000 in 1993. The pattern of known deaths from AIDS is different, showing a rise from a negligible number in 1981 to more than 25,000 in 1988. But 1991 saw a fall to just over 15,000. However, it should be noted that the first 100,000 cases were reported between June 1981 and August 1989; while the second 100,000 cases were recorded between September 1989 and November 1991. It is estimated that more than 1 million individuals in the United States are infected with HIV, and that more than 40,000 adults and some 2,000 babies will be infected per year.

The northern states show the lowest incidence; the highest is right across the southern half of the United States. Initial awareness of HIV/AIDS brought a renewed willingness by men to use condoms, and a decrease in the 'promiscuity quotient' of American women, but polls have indicated that among teens and college-aged men, condom use and concern has not increased with public awareness of AIDS.

3

BODYCARE

4

Skin

Skin covers the surface of the body. It is the largest organ of the body, accounting for about 16% of total weight. The skin of an average man covers an area of about 20 sq ft (61 sq m). The skin is a major organ of the body. It presents an impermeable barrier against invasion by bacteria and other foreign organisms from the outside. The sweat and sebaceous (oil) glands, and the tear ducts secrete strong antiseptics. It is self-repairing and self-regenerating when damaged.

The skin also protects the body from exposure to harmful ultraviolet rays from the sun by producing melanin, a dark pigment, which forms a layer to absorb ultraviolet light. Peoples living in regions that are exposed to strong sunlight for long periods every year have adapted to their environment by laying down permanent melanin pigmentation in their skin. Albinos have an inherited condition in which there is no melanin in their skin, so cannot adapt to sunlight by turning brown. They have white hair and skin and very pale eyes.

In the presence of sunlight, the skin manufactures vitamin D. The skin is an impermeable membrane, preventing the body fluids from evaporating, but it also has an active role in the body's water and heat balance. The body hairs become erect in the cold, trapping warm air close to the skin; and the sweat glands secrete sweat to cool the body when it is too hot.

The skin is a major source of information about the outside world, transmitting information about touch, pressure, pain and temperature to the brain via surface sensors.

The Structure of the Skin

Skin is made up of several layers of different cells. The top layer is made of dead, flattened cells bound together to form a tough, flexible and waterproof surface that is constantly being rubbed off and replaced by the living layers below. About 40lb (18kg) of dead skin is shed by an average adult in his lifetime. The lower layer, called the dermis, is made of living cells. It contains the sacs, called follicles, in which hairs are synthesized. Apocrine glands, which secrete sweat containing waste products from the body, open into the hair follicles. Sweat glands open elsewhere on the skin's surface and secrete a salty liquid. Sebaceous glands, which secrete sebum, an oily, lubricating substance, open both into hair follicles and on to the surface of the skin.

The skin is more richly supplied with nerve endings than any other part of the body. The sensations of touch, heat, cold and pain, are each served by different nerve endings. When stimulated, they transmit electrical impulses along the peripheral nervous system to the spinal cord and the sensory centers in the brain.

The epidermis and dermis together form a layer which averages 1-2 millimeters thick, but on the eyelids it is only 0.5 millimeters and on the palms of the hands and soles on the feet, where it is dense and ridged to increase gripping powers, it is up to 0.6 millimeters thick.

The skin is attached to the deeper tissues by connective tissue made of elastic fibers called collagen. This enables it to move about to some degree to allow the joints to function. The skin grows constantly with the body, but as the body ages, those parts, such as the face, neck, and hands, that have been exposed to the ageing effects of sunlight, lose elasticity. This is caused by the breakdown of the collagen fibers, which causes bagginess and wrinkles.

Cross section of the skin

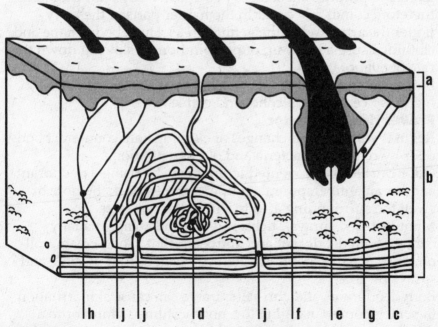

a Epidermis

b Dermis

c Subcutaneous fat

d Sweat gland

e Hair follicle

f Hair shaft

g Erector muscle

h Nerve

j Blood capillaries

The Nails

The nails protect the tip of each finger and toe from wear and damage. They can also be used as weapons of self-defence. They are made of keratin, a hard protein which occurs in the outer layers of the skin and in the hair.

Perspiration and Body Odor

Perspiration is a term used to describe the fluid produced by the sweat glands (sweat), and its production. Sweat is composed of 99% water and 10% dissolved salts, urea and waste products. An average 1½ pints of sweat is produced in one day in temperate conditions. Perspiration helps keep the body temperature normal in hot conditions because heat is lost when the sweat evaporates from the surface of the body. Perspiration increases during exercise and anxiety.

Fresh perspiration produces very little smell in a healthy person. Stale perspiration results in body odor because bacteria that live on the skin act on the sweat produced by the apocrine glands to produce substances that smell. Body odor problems therefore commonly occur in the hairier parts of the body – under the arms and in the genital areas. Here, body shape and clothing cause a build-up of perspiration by slowing down the rate of evaporation.

Both sweating and body odor can be aggravated by obesity, highly spiced foods, alcohol and coffee.

Preventing body odor

Regular washing and changes of clothing help counteract body odor by removing bacteria and old perspiration.

Odor can also be prevented temporarily by using a deodorant and/or an antiperspirant. Antiperspirants block the pore or swell the surrounding area to shrink the pore size.

Manufactured sprays, sticks, roll-ons and creams usually contain both deodorant and antiperspirant. Good cream, roll-on, or stick anti-perspirants reduce sweat output by 40%, and sprays by 20%.

Both deodorants and anti-perspirants can cause skin irritation in some people. Changing to a non-perfumed brand or to a different type often eliminates the problem.

Foot odor

Foot odor is commonly caused by perspiration being concentrated in a constricted area, since shoes and socks create warm airless conditions. To prevent foot odor the feet should be washed every day, thoroughly dried, especially between the toes, and sprayed with foot deodorant. It is essential to change socks and shoes daily – or more often, and to wash socks and air shoes after wear to prevent a build-up of bacteria. When foot odor is a serious problem, it may be necessary to wash the feet more than once a day, dust them with anti-bacterial powder and spray the shoes with a shoe deodorant.

Skin Color

The most important of the skin-coloring pigments is melanin, a brown pigment found in skin cells called melanoblasts. The melanoblasts of dark-skinned people contain more melanin granules than those of people with lighter skins. The concentration of melanin in an individual's skin is largely determined by heredity.
Tiny blood vessels near the surface give white skins a pinkish color. White-skinned people other than albinos have melanoblasts in their skin, which darken the color of the skin when it is exposed to sunlight.

4

Skin and Sun

Exposure to the ultraviolet rays of the sun produces an increased concentration of melanin (see p 168) in the skin. In fair-skinned people this produces freckles and tanning. Freckles are brown spots formed by patches of melanin. A suntan results from a more even increase in the skin's melanin content. The sun often improves acne (see p 175). If you are unused to the sun or have a very fair skin, it is essential to sunbathe with moderation. Gradually building up sunbathing time, and using sunblocks formulated to the correct factor for the prevailing sunlight, are effective precautions.

Overexposure
Overexposure to sunlight has the same effect as superficial thermal burns, but with some hours' delay. Cooling, moisturizing lotions are sufficient treatment in mild cases. In more serious cases, treatment in a hospital burns unit may be necessary.
Overexposure in intense heat can lead to heat stroke or heat exhaustion. Repeated overexposure over a long period causes breakdown of the collagen fibres beneath the skin, and consequent wrinkling. It can also result in the production of

wart-like growths called solar keratoses. More important, the risk of skin cancer is seriously increased.

Overexposure to strong sunlight is especially dangerous in parts of the world, such as Australia and New Zealand, where the protective ozone layer has thinned or vanished.

Lupus erythematosus is one of a few diseases that can cause photosensitivity – an abnormal sensitivity to light that results in a skin rash.

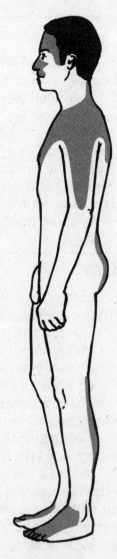

 Sunburn danger areas

Birthmarks

Any of several different skin blemishes may be present at birth. Strawberry marks are red, slightly raised, spongy areas of skin containing enlarged blood vessels. They are usually fairly small and often disappear without treatment. If a strawberry mark persist, it may be shrunk by injections or removed surgically.

Port wine stains are dark red, flat areas of skin containing enlarged blood vessels. They tend to be extensive and often occur on the face and neck. They can be faded by laser treatment or bleaching, or concealed by cosmetics.

In vitiligo, an area of skin always remains white whatever the color of the skin around it. It can be concealed, but there is no treatment. Liver spots are dark patches of skin resembling large freckles. They are caused by concentrations of the skin pigment, melanin. They can be bleached and faded.

Moles and Warts

4

Moles are raised brown skin blemishes made of a mass of cells with a high concentration of melanin. They may be present at birth, but some develop later. Pregnancy often causes an increase in their size or number. Some moles have a growth of hair, which should not be plucked because of the risk of infection. Moles should be removed under medical supervision. Most moles are harmless, but they should be watched for changes. It is possible for moles to develop into a very fast-growing form of cancer called a melanoma. A doctor should be consulted without delay if a mole changes character and enlarges, ulcerates or bleeds.

Warts are small benign skin tumors. They are common on the hands, and verrucas and plantar warts occur on the feet. Many warts vanish without treatment, but persistent warts can be 'frozen' and removed, or removed chemically.

Cuts and Bruises

Bruises develop when small blood vessels under the skin are ruptured. Blood seeps into the surrounding tissue to give the bruise its color – usually black or blue at first, often changing to purple, green, and yellow as the blood cells are broken down and their constituents reabsorbed. Cold, wet compresses speed healing and ease pain, but even without treatment most bruises disappear after about a week. A severe bruise that remains painful may be a sign that a bone is broken.

When the skin is cut, healing begins at once:

1. The capillary blood vessels contract to stop the flow of blood and prevent the entry of bacteria. Then, clotting substances

from the blood vessels form fine threads which knit the sides of the wound together.

2. During the first day, white blood cells enter the wound to break down and later absorb any foreign particles. At the same time, the epidermal cells begin to multiply.

3. By the second day, a scab has formed over the wound. Beneath the scab, epidermal cells on each side of the wound join up to form a continuous layer.

4. About a week later, the scab falls off, leaving new epidermis beneath.

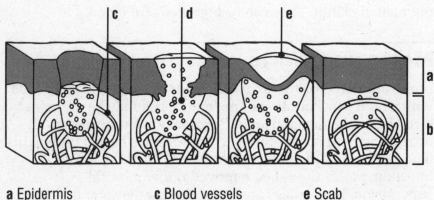

a Epidermis   **c** Blood vessels   **e** Scab
b Dermis   **d** Blood cells

Blackheads and Whiteheads

A blackhead or whitehead appears when a skin pore becomes blocked by dust, dirt or sebum. The waxy plug that blocks the pore is called a comedo. This forms a blackhead when it is exposed to the air: oxidation turns the head of the comedo black. If it is not open to the air, a whitehead is formed. A pore may be cleaned by gently pressing out the plug, but unless this is done soon after the plug is formed, the spot is probably best left to heal itself. When cleaning out pores, it is important to avoid damaging the skin or spreading infection. A preliminary wash with warm water will loosen the plugs, and the skin should be bathed in a mild astringent, such as witch hazel, afterwards.

People prone to blackheads should wash their faces daily with an antiseptic face wash. A diet low in greasy food and high in fresh fruit and vegetables helps correct excessive sebum production. Skin cosmetics can cause an outbreak.

Acne

This is a skin disease in which blackheads, whiteheads and pus-filled spots affect the skin, commonly of the face, neck, chest, and back, but it may also affect the upper arms. Acne is very common in adolescents. One late-1980s survey in Scotland found a prevalence of 93% in boys by age 17. The condition usually clears up by the mid-20s, but can persist through life into middle age. Acne is a disorder of the sebaceous (oil-producing) glands of the skin. It is not caused by poor hygiene or diet. Washing the affected skin excessively can aggravate the condition. People prone to acne should follow a well-balanced, healthy diet. Chocolate is a fatty food and should never be consumed in excess, but there is no need for people affected by acne to cut chocolate out of their diet. Chocolate does not affect the condition, as is commonly believed.

Acne needs expert medical treatment. A physician will grade the acne according to its severity and type (i.e. its extent), the presence of blackheads and whiteheads, cysts, deep-seated inflamed pustules, etc. The grading will eliminate factors such as shaving rash, which may make the acne appear more serious than it is. Grading is also a guide to treatment. Several new drugs have been developed in recent years that are very effective in treating acne: benzoyl peroxide is most effective in treating acne that is not inflamed; tretinoin in treating painful, inflamed acne or in extreme cases isotretinoin if other treatments prove ineffective, however this last drug can have side effects. Treatment may also include exposure to ultraviolet light, tetracycline antibiotics, and hormone treatment. People affected by acne often lose confidence and become socially isolated. In recent years support groups have formed to provide information, advice, support and, if necessary, counselling.

Dermatitis (Eczema)

'Dermatitis' is a general term for skin inflammation. It is often caused by exposure to skin irritants, but may have a nervous origin.

Some chemicals irritate everyone's skin, but others affect only people who are hypersensitive or 'allergic' to them. Common allergens are cosmetics, paints, detergents, insecticides, metals, textiles, rubber and some plants. After contact with an allergen, the blood vessels dilate and become porous, so that cell fluid collects in the skin and forms blisters, which eventually burst. The fluid then dries out and the skin becomes encrusted. It thickens around the sores and flakes off in scales. There is a serious risk of infection if the affected area is either scratched, or left untreated.

Recurrence can be prevented by identifying the cause, then avoiding or protecting against the substance. However, identification can be a long process involving many tests. Good Chinese herbalists can prepare ointments which are recognized by many doctors as extremely effective in treating dermatitis and related conditions and some suffers have found homeopathic remedies helpful.

Hives

A common allergic reaction, also called nettle rash and urticaria. It causes a painful, irritated skin welt. It is often caused by a food allergy: citrus fruits, shellfish, wheat products and chocolate are all known allergens. Antibiotics, dust, pollen and stress can also produce it. Sensitive skin tissues react to the allergy by releasing the chemical histamine, dilating the blood vessels, increasing the flow of blood to the skin, which creates welts. Hives is not a serious condition and it may be helped by soothing lotions. Seek medical attention if large swellings near the mouth and throat affect breathing.

Boils

These are painful, pus-filled lumps caused by bacterial infection of a hair follicle, a sebaceous or sweat gland, or a break in the skin. They commonly occur around sites of friction with clothing, such as the neck or wrist, and may be an indication that a person is run down. Only after the dead skin that forms the core has been excised will the boil disappear. Boils should be treated by bathing in very hot water and lanced when they appear to have reached their full size. If several boils occur, a physician should be consulted.

Psoriasis

Psoriasis is a chronic skin complaint characterized by red spots and patches covered with loose, silvery scales. The skin of the elbows, forearms, knees, legs and scalp is most usually affected, but psoriasis can occur anywhere on the body. The condition results from large-scale production of an abnormal type of keratin. It takes 28 days for normal skin to produce a mature keratin cell, but only 4 days for a person with psoriasis. The cause is unknown, but there may be a genetic link. Psoriasis is not infectious and does not affect general health. The condition comes and goes intermittently. Treatment is with exposure to ultraviolet light, especially when combined with a plant derivative called psoralen; coal tar, dithranol and corticosteroid ointments, and a cytotoxic drug (which kills cancer cells) called methotrexate.

Chilblains

Body temperature decreases toward the extremities of the body. In cold weather, good blood circulation is necessary to keep the hands and feet warm. If the circulation is poor, the skin tissue of the fingers, toes and ears especially may be injured as a result of insufficient blood supply. This causes swollen areas, redness, itching and pain. If the skin becomes white and numb through cold, it should be warmed slowly by bathing in tepid, then warm water, or by rubbing. Direct heat should not be applied. The itching and other symptoms may be helped by regularly massaging the area with a dry skin cream, and brisk walking or other exercise every day. Recurrence should be prevented by wearing warm socks, shoes, gloves and a hat that covers the ears, and by avoiding extreme cold.

Frostbite

Exposure of a part of the body to extreme cold causes the blood vessels to contract. This leaves the surface areas vulnerable to freezing. Although cold is painful, freezing causes no sensation. The tissues are damaged by expanding ice crystals that form beneath the skin, and their blood supply is cut off. The tissues die and gangrene may result in loss of fingers and toes. Frostbite is especially likely to affect the hands, feet, ears and nose. A person suffering from frostbite must be moved immediately to warm, but not hot, conditions to thaw. However, if freezing has been severe and of short duration (for example, if someone were shut in a cold store), rapid rewarming can be carried out by immersing the frozen parts in warm water. Antibiotics may be needed to prevent infection if the tissues are damaged. If the tissues are dead, amputation of the affected part may be necessary.

Athlete's Foot

This is a fungal infection, *Tinea pedis,*which usually begins with splits and flaking skin between the toes. It occurs twice as often in men as in women. If untreated it may spread to the soles of the feet. Some types of fungus can cause irritating, white, flaking sores on the legs and hands, which extend outward while the centre heals. Sweat helps the fungus grow, so the infection is more common in hot weather. Treatment of athlete's foot and other skin fungus infections has been greatly improved by the introduction of the imazole drugs. Other forms of *tinea* include 'jock itch' *(Tinea cruris)* which produces a reddened, itchy area spreading from the genitals over the inner side of the thighs.

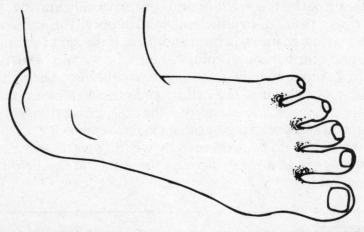

Using Cosmetics

Ranges of cosmetics for men include useful pencils and sticks of foundation make-up to hide blemishes, such as birthmarks, and the disfiguring scars caused by some skin diseases, such as acne. Before buying, try them on the skin inside your wrist to make sure they blend with your skin tone. Ask for advice if you are not sure about a preparation.

Ranges of men's cosmetics contain moisturizers. It is especially worth considering using these if you have dry skin. Dry skin tends to be flaky in texture, and may be itchy and painful; in cold weather it tends to redden and be sore. Medicated face washes are excellent preventives against breaking out if you have oily skin and tend to have blackheads and spots.

Oily skin is coarse in texture, with open pores around the nose and on the chin; a tissue held against the face will be slightly greasy when it is removed.

These days, many moisturizers contain a sun block, which protects against ultraviolet light damage to the skin. These have become very necessary for men who spend a lot of time outdoors, especially those who live in a hot, sunny climate or in regions affected by the holes in the ozone layer.

Cosmetic Surgery

Minor facial disfigurements, such as a baggy chin or sticking out ears, can be corrected surgically to improve the appearance. Such operations are common and very safe – but make sure you consult a surgeon with a good reputation. Any operation can go wrong.

All cosmetic surgery is expensive. It can also be painful for some time afterwards, and it may take a while for evidence of surgery, such as swelling and bruising, to vanish. Many cosmetic operations are carried out under local anaesthetic these days.

For many people, cosmetic surgery can improve self-confidence and relieve anxiety.

4

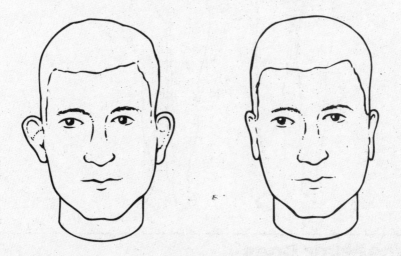

Ear surgery can correct ears that stick out too far. An ellipse of skin is removed from the back of the ear, and the cartillage beneath is trimmed.

Hair

Hair is found over the whole surface of the human body except the palms, soles and parts of the genitals. There are three types of hair: scalp hair, body hair and sexual hair. Scalp hair resembles the body hair of other mammals. Human body hair is very fine and usually less pigmented. Sexual hair develops around the genitals, the armpits and (in men) the face. Its growth is dependent on the male sex hormones produced by both sexes in puberty. The number of hairs on the body varies between individuals, but on average there are about 100,000 hairs on the head.

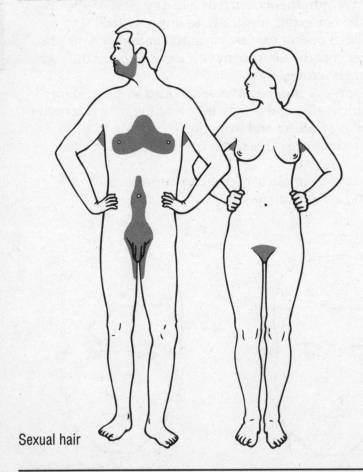

Sexual hair

What Hair Does

Hair acts as a protective barrier. The eyelashes protect the eyes, and hairs in the nostrils and outer ears trap and prevent the entry of foreign bodies. The eyebrows prevent sweat dripping into the eyes.

Hair also acts to conserve heat. Air trapped between hairs insulates the skin and stops heat loss. The straighter the hair stands the more air can be trapped. Attached to each hair follicle is a strip of muscle which makes the hair stand on end when it contracts causing 'goose flesh'. These muscles are stimulated by cold or emotional stress.

Hair Growth

Hair is made out of keratin, a tough type of protein.
It grows out of follicles in the skin. All these follicles are established at birth and no new ones are formed later in life. The root of the hair is the only live part of the hair: it grows and pushes the dead hair shaft out of the skin. Hair growth is cyclical with a growth phase followed by a rest phase in which the hair is loosened. A new hair then pushes it out. Some 30-100 hairs are lost from the scalp each day. In an adult scalp the growth phase is about 3 years and the rest phase is 3 months. Hair growth is irregular and at different stages all over the body. Head hair rarely exceeds 3ft in length.

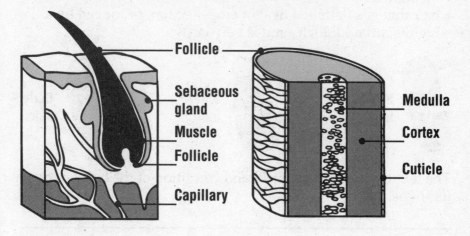

Hair Color

Hair color is determined by how much pigment it contains. Melanin, the skin pigment, is produced in the hair follicle. Pigment production in the hair follicle slows down with age and often ceases, so that eventually each hair becomes colorless. Gradual 'graying' occurs because a few hair follicles slow down pigment production at a time over a number of years. A gray hair contains a reduced amount of pigment; a white hair contains no pigment at all – albinos have pure white hair. As the hair turns gray, the skin also loses pigment and lightens in color.

In some people the 'graying' process begins as early as their twenties and they may turn gray within a few years. Others retain their hair colour well into middle age. The graying process is determined by genetics; the hair cannot turn gray or white overnight or even over a few weeks due to stressful events, as is often suggested in fiction. There is no known way to stimulate pigment production once it has ceased; however, various cosmetic preparations are available which will restore hair color if regularly applied.

Hair Type

There are three principal hair types:
- hair that is round in cross-section and falls straight
- hair that is kidney-shaped in cross-section and is wavy, the degree of waviness depending on the extent of the curve of the follicle
- hair that is a flattened oval in cross-section, produced by a highly curved follicle, and is very curly.

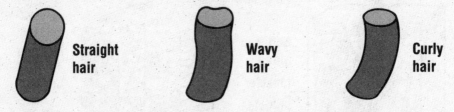

Straight hair   Wavy hair   Curly hair

The texture (fine, wiry, thick) and condition of the hair affect its shape.

Hair Care

- Keep the hair clean. Oily hair should be washed every 2-3 days, dry hair every 5-6 days. Choose the shampoo according to type and condition of your hair.
- Ensure that the comb is clean and well made. Unclean combs spread bacteria and infection. Sharp edges damage the structure of the hair.
- Take care when the hair is wet: it is more vulnerable and prone to pulling and splitting in this state. Comb gently.
- Check the condition of the scalp, looking for itching,

inflammation, scaling, dandruff or degeneration. Visit a
physician or dermatologist if worried.
- Protein, the B vitamins, iron, copper and iodine are all
essential for strong, healthy hair.

Flaking and Dandruff

Flaking is usually attributed to dandruff, but it may be caused
by a dry scalp, and dandruff shampoos and treatments can
worsen it. If your skin is dry and you find fine, dry scales on
the shoulders of your clothes, you probably have dry scalp.
Your hairdresser will advise if you are not sure. There are
many effective treatments, ranging from using a shampoo and
a conditioner for dry hair, to professional hot oil and massage
treatments. Brushing the hair with a brush that is not too stiff
for your hair texture stimulates the sebaceous glands to
produce more sebum.

Dandruff
Thick flakes of dead skin can be seen in the hair and fall onto
the shoulders. The flakes are fairly oily. The scalp sheds skin
cells as a normal part of its growth. Excessive scaliness may be
caused by infection by a fungus, Malassezia furfur. Dandruff
responds well to the regular use of selenium shampoos
specially formulated to treat it.

Fungal Infection

The scalp can be infected by several different fungi in a
condition that is often called 'ringworm', because the infection
causes a scaly rash which tends to move outward from the
original site of infection. Ringworm causes the scalp to itch. It
is treated with a drug called griseofulvin, or by fungicidal
creams, such as imidazole.

Hair Lice

Two species of lice affect humans: *phthirus pubis*, found in the
pubic hair (see Infestations) and *pediculus humanus*, found in
the hair on the head. The latter can be acquired not only by
contact with an infected person, but also via objects such as
combs and hats. The infestation causes severe itching. It is
most easily diagnosed by examining the scalp for the tiny eggs
('nits') attached to the hair shafts. The lice are more difficult to
find.

They are attracted to clean hair and cannot be removed by washing the hair with ordinary shampoos. Suitable treatment should be obtained from a physician or pharmacist: it will include a shampoo and often also a scalp emulsion. The eggs are hard to kill, and treatment should be repeated at intervals until completely successful.

Hair Loss

If the hairs lost every day from the scalp are not replaced by normal hairs but by fine, downy hair; then baldness will result. This happens in varying degrees to nearly all men and women. Hair can be lost for various reasons. Physical ailments that cause hair loss include: scars or burns that destroy the hair follicles; skin disturbances, such as dermatitis, psoriasis or allergic reactions; general bodily ailments, such as serious anemia; and chemical pollution of the body (as in mercury poisoning).
Hair loss can also be caused by mental stress. This is because hair growth is linked with hormonal production, which in turn is closely linked to one's emotional state. The hair grows back when the period of stress is over. In the above cases, by treating the illness, hair will usually be restored. But the commonest type of hair loss is male-pattern baldness. This is caused by a male hormone influenced by hereditary aging factors. Nothing, short of castration, can be done about this condition. Not only can it not be reversed but it cannot be stopped or even slowed down by any means so far discovered.

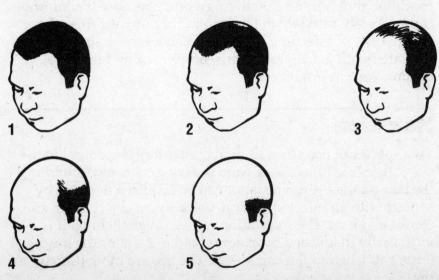

1 2 3

4 5

Effective treatment

The drug Minoxidil (proprietary name Regaine, or Rogaine) has been found to be effective in some cases in restoring thinning hair. It is available in the form of a lotion which has to be applied daily to the hair. It works well as long as it is used regularly, but the hair will begin to thin as soon as it is stopped. The drug is expensive.

Short of castration, nothing else can be done to slow, stop or reverse the condition. Other treatments in the form of creams, lotions, massage, shampoo, and ultra-violet and infra-red radiation do not work and are sometimes harmful.

Surgery

A developing bald spot can be reduced by a procedure of cosmetic surgery involving implantation of hairs from elsewhere on the head (see overleaf).

4

Hairpieces

This is the traditional way of concealing hair loss.

The hairpiece is built from a base shaped to the bald area. Hair is attached to this base and cut to match the rest of the hair. The base can be hard or soft. The hard type is made from fiberglass or plastic. The soft type is made out of silk, cotton, Terylene or nylon netting.

Human hair is usually used but animal hair can be added to give a special color or texture. The hairpiece is fixed onto the scalp with strips of double-sided sticky tape. This makes it unlikely to move accidentally. Two hairpieces are usually needed: one to wear when the other needs to be cleaned or repaired. This adds considerably to the cost. The main advantages of wearing a hairpiece are – hopefully – a more youthful appearance and a gain in confidence. Hairpieces also serve some of the true functions of hair: keeping the scalp warm and protecting it from the sun. The disadvantages of wearing a hairpiece are: discomfort from perspiration; fear of the hairpiece getting unstuck, or being disarranged by the wind – and embarrassment if it does; having to protect the hairpiece from strong sunlight, in case it fades or changes color; and the time and expense involved in its care. A good hairpiece has to match the color and texture of the surrounding hair, fit the scalp perfectly, look natural, stand up to sunlight and rain, stick firmly to the head, be easy to clean, and last for several years. A bad hairpiece reveals itself to observers by a bad color match, unnatural parting, or hard front hairline.

Hair Transplant

This is a recent technique. Hair follicles are surgically removed from parts where there is abundant hair, and implanted into the bald areas. But there is no guarantee that they will grow in their new location.

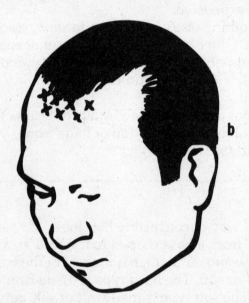

a Recipient site
b Donor site

Hair Weaving

This is another way of covering up baldness. It is also known as hair linking, hair extension, and hair replacement.
There are two methods. In the first, a hairpiece is made in the normal way, and then attached to the scalp by stitching the sides of it to the normal hair.
In the second, threads are strung across the bald area, from one side to the other, and pieces of hair, sewn together in clumps, are woven directly into this. In both cases, around the edge of the area to be concealed, the existing hair is gathered and woven into a strengthened line, to take the strain of the hairweave. The fitting takes from 2 to 4 hours.
In addition, as the existing hair grows, the hairweave gets looser, and so about every 6 weeks – sometimes more often – it has to be taken off and refitted. The basic cost, and the need for frequent return visits, make the process expensive. Also the continual pulling of the hairweave on the natural hair can help speed up hair loss.Washing of the hairweave can be a lengthy business as it tends to get tangled and cannot be combed hard.

Because of this difficulty, the hair is often not washed enough, which means that the scalp is irritated by dirt, dead skin and soap not washed out.

Hairweaving

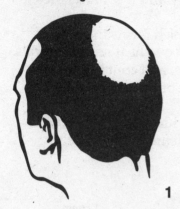

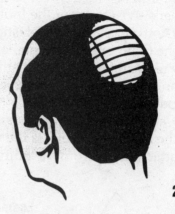

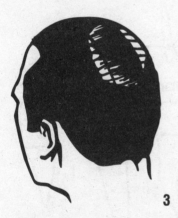

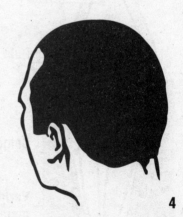

Teeth

Teeth are hard structures set in bony sockets in the upper and lower jaws. Their main function is to chew and prepare food for swallowing. They also help in the articulation of sounds in speech. In humans there are three main types of teeth.

Incisors are sharp, chisel-like teeth at the front of the mouth, used for cutting into food.

Canines are round pointed teeth at the corners of the mouth, used for tearing and gripping food.

Molars are square teeth with small cusps, which grind food at the back of the mouth.

A tooth consists of two parts: the root is embedded in the jaw; the crown projects out of the jaw. Where the root and crown meet is called the neck.

Each tooth is made up of enamel, dentine, pulp and cementum. **Enamel** is the hardest tissue in the body and it protects the sensitive crown of the tooth.

Dentine is a slightly elastic material which forms the bulk of the tooth under the enamel. It is sensitive to heat and chemicals.

Pulp is the soft tissue inside the dentine, and contains nerves and blood vessels, which enter the root of the tooth by a small canal.

Cementum is a thin layer of material which covers the root of the tooth and protects the underlying dentine. It also helps attach fibers from the gum to the tooth.

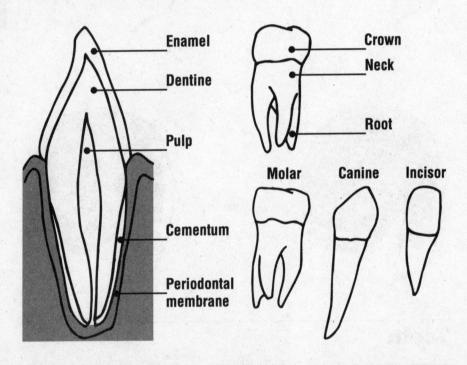

Enamel • Dentine • Pulp • Cementum • Periodontal membrane • Crown • Neck • Root • Molar • Canine • Incisor

The Teeth We're Given

In humans there are two successive sets of teeth. The primary or 'milk' set arrive 6 to 24 months after birth. Later they gradually fall out, from the age of 6 on, as the permanent teeth appear. Most of these are out by the age of 13, but the 3rd molar or 'wisdom tooth' can erupt as late as the age of 25, or never. Human teeth do not keep growing, but reach a certain size and then stop. Also, when the permanent teeth fall out, they are not replaced by a new set. But in some animals, such as the rabbit, the incisors keep growing, as they are worn down by use, while the shark grows set after set of teeth to its great advantage!

Age of Appearance

These are average figures only: actual dates vary greatly from child to child.

Primary Teeth

Central incisors	6 to 8	months	1
Lateral incisors	9 to 11	months	2
Eye teeth	18 to 20	months	4
FIrst molars	14 to 17	months	3
Second molars	24 to 26	months	5

The key numbers give the typical order of appearance.

4

Primary teeth

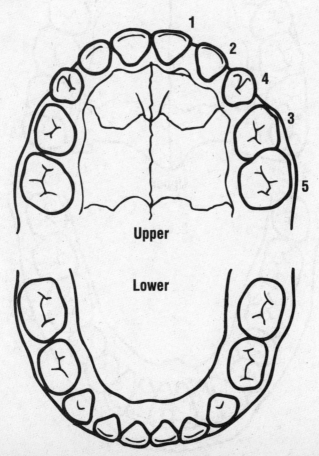

Upper

Lower

Adult Teeth

Central incisors	7 to 8	years	2
Lateral incisors	8 to 9	years	3
Canines	12 to 14	years	6
First premolars	10 to 12	years	4
Second premolars	10 to 12	years	5
First molars	6 to 7	years	1
Second molars	12 to 16	years	7
Third molars	17 to 21	years	8

The key numbers give the typical order of appearance

Adult teeth

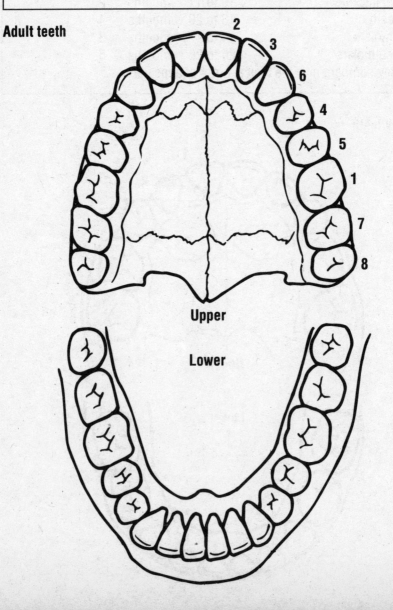

Upper

Lower

Sequence of appearance
(upper jaw)

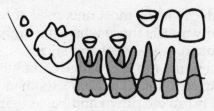

5 years

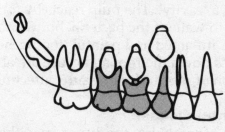

8 years

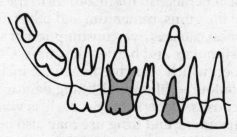

9 years

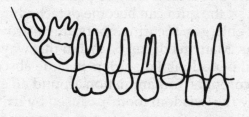

11 years

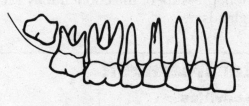

13 years

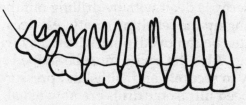

Adult

4

Dental Disorders

Tooth decay is the most universal of human diseases. It especially affects those who eat a highly refined diet which is overcooked, soft, sweet and sticky.

Bacteria in the mouth change carbohydrates in the food into acids strong enough to attack tooth enamel. Gradually the enamel is broken down and bacteria invade the dentine, forming a 'cavity'. The pulp reacts by forming secondary dentine to wall off the bacteria, but without treatment the pulp becomes inflamed and painful (toothache). The infection may then pass down the root and cause an 'abscess' – a painful collection of pus under pressure, affecting the gum and face tissues.

Peridontal disease

This is a general term for disorders in the supporting structures of teeth: the gums, cementum and other tissues. The commonest cause is overconsumption of soft food, which cannot stimulate and harden the gums. Other causes include sharp food which scratches the gums, inefficient brushing, badly contoured fillings, ill-fitting dentures, irregular teeth and teeth deposits. General factors such as vitamin deficiencies, blood disorders, and drug use may also be involved. Periodontal diseases may be painless, but, if allowed to progress, the gum can become detached from the tooth. The socket enlarges, securing fibers are destroyed, and the tooth loosens. Many teeth can be lost in this way.

Painful periodontal disorders include abscesses in the gum and 'periocoronitis' (inflammation around an erupting tooth, usually the 'wisdom tooth'), caused by irritation, food stagnation, pressure or infection. It may accompany swollen lymph glands.

Dental Treatment

Filling cavities

Tooth decay is dealt with by drilling out the decayed matter and filling up the resulting cavity. All decay and weakened areas must be removed, otherwise decay will continue beneath the filling. Also the cavity must be shaped so that the filling will stay in securely and withstand pressure from chewing. High-speed ultrasonic drills are now usual, and so is the use of injected local anesthetic to make the procedure painless.

A lining of chemical cement is put in the prepared cavity to protect the pulp from heat and chemicals. The filling, placed on top of this, is usually an amalgam of silver, tin, copper, zinc alloy and mercury. Alternatively, translucent silicate cement is used for its natural appearance, but since it can wear away, this must be given a further translucent coating if used on grinding surfaces. However, it has recently been discovered that mercury, thought to be sealed within the filling, leeches out of a tooth filled with amalgam. Since mercury is a poison, substitutes for amalgam fillings are increasingly being used, and the discovery has given new impetus to research into new materials for fillings.

Other restorative work
Some other replacement work can be prepared outside the mouth and then cemented into place. Inlays are cast gold fillings, shaped to fit a cavity in the crown of a tooth. A wax impression of the cavity is made and the resulting mold filled with molten gold. Crowns are extensive coverings to the crown of a tooth, made of porcelain on gold. The whole of the enamel of the tooth is removed, an impression made, and the crown made from a model.

Pulp and root-canal treatment
This is carried out when the pulp is dead or incurably infected. The pulp is removed and replaced with antibiotic paste, the tooth sealed, and a temporary filling left for a week. Once the cavity is sterilized, it is filled with paste and/or tapering, metal oxide 'points', and the tooth sealed.

Treatment of gum disorders
Acute conditions are treated by pus drainage, antiseptic mouth washes, antibiotics and tooth extraction if necessary. Surgery may be needed to cut away the diseased gum. Long-term treatment aims at eliminated as many causative factors as possible, by improving oral hygiene, diet and general health.

4

The progress of dental decay
Different stages are shown in different teeth. For example, tooth decay is only a spot in the incisor of the far left. In the center tooth (a molar), it has reached the dentine; in the next, the pulp; and in the last, the roots

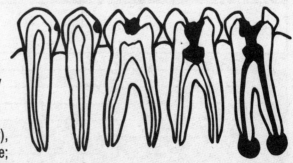

Extraction

Teeth need to be removed if they are irretrievably decayed, or so broken that they cannot be repaired, or if new teeth are erupting and have no room.

Forceps are used. They grip the tooth at the neck, while the blades of the forceps are inserted under the gum. The tooth is then moved repeatedly to enlarge the socket and can be pulled out. Local or general anesthetic, by injection or gas, usually makes extraction painless.

The Teeth We Lose

Here we show the average fate of western teeth. For example, upper right 3 is sound in over 60% of adults, treated in over

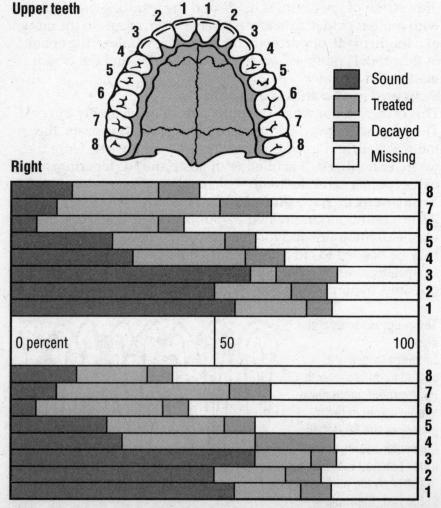

10%, decayed in about 5%, and missing in the remainder.
Upper right 6, in contrast, is missing in about 55%.

Lower teeth

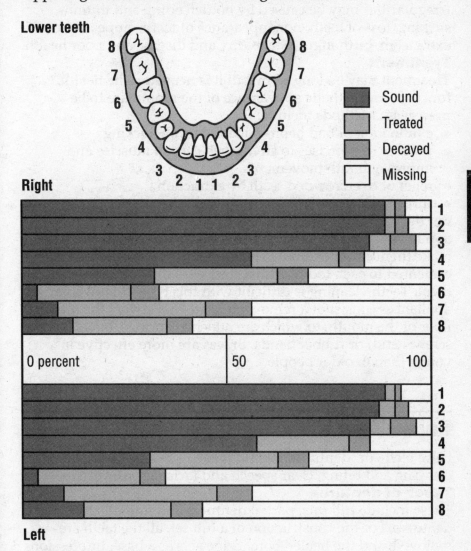

Sound

Treated

Decayed

Missing

Right

0 percent 50 100

Left

Orthodontics

This is the branch of dentistry concerned with preventing and
correcting irregularities of the teeth, such as variations in the
numbers of teeth and abnormalities in their shape, size,
position and spacing. All these can cause defects in eating,
swallowing, speech and breathing.
Malocclusion is the typical example. This means that the teeth
are not in the normal position when the jaws are closed,
relative to those in the opposite jaw. Teeth may stick out or in,

or there may be spaces between the biting surfaces due to uneven growth of the teeth or jaws.

Irregularities may be caused by bottlefeeding and thumb-sucking, loss of teeth, nonappearance of teeth, appearance of extra teeth, birth injuries, heredity and disease and poor health.

Treatment

Treatment may be long term, but it is needed if the health, function, and esthetic appearance of the mouth are to be preserved. Methods include:

- elimination of bad habits such as thumb-sucking
- practice of exercises to strengthen certain muscles and improve mouth movements
- relief of overcrowded teeth by extraction
- surgery on the soft tissues or bones to recontour the jaws.

But the commonest technique is to attach 'braces' or similar appliances to the teeth, to apply continual pressure, and so make them shift position. Fixed appliances consist of brackets, cemented to each tooth, with a steel wire threaded through them. Teeth-cleaning is difficult with this type. Removable appliances consist of a removable plate that covers the roof or floor of the mouth, to which are attached springs, bows, screws, and/or rubber bands. Braces are more effective in young than in older people.

False Teeth

False teeth, or 'dentures' should ideally preserve normal chewing and biting, clear speech and facial appearance.

Types of dentures

These include full sets, partial dentures and immediate dentures. For the construction of a full set, all the teeth are removed, and the healed bony ridge acts as a base. Impressions of both jaws are made in warm wax, and these give the basic patterns from which the dentures are made up.

Partial dentures are attached to surviving natural teeth to keep them anchored. If the anchoring teeth are not immediately alongside, they are linked to the false teeth by a bridge.

Immediate dentures are prepared before the teeth being lost have been removed. After extraction, the empty sockets are immediately covered with the new dentures, and healing takes place beneath. A new set is needed after about 6 months, as the ridge from which the teeth have been extracted shrinks.

Using dentures

Dentures can be uncomfortable. To prevent gum soreness when dentures are new, eat only small amounts of soft foods at first. If soreness occurs, consult a dentist. Do not leave the dentures out of the mouth for more than a day or two, or the remaining natural teeth may begin to shift position.

Brush false teeth after every meal. Soak detachable dentures overnight in water containing salt or denture cream.

At first, denture wearers often find it difficult to speak. This is easily overcome by practice.

New teeth for old

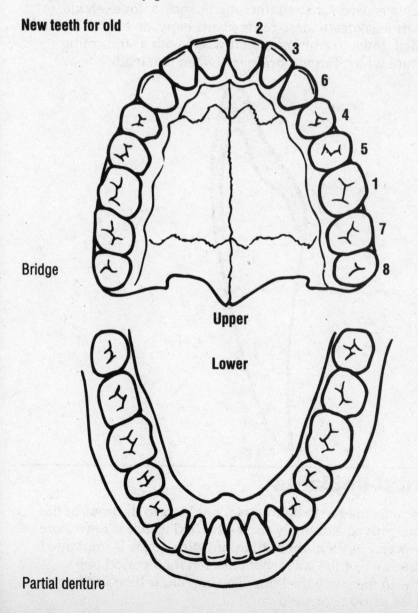

Bridge

Upper

Lower

Partial denture

Crowns and Bonding

These techniques can be used for cosmetic reasons or to prevent decay. In crowning, the visible part of the tooth is filed down to a small stub, which is then used as a base on which to construct a synthetic tooth. In bonding, a sealant is used to attach plastic or porcelain to fill gaps or cracks, or level off chipped teeth. However, it may not be as strong as a crown, and may need renewal every few years.

Bridges

Bridging is used for strengthening purposes, for example, to support weak teeth, or to bridge gaps between teeth. The teeth are filed down to stumps and crowned with a supporting structure which forms a bridge between two teeth.

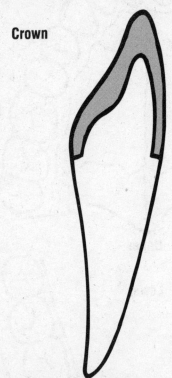

Crown

Dental Implants

A recent technique to bond metal implants to the bone of the jaw has proved extremely successful and its use is now more widespread. A titanium or titanium alloy screw is implanted into the bone of the jaw, where it is left for a period of 6 months to fuse with the bone. The implant is then used as the basis for a bridge or a crown.

Preventing Dental Trouble

Diet

At any age, the ideal diet for dental health should be:
- well balanced and adequate, so that general health is maintained
- chewable enough to stimulate the gums
- low in sugar content to reduce acid attack.

The balance and adequacy of the diet is especially important for expectant mothers and growing children, so that strong teeth form. Proprietary toothpastes are now formulated to inhibit acidity and plaque formation.

Oral hygiene

Teeth should be cleaned at least twice a day. After every meal is best. This polishes the teeth, removes debris, and inhibits acid attack. Brushing also stimulates the gums and cleans effectively. Methods of cleaning vary from culture to culture. To use the toothbrush effectively:
- backward and forward strokes are good for the tops of molars, and the back of the front teeth;
- for the side teeth, brush sideways repeatedly in one direction – upward on the bottom teeth, downward on the top ones.

In addition to brushing the teeth, toothpicks made of soft wood can be used to dislodge food.

Removing plaque

Plaque, or tartar, is a sticky deposit that forms on the surface of teeth and causes decay by harbouring bacteria and encouraging acid attack. If not removed it hardens to form a coating around the neck of the tooth. Plaque can be removed by brushing the teeth with specially shaped brushes.

Disclosure tablets show the extent to which you need to brush the teeth to remove plaque. A tablet is chewed and so spread by saliva on to all tooth and gum surfaces. After rinsing with water, all areas of plaque are stained red. The plaque can then be removed by brushing.

Dental floss or tape should also be used regularly to clean and removed plaque from between the teeth.

Dental chewing gum

Sugarless chewing gums have been formulated to prevent the formation of acid in the mouth immediately after eating.

Visiting the dentist

Regular 6-monthly visits to the dentist ensure that any accumulated plaque is removed and the teeth polished, and that any problems are dealt with in their early stages, preventing more drastic treatment in the future.

Fluoride

This is a tasteless, odorless, colorless chemical which, if added to drinking water in small amounts, reduces tooth decay in children by 60 percent. (Excessive amounts can cause the enamel to become mottled). In the US, 60 million people now drink water with fluoride added, and 7 million others drink water that naturally contains fluoride. Some toothpastes also contain fluoride, and tablets can be bought to add to the unfluoridated water. So far, no ill effects of the use of fluoride in these quantities have been established, but it only benefits the teeth of children under 14.

Cleaning the teeth

Backward and forward strokes with the brush are good for the tops of the molars (**a**), and the back of the front teeth (**b**).

But on the side teeth, use the brush sideways in a repeated stroke in one direction upward on the bottom teeth (**c**), and downward on the top ones (**d**).

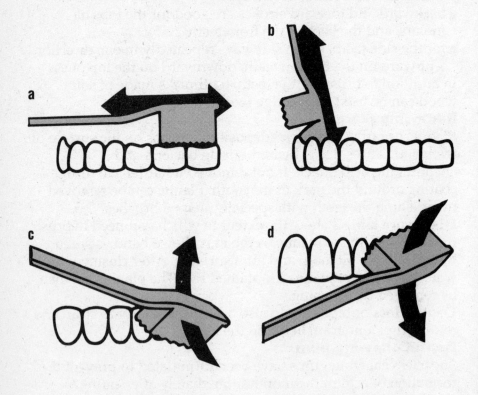

Temperomandibular Joint Syndrome

This is pain in the jaw, face and head that is thought to be caused when the jaw joints and the muscles and tendons controlling them do not to work together properly. Clenching and grinding the teeth, usually due to emotional tension, perhaps aggravated by an incorrect bite, may produce a spasm of the chewing muscles leading to this pain. It can also be the result of displacement due to injury.

Treatment

Treatment with moist heat, massage or drugs to relax the muscles and relieve pain may be supplemented by application of a splint device at night to prevent clenching and grinding. Teeth braces or selective grinding may be necessary to correct the bite.

4

MIND AND BODY

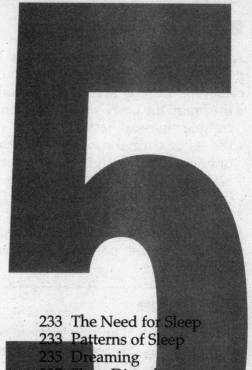

Brain and Body

All parts of the body are connected to and controled by the
nervous system. The central nervous system is the control
center for all body systems. This consists of:
- the brain: the body's central organ and its largest and most
  complex mass of nerve tissue
- the spinal cord: the extension of the lower part of the brain,
  or brainstem, through the vertebral column. The spinal cord
  acts as a central junction for the transmission of nerve
  impulses between the brain and the rest of the body.

The peripheral nervous system is the collective name for all the
nerves that carry information from the brain and spinal cord to
and from all other parts of the body.

The Brain

The brain's 14,000 million or more cells are organized into two
main divisions, the cerebrum and cerebellum, and several
subdivisions as illustrated opposite:

1 cerebrum or forebrain, the largest part of the brain, divided
into right and left hemispheres, consisting of:

a cerebral cortex a 3-millimeter thick layer of gray nerve cells,
which carry out the higher functions

2 diencephalon or interbrain, the central part of the cerebrum,
connecting the cerebrum and the cerebellum, consisting of
gray cells which control muscle contraction; the pituitary, the
central, controling hormonal gland; and

b the thalamus which collects and coordinates information
from the eyes and ears;

c the hypothalamus where the nervous and hormonal systems
interact;

d cerebellum or hindbrain coordinates and controls posture,
balance, and voluntary movements.

3 brainstem connects the cerebrum to the spinal cord. It
consists of:

e midbrain is the continuation of the spinal cord into the brain,
and contains neural pathways along which nerve impulses
travel between the hind (lower) to the fore (upper) brain
centers. It controls reflexes, such as keeping the head the right
way up and turning it in the direction of a sound.

f pons conducts nerve impulse between the medulla oblongata
and the higher brain centers, and controls some aspects of
respiration.

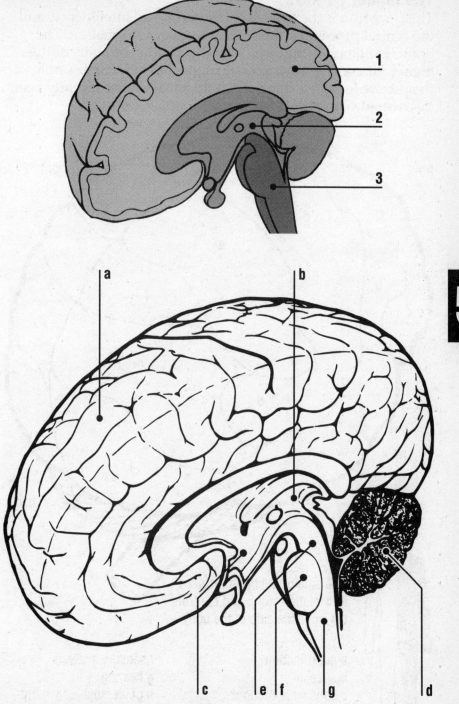

g medulla oblongata contains the control centers for respiration and heartbeat, and reflexes such as sneezing, coughing, vomiting and swallowing.

The higher centers

The cerebrum is the location of memory and intelligence, and the central processing area for all sensory information. The brain is still being 'mapped', but the location of many of the higher functions is now known in great detail. For example, the precise locus for color vision information has recently been discovered within the visual center.

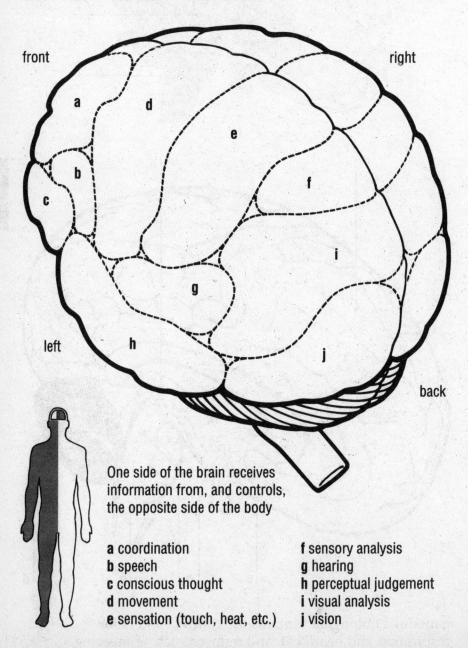

One side of the brain receives information from, and controls, the opposite side of the body

a coordination
b speech
c conscious thought
d movement
e sensation (touch, heat, etc.)

f sensory analysis
g hearing
h perceptual judgement
i visual analysis
j vision

Mind over matter

Differing proportions of brain tissue are dedicated to controling different parts of the body. The drawings below represent the importance the brain gives to conscious control of different parts of the body, and to the organs of information.

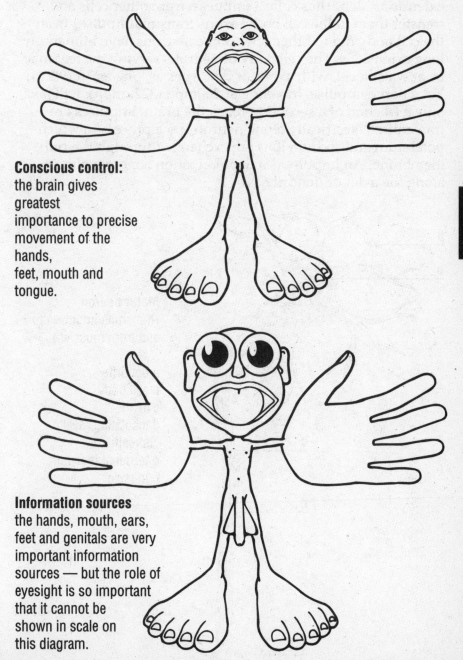

Conscious control:
the brain gives greatest importance to precise movement of the hands, feet, mouth and tongue.

Information sources
the hands, mouth, ears, feet and genitals are very important information sources — but the role of eyesight is so important that it cannot be shown in scale on this diagram.

5

Nerves

Information is transmitted from the central nervous system to all parts of the body along nerve cells, called neurons. A neuron is a single, microscopic cell body, with many extensions: dendrites collect impulses from other cells and transfer them to the cell body; axons transmit impulses from the cell body out to other cells. Some neurons have immensely long extensions. The cell body of neurons serving the feet may be at waist level, with axons or dendrites as long as 3ft (90cm). Yet a nerve impulse, traveling at 200mph (322kmph), will take only a fraction of a second to reach the brain. Impulses are transmitted electrically along neurons by a process in which potassium and sodium ions are exchanged through the cell membrane. An impulse is a depolarization zone traveling along the axon or dendrite.

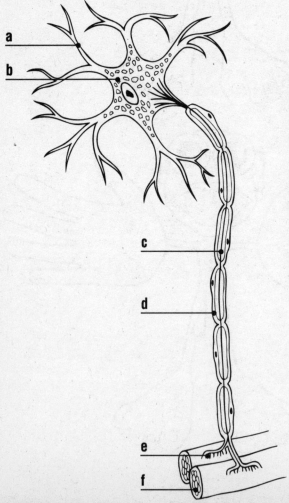

Motor neuron
(transmits impulses to
and from muscles)

a dendrite
b cell body
c axon
d insulating myelin
   sheath
e terminal receptor
f muscle

The Synapses

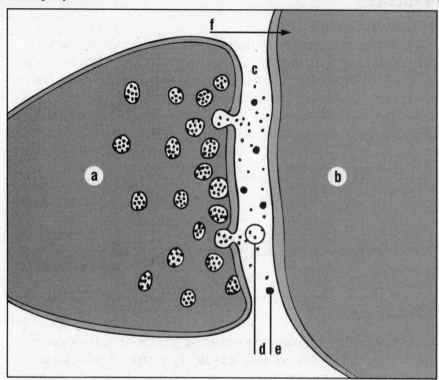

a axon terminal   **d** acetylcholine
b dendrite   **e** inhibitor
c synapse   **f** direction of nerve impulse

Synapses

The junction where the axon (transmitter) of one neuron meets the dendrite (receiver) of another is called a synapse. The arrival of the nerve impulse at the terminal stimulates the release of a chemical transmitter into the gap, which acts as a bridge for the nerve impulse. There are many different stimulating chemicals. They are called neurotransmitters:

- acetylcholine transmits impulses through the peripheral nervous system and from nerve to muscle
- dopamine transmits emotional responses
- serotonin transmits sensory impulses

At the release of the neurotransmitter, a second chemical is also released, which will destroy it and so terminate the impulse.

Inhibitors – enkephalins, endorphins, gamma amino butyric acid, and dynorphin – are released to prevent the transmission of painful impulses.

Vision

The optic nerve

Most nerves contain fibers that carry sensory information to
the central nervous system, and others that carry instructions
from the brain to activate muscles and glands. The optic nerves
are rare specialist nerves, dedicated to carrying sensory
information to the brain's visual centers. They extend directly
from the brain to the back of the eye.

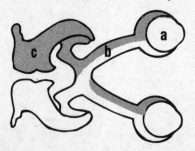

a Eyeball
b Optic nerve
c Brain

The Eyeball

a conjunctiva the membrane covering the front of the eyeball
and the inside of the eyelids. It is richly supplied with blood
vessels and is very sensitive.
b cornea the eye's principal lens, which forms the outer
transparent layer of the eye, covering the colored iris and the
pupil, or central hole, which lets in the light.
c iris the colored diaphragm surrounding the pupil – the central
opening through which light enters the eye. Circular muscle
fibers enable the iris to contract, and so reduce the size of the
pupil; radial fibers enable it to dilate or enlarge the pupil.
d crystalline lens the inner lens, which adjusts focus. The
crystalline lens is transparent, with a concave and a
convex surface, which bends rays of light that fall on it so that
they diverge or converge on the retina. It is contained in a
fibrous capsule.
e suspensory ligaments hold the crystalline lens in place.
f ciliary body at each edge of the lens contains a 'focusing
muscle' – muscle fibers that contract or relax to change the
shape of the lens and so bring near or distant objects into focus.
g anterior chamber between the crystalline lens and the cornea
is filled with a clear watery fluid called the aqueous humor.
h sclera the dense white tissue which is visible around the iris,
but which completely surrounds the eyeball, except where the
optic nerve enters at the rear.
i choroid a layer of tissue lying just beneath the retina, colored

brown or black because it is very densely packed with blood
vessels that supply the retina.

j retina a membrane of light-sensitive cells, called
photoreceptors, that lines the inside of the back of the eyeball.
Light rays focussed on it by the lenses are converted into nerve
impulses.

k fovea a small depression in the retina on the visual axis of
the eyeball, where vision is sharpest. It contains only color
receptors, called cone cells.

l optic nerve a bundle of nerve fibers extending from the optic
disk in the retina to the brain. The nerves from the left sides of
the two retinas travel to one side of the brain; those from the
right sides to the other. The two visual centers receive
composite images from both eyes, mixed 50:50.

m vitreous body a transparent gel that fills the interior of the
eye behind the crystalline lens, maintaining the eye's shape. It
contains minute specks which may be seen by staring at a
white surface. They are called 'floaters'.

n optic disk is the head of the optic nerve where it enters the
eyeball. It has no light-sensitive cells and so forms a blind spot
in the vision. The eye is sometimes aware of it as a black dot on
the periphery of vision.

5

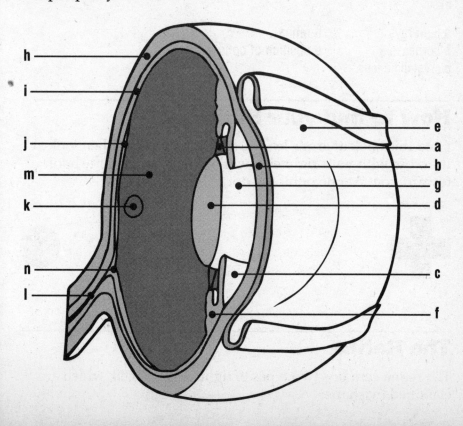

The mechanism of sight

When light rays reflected from an object enter the eye they are bent ('refracted') by the cornea, the eye's outer lens, and by a second, crystalline lens inside, and to some extent by the clear fluids within the eye. This refraction focuses the rays of light on the retina, a group of light-sensitive cells at the back of the eye, forming an upside-down image.

Light stimulating the retina triggers an impulse, which travels down the optic nerve to the visual centers of the brain. Here, the impulses are imaged and interpreted as moving colors, shades and shapes.

Refraction: The crystalline lens changes shape to focus on objects at different distances.

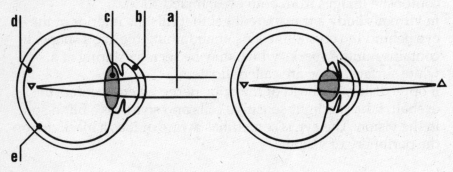

a light rays   **d** retina
b cornea   **e** position of optic nerve
c crystalline lens

How to find your Blind Spot

Hold this book at arm's length, shut your left eye, then look at the cross with your right eye, while slowly moving the book toward you. At one point the dot will disappear.

The Retina

The retina contains two types of light-receptor cell, which are classified by shape:

rods are sensitive to low light levels, giving humans sensitivity to black, white and gray, and good night vision. They are not color-sensitive. There are about 125 million rods in each retina, each less than one four-hundredth of an inch (0.6mm) long and one-hundredth of an inch (.25mm) thick. They contain a purple photosensitive pigment called rhodopsin. Light striking the rod is absorbed by the photopigment, and undergoes a very fast chemical reaction in which the pigment breaks down. This stimulates nervous impulses, which are transmitted along the optic nerve to the brain. The chemical reaction that takes place causes increased transmission in the dark and reduced transmission in the light.

Once the electrical impulse has passed to the brain, enzymes cause the rhodopsin to regenerate. The eye is therefore like a film projector. It does not sent a continual, moving picture to the brain, but an unending series of 'stills' at intervals of 8 per second.

cones are shorter and thicker for most of their length than rods. They are clustered in the center of the retina and are activated at higher light levels, so they give more accurate visual information than rods and are sensitive to the wavelengths of colored light.

The mechanism whereby cones transmit color information to the brain is broadly the same as that for rods, with the difference that each cone absorbs light in a different part of the spectrum: one type is mainly sensitive to light in the longer red and yellow wavelengths, but also senses light in other wavelengths. A second type absorbs mainly light in the shorter blue wavelengths. And a third type absorbs light in and around the green wavelengths of the middle spectral range. The nature of the signal transmitted to the brain varies according to the wavelength and intensity of the light source, so our perception of color is based on the interpretation of signals supplying different information from all three types of cone.

People with color defective vision have a reduced number of cone cells of one particular type. This visual disorder is usually hereditary. The faulty gene is transmitted by women, but the disorder only appears in men. Consequently, 99% of women have normal color vision, but only 90% of men.

In general, men tend to have a lower color vision acuity than women – for this reason women have traditionally been employed for work such as grading colored lenses.

5

Color Vision

Any color can be produced by mixing blue, red and green light in different proportions. The cone cells in the retina of the human eye are sensitive principally to yellow-red light of 560 nanometers wavelength; green light of 530 nanometers; and blue light of 420 nanometer wavelength, although each is stimulated to a lesser degree by light of other wavelengths. Thus, for every color perceived by the eye a three-parameter coding is transmitted to the brain.

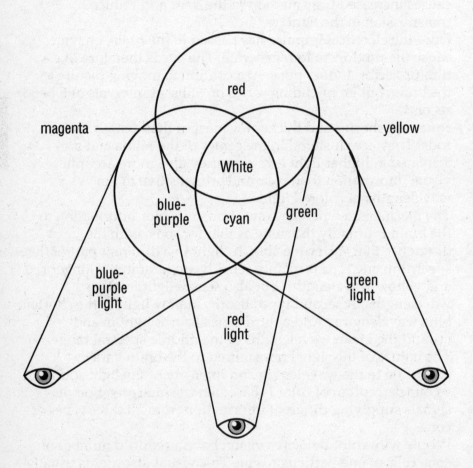

Perception

The ability to perceive objects, colors and distances is learnt by experience. To the newborn child, the images he receives are meaningless and confused. It takes time for him to learn to use his eyes and correlate past with present information to bring about recognition. This dependence of perception on the brain's judgements can be shown by presenting the eye with trick pictures: ones that allow alternative interpretations, or that give evidence that seems contradictory. Perception will then shift or struggle between the alternative interpretations. The same process can be observed naturally, in unfamiliar surroundings or moments of confusion – such as waking up in a strange room. A series of alternative pictures then flashes through the brain, as it tries to make familiar sense of the data it is receiving. Each eye sees a slightly different view of the same object. The further away the object is, the less the discrepancy between the two views. This, plus the amount of tension needed to focus and the amount of blurring, forms the basis of judgment of distance.

5

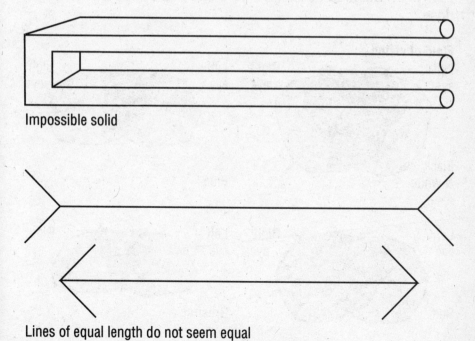

Impossible solid

Lines of equal length do not seem equal

Eye Movement

Movement of the eye is controlled by six muscles attached to the outside of the sclera (white of the eye).

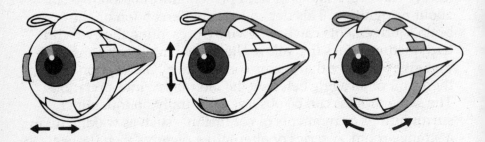

Visual Scope

The field of vision is the area that can be seen by an eye without moving it. The size of the field varies with different colors. White has the largest, then yellow, blue, red and green. However, the field of vision is also affected by the size of the nose.

Field of vision

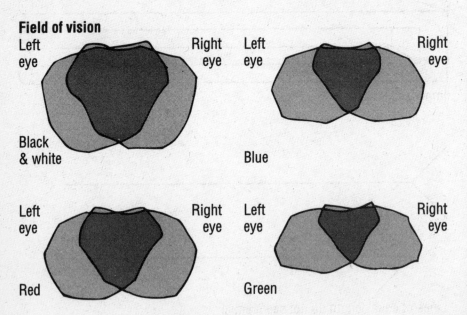

Left eye   Right eye

Black & white

Left eye   Right eye

Blue

Left eye   Right eye

Red

Left eye   Right eye

Green

The range of movement of the eyeball with the head still is also limited. The human eyeball can tilt 35° up, 50° down, 50° in (i.e. toward the other eye), and 45° out. The greater angle available when turning in allows an eye to focus on an object that is just within the other eye's outer range.

The area of vision is the total range through which a creature can see without moving head or body. It is determined by: the position of the eyes in the head; the shape of the eyes; range of movement; and, at the edge, by the eye's field of vision.

Areas of vision

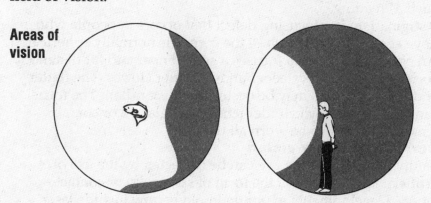
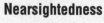

Vision Defects

Nearsightedness (myopia) is due to the refractive power of the eye being too strong (eg the crystalline lens may be too thick) or to the eyeball being too long. In both cases, the light rays are focused in front of the retina, giving a blurred image. Concave corrective lenses are needed to focus on distant objects.

Nearsightedness   **Concave lens**

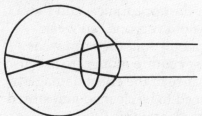
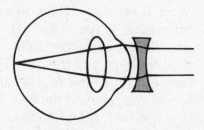

Farsightedness (hypermetropia) is due to the eye's refractive power being too weak or the eyeball too short. The light rays are focused behind the retina, again giving a blurred

Farsightedness

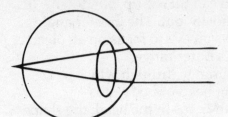

Convex lens

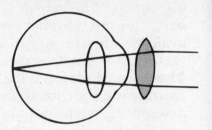

image. Convex corrective lenses are needed for close work such as reading.

Astigmatism is a focusing defect that occurs in people who have egg-shaped corneas — the cornea is normally spherical. An egg-shaped cornea focuses a spot at near and far distances, corresponding to its steeper and its flatter curves. The flatter and steeper curves may be occur in any meridian. The focus can be corrected by cylinder lenses, but glasses or contact lenses may have to be worn all the time.

Correcting faulty vision

Faulty focussing of the eye can be corrected by the use of artificial lenses either in the form of spectacles or contact lenses. Developments in ophthalmology now include laser surgery to correct short and farsightedness but this treatment is not suitable for the increase in long-sightedness which develops with aging in most people and requires them to use reading glasses.

Contact Lenses

Contact lenses are thin, round disks of plastic that rest directly on the surface of the eye. Since they were introduced in the 1980s, they have taken over from glasses as the most popular form of eyewear. They do not alter the appearance, and they often give better vision. However, not everyone can wear contact lenses successfully. Some people find they can wear them only part of the day. They also require more care because they are small and fragile, and because of the effect damaged lenses can have on the eye. They need to be cleaned and stored in a special fluid when not being used, and this fluid sometimes causes allergies.

Types of lens

Contact lenses are of three different types: 'hard', 'hard gas-permeable', or 'soft'.

Hard lenses are made of acrylic PMMa (perspex), or CAB

(cellulose acetate-butyrate). The type of hard lens normally prescribed today is the 'corneal' lens, which rests on the center of the eye, floating on a film of tear fluid. There is another type of hard lens called a 'scleral' lens, which covers the whole of the visible part of the eye, but this is now only prescribed to treat specific medical conditions.

Soft lenses are are made from HEMA (hydroxyl-ethyl-methacrylate) or hydrogel, which, when wet, is flexible and jelly-like, but becomes hard and brittle if allowed to dry out. Soft lenses are easier to fit than hard lenses and easier to adjust to. Soft lenses remain soft while being worn because they absorb water from the tear fluid. They are larger in diameter than the cornea. Disposable lenses for one use only are now available.

Hard and soft lenses compared

Soft lenses are immediately comfortable, easy to get used to, can generally be worn all day, can be left off for several days and then worn again without discomfort, and can be worn with little discomfort in a dirty atmosphere.

Hard lenses are comparatively cheap and difficult to damage; last for perhaps 6-8 years (only 2-3 years for soft lenses with routine wear and tear, and often less than a year if damage occurs); and are more suitable for most prescriptions, since they are capable of altering the shape of the cornea slightly – and so adjusting the eye's focus. They may give clearer vision than soft lenses, are easier to keep free from bacteria, and much easier for an optician to adjust if difficulty arises.

Gas-permeable lenses

Gas-permeable lenses are made of a mixture of materials. They have similar qualities to hard lenses, but are more comfortable, because oxygen is able to pass through them to the cornea. This is important because the cells of the cornea get the oxygen they need from the air, via the tear fluid that bathes the eye. The cells of the cornea are transparent and so have no blood vessels to supply oxygen. Both hard and soft contact lenses reduce the amount of oxygen diffusing through the tear fluid and reaching the cornea. If this persists for many hours, the outer protective layer of cells in the center of the cornea dies, and is torn off when the lens is eventually removed. For some hours, until new cells regenerate, the exposed corneal nerves are excruciatingly painful.

Gas-permeable lenses can be worn for longer than hard or soft lenses, but must still be removed at the end of the day. They do not last as long as hard lenses (perhaps up to 5 years), and they are more expensive.

5

Continuous wear lenses The production of very thin soft lenses with a very high water content — and some are over 80% water), brings closer the possibility of lenses that need not be removed, even at night. Such lenses would be a boon to patients with illnesses that prevent them from inserting their lenses without assistance, and to people who have had cataract operations.

Wearing contact lenses continually carries the risk that the corneas may become waterlogged and wrinkled – like any skin that has been in water too long. This is a serious condition, which may damage the vision. Another risk is that of tiny blood vessels growing into the cornea and interfering with vision. There is also a risk of *Acanthameba polyphaga*, a commonly occurring ameba, infecting the corneas, and of recurring infection if the lenses become infected.

Continuous-wear lenses can cause the corneas to change shape, exacerbating the original focussing problem; and the lenses may be contaminated by deposits of protein, fat, or mineral deposits on their inner surfaces, which are difficult and expensive to remove.

The Eye's Protective Structures

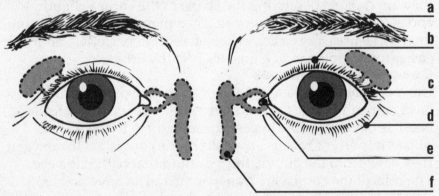

The organs of sight are protected from injury by their position within deep hollows in the skull, and by several other surrounding structures:

a eyebrows prevent sweat, water and particles of solid matter from running down into the eye from above

b eyelids – folds of skin – close to completely cover and protect the eyes. They also form a seal that protects the eyeball from invasion by foreign bodies – the inner membrane of each eyelid is a continuation of the conjunctiva. Blinking is a protective action of the eyelid, which spreads the lacrimal fluid over the front of the eyeball, thus cleaning it. Blinking is a reflex controlled by the brain. It occurs every 2 to 10 seconds, and the rate increases under stress, in dusty surroundings or when tired, and decreases during periods of concentration.

c conjunctiva, the transparent protective layer that covers the front of the eyeball.

d eyelashes – long, thick hairs growing outward from each eyelid. They prevent foreign bodies from entering the eye and trigger the protective blinking mechanism when touched unexpectedly.

e lacrimal glands produce a watery, salty fluid that cleans the front of the eyeball and acts as a disinfectant. It also lubricates the eyeball, so that the eyelid can move over it. The glands can produce quantities of tears – excess fluid – if irritated or stimulated by strong emotion.

f lacrimal ducts – drain the fluid from the eye surface into the lacrimal sacs, which lead into the nasal passage. When the ducts cannot clear the fluid fast enough, it overflows and falls down the face as tears.

5

Eye Care

Injuries to the eye and the immediate surrounding area should receive expert medical attention. Infection is a danger even if there is no significant damage. The eyes are tough but vital, and should be treated with care.

Small foreign bodies that get stuck in the eye can usually be removed by blinking. If this fails, pull the upper lid outward and downward over the lower lid. When the upper lid is released, the particle may be dislodged. A particle can also be removed with the corner of a handkerchief or by blowing it toward the edge. If none of these measures is effective, get medical attention quickly to avoid scratching the eye and possible infection.

Black eyes are bruises of the eyelids and the tissues around the eye. They can be treated by applying a cold compress. If a black eye appears after a blow elsewhere on the head, see a doctor for an examination.

A stye is an inflammation of the sebaceous gland (see p 168) around an eyelash, and is caused by bacterial infection. It occurs most commonly in adolescents. A large area of the eyelid may become infected. To treat a stye, remove the infected eyelash and bathe the eye with hot water regularly several times a day until the stye bursts. Antibiotics should be used only in extreme cases.

Conjunctivitis is inflammation of the conjunctiva. It can be caused by infection or irritation. Infection is treated with antibiotic eye drops. An irritant, such as an ingrowing eyelash, is removed. Bathing the eye with warm water and lotions will help healing. Bandages and pads encourage the growth of bacteria, but dark glasses or eyeshades protect the eye from further irritation by light, dust and wind. Conjunctivitis should be treated as early as possible to prevent complications, such as ulceration of the cornea. Trachoma, infection with the organism chlamydia trachomatis, is a serious tropical disease of which conjunctivitis is a major symptom.

Cataract is the whitening of the internal crystalline lens of the eye, due to coagulation of protein within the fibers from which it is made. Cataract often occurs spontaneously with advancing age. It can also be caused by injury to the eye, by severe malnutrition, electric shock and a number of drugs. Rubella (German measles) and other illnesses during pregnancy can result in cataract as a birth defect, and it can be caused by diabetes. Changes in color vision, increasing short-sightedness, clouding of the vision, and light-scattering are the main symptoms. Cataract causes deterioration of vision but not blindness, and can affect one eye or both. Removal of the lens is the only treatment. Afterwards, short-sighted people may find their vision improved, but others need to wear glasses to restore accurate focus.

Glaucoma is a rise in the pressure of the aqueous humor, the fluid which fills the outer chamber of the eye, between the cornea and the crystalline lens. The cause is often a blockage in the channels that drain the eye of excess fluid. Glaucoma usually occurs gradually, with few symptoms, and is often only noticeable when loss of parts of the visual field occurs. If untreated, glaucoma causes blindness. It can be treated in the early stages with drugs to inhibit fluid production and increase drainage, and in later stages by surgery. Glaucoma affects mainly older people, and from the age of 40 it is advisable to see an optician for a test for pressure within the eyeball. Glaucoma also occurs in acute (sudden) form, and symptoms include repeatedly seeing blue, green, orange, yellow and red concentric circles around lights; a dull ache in or around the eye; misty or fogging of vision; reddening of the eye. These symptoms should be reported to an ophthalmologist.

Retinal detachment is the separation of part of the retina from the layer of pigmented cells behind it. Retinal detachment is often caused by a tear or a hole, which fills with fluid, but it can also be caused by a blow to the head. Extremely short-sighted people are prone to this condition, and there is a hereditary element. Retinal detachment is often preceded by flashing lights and dark spots before the eyes, but the major symptom is the perception of a dark curtain falling across the field of vision. When this happens, acting correctly can prevent permanent loss of sight:

- if the black curtain comes down from above, the retina is, in fact, detached from below. The affected person should keep his head upright or lie on his face
- if the dark curtain comes across from the left, the detachment is occurring on the right side of the retina, and the person affected should lie on the right side.
- if the dark curtain comes across from the right, the detachment is occurring on the left side on the retina and the person should lie on the left side
- if the curtain comes up from below, the retina is detached above. The person should lie face down.

The next step is to get emergency treatment by an ophthalmologist as soon as possible. An examination is necessary to locate all holes and tears, and an operation to seal them off using cryosurgery and microsurgical techniques. As long as the central part of the retina, called the macula, is not damaged, good vision can be restored.

5

Hearing

When a solid object vibrates in air, it passes on this vibration to the surrounding air molecules. Sound waves are the vibrations of air molecules. Sound has three qualities:

- Pitch is the sharpness of a sound, it depends on the 'frequency' of the sound waves (i.e. the number of vibrations per second). High-pitched (piercing) sounds have a high frequency. Low-pitched (deep) sounds have a low frequency. The human ear can distinguish one sound from another because different frequencies stimulate different parts of the organ of Corti in the inner ear (see p 225). The ear can detect sounds ranging in pitch from 20 cycles per second (low) to 20,000 cycles per second (high). Frequencies above this, called ultrasounds, can be heard by some animals but not by humans.
- Intensity is the loudness of a sound and it depends on the amount of energy in the sound waves – how widely they vibrate. Intensity is measured in decibels. The human ear can

hear sounds ranging in loudness from 10 to 140 decibels, but after 100 decibels sound becomes painful, and damages the ear. On the decibel scale, a 10-unit increase means 10 times the loudness.

- Timbre is the quality of a sound. Sounds with the same pitch and intensity can be distinguished by their timbre. Timbre is created by the subordinate notes that accompany the main pitch.

The Ear

Outer ear

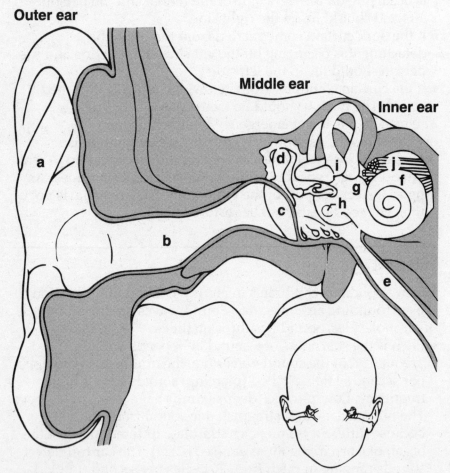

Middle ear

Inner ear

a Cartilage flap	**f** Cochlea
b Ear canal	**g** Oval window
c Eardrum	**h** Round window
d Ossicles	**i** Organ of balance
e Eustachian tube	**j** Auditory nerve

The structures of the ear can be divided into three groups:

1 The outer ear includes the external flap of cartilage (the 'pinna' or 'auricle') and the ear canal (the 'meatus'). Sound waves are collected by the pinna and funneled into the ear canal.

2 The middle ear includes: the eardrum (the tympanic membrane); three small bones called the ossicles, which have descriptive names – the hammer (the malleus), the anvil (the incus), and the stirrup (the stapes); the eustachian tube, which opens into the back of the throat and keeps the air pressure in the middle ear equal to the pressure outside. The eardrum vibrates in times with the sound waves. This vibration is passed along the ossicles to the oval window. The lever action of the ossicles increases the strength of the vibration, so that it is transmitted from the air in the outer and middle ear to the fluid in the inner ear.

3 The inner ear includes: the cochlea, a spiral filled with fluid, containing the organ of Corti, the oval window; the round window; and the organ of balance. The vibrations of the oval window make the fluid in the cochlea vibrate. The pressure changes in the fluid are picked up by specialized cells in the organ of Corti and transmitted to the brain. Meanwhile, the vibrations pass on through the cochlea and back to the round window, where they are lost in the air in the middle ear and eustachian tube.

5

Auditory Nerve

The organs of Corti are the dendrites (nerve receptors) of the auditory nerve. Wave vibrations transmitted into the inner ear through the oval window stimulate hair cells of the organ of Corti, which are converted into nerve impulses and transmitted along the dendrite to the hearing centers of the brain (see p 207).

Direction The slight distance between the ears means that there are minute differences in their perception of a given sound. The brain interprets these differences to tell from which direction the sound came. But if a sound comes from directly behind or in front of the listener, both ears receive the same message, and the listener must turn his head before he can pinpoint the location. Decline in hearing progresses with age.

Balance

The organ of balance is in the inner ear next to the cochlea. It consists of three U-shaped tubes ('semi-circular canals'), at right angles to each other. They are filled with fluid, which is set in motion when the person moves. Hairs at the base of each canal sense this movement and send messages to the brain, which are interpreted and used to maintain the person's balance. The organ also contains two other structures, the saccule and the utricle. These have specialized cells which are sensitive to gravity, and so keep a check on the body's position.

Ear Care

The outer ear should be kept clean and dry to prevent water and bacteria from collecting in the ear canal and causing infection. However, the wax that forms in the ear is an important protection. The ear should not be cleaned so thoroughly that very little wax is left. It is not necessary to clean the ear by swabbing the ear canal with cotton buds; sticks and other rigid objects should not be poked into the ear.

Syringing Should excess wax accumulate in the ear canal, it should be cleaned out by a nurse using a syringe and ear solvents. Syringing is also used to remove foreign bodies from the ear canal. A large glass or metal syringe is used, with a blunt end not more than 1 inch (2.5cm) long so that it cannot hurt the eardrum. The syringe is filled with warm water containing an antiseptic and/or a wax-dissolving agent. The fluid is directed along the upper wall of the canal and flows out along the lower.

Examination A beam of light from a flashlight is shone down the ear canal to examine the outer ear.

The inner ear is tested by using a tuning fork. If hearing is acute, the fork should be clearly audible when it is held in front of the ear. If it is more clearly audible when placed on the bone behind the ear, the outer ear is blocked with wax, or something is wrong in the middle ear, since sound vibrations are being heard more clearly through the skull. If hearing is still poor when the fork is placed on the bone behind the ear, something is wrong in the inner ear or with the auditory nerves.

Hearing loss It is crucially important to protect the ear against hearing loss. Sudden loud noises, such as gunfire, alarms, heavy road vehicles without silencers passing by; and persistent loud noises, such as loud music, especially through stereo headphones, chain-saws, snowmobiles and loud workplace noise will all damage the hearing. Try to get used to listening to music at a lower volume than you think of as normal; always wear ear protectors if you are issued with them at work; and cover your ears if you are subjected to loud noises in the street. Complain about noise in the environment. Loud noises damage the organs of Corti in the inner ear; once destroyed, they will not regenerate. Hearing loss is not detectable until it is too late.

Ear Disorders

Earache is usually caused by infection and inflammation in the ear. Infection in the outer ear can be caused by physical damage, boils, or eczema (pp 175-6). Large wax deposits can also cause earache. Germs from throat infections may spread up the eustachian tube and cause inflammation of the middle ear. This is especially common after tonsilitis, flu and head colds, and it can be painful.

Earache sometimes occurs in the absence of ear disorders as a result of disturbances affecting the nerves it shares with other parts of the head. Tonsilitis, bad teeth, swollen glands and neuralgia can all cause earache in this way.

Fungal infections sometimes affect the outer ear. They are most common in tropical climates. There is persistent irritation and discharge, which is treated with antibiotics and antiseptic cleaning of the ear canal.

Discharges are sometimes caused by boils or other infections.

Tinnitus is sound originating in the head and perceptible only by the affected person. It may take the form of a pure musical note, hissing, whistling, clicking or ringing affecting one or both ears, or emanating from the center of the head. It is usually accompanied by deafness or a lesser degree of hearing loss. It is caused by anything that damages the hearing, such as loud noises, by diseases such as Ménière's disease and otosclerosis, and by certain drugs:

- the aminoglycoside antibiotics which include Streptomycin, Neomycin, Framycetin, Kanamycin, Gentamycin (also called Garamycin), Tobramycin, Amikacin, Vancomycin and Polymyxin B.
- certain diuretics when taken in large doses: Frusemide (lasix), Ethacrynic acid (Edecrin), and to a lesser extent, Bumetanide and Acetazolamide (Diamox).

- aspirin in large doses (which also causes high tone deafness).
- Vancomycin, Chloromycetin, Ristocetin, Viomycin, Pharmacetin, Colistin, Ampicillin, Mefenamic acid, Oil of Chenopodium, Bleomycin, nitrogen mustard, cis-platinum, Pentobrbital, Hexadine, Mandelamine, Practolol, carbon monoxide, mercury, nicotine, gold, lead, arsenic and aniline dyes.

Giddiness (vertigo) can be caused by infections of the inner ear that affect the organ of balance.

Otitis externa is infection and inflammation of the outer ear, due to fungus infection, physical damage, allergy, boils or spread of inflammation from the middle ear. There is itching and often a discharge, which may cause temporary deafness if it blocks the ear canal. Treatment is by antiseptic syringing and use of soothing lotions. Hot poultices and aspirin may relieve the pain.

Otitis media is middle-ear infection, usually due to bacteria arriving via the eustachian tube. The eardrum becomes red and swollen, and may perforate. Pressure and pain increase as pus fills the middle ear. There is often temporary deafness and ringing, and sometimes fever. Treatment is with antibiotics. A form of otitis in which a sticky substance is discharged in the middle ear is common in children. The ossicles cannot function, and in severe cases permanent deafness results.

Mastoiditis is a middle-ear infection that has spread to the mastoid bone – the part of the skull just behind the ear. Infection swells the bone painfully and the patient is feverish. Treatment is by antibiotics or the surgical removal of the infected bone (mastoidectomy).

Ménière's disease affects the inner ear, and results in too much fluid in the labyrinths. Its cause is not known. It tends to occur in middle age, usually affecting more men than women. The symptoms are attacks of giddiness and sickness, followed by deafness with accompanying tinnitus. Treatment is with drugs and control of fluid intake (not more than 2½ pints a day). In extreme cases the labyrinths or their nervous connections are destroyed.

Deafness

Types of deafness

'Conductive deafness' refers to any failure in those parts of the ear which gather and pass on sound waves, eg blockage of the ear canal, eardrum damage, ossicle damage, etc. 'Perceptive deafness' refers to any failure in: that part of the ear which translates the sound waves into nerve impulses (the cochlea); the auditory nerves which transmit the impulses to the brain; or in the auditory centers of the brain which receive the message. Perceptive deafness may not mean that the person can perceive no sound. It may be that sound is received, but so scrambled as to be unintelligible.

Causes of deafness

Disease. Some disorders can end in deafness.

Noise-induced. Any exposure to extremely loud noise, or continued exposure to moderately loud noise, can damage the eardrum and middle ear, causing hearing decline and eventually deafness. The main victims are those who work in very noisy surroundings, and also the fans – and performers – of loud popular music.

Congenital deafness. Deformities at birth range from complete absence of the ears, to minute mistakes in the internal structure. The latter can often be cured surgically. Congenital deafness can be due to heredity (genetic defects). It can also result from certain infections in the mother in the first few months of pregnancy including German measles, flu, and syphilis. If there is anything in your child's response to sounds that gives rise to worry, consult your doctor.

Otosclerosis. This is a condition in which the stirrup becomes fixed within the oval window, due to deposits of new bone. About one person in every 250 suffers from this, and it is more common in men than in women. Surgical treatment can give improvement, but there is no way of halting the process responsible (though it may stop spontaneously).

5

Hearing Aids

Hearing aids work by amplifying sound. If the amplification is loud enough, it can overcome the blockage or damage that causes conductive deafness, and allow the sound to reach the inner ear. Amplification also seems to help in many cases of perceptive deafness. However, sometimes the aid does not allow speech to be distinguished: it only makes the person more aware of unintelligible noise. The performance of a hearing aid depends on:

- The frequency response. Normal speech usually lies between 500 and 2000 cycles per second.
- The degree of amplification.

- The maximum amount of sound that the aid can deliver. Too much sound can make speech unintelligible, and/or damage the ear mechanisms.

Insert receivers are the most common type of aid. They are molded to fit into the ear canal and form a perfect seal. No sound escapes, there is little or no acoustic feedback and background noise is at a minimum. They can also be very small and, if transistorized, need no wires or attachments. A high degree of amplification is possible. One problem with hearing aids is 'acoustic feedback'. This is the re-amplification of sound vibrations that have already passed into the ear but have partly leaked out again.

Flat receivers fit against the external ear cartilage, and are kept in place by a metal band. They are usually used only if there is a continuous discharge from the ear, or if there has been a serious mastoid operation. Because of the bad contact, many sounds escape, and acoustic feedback produces much background noise.

Bone conductors amplify the sound waves and send them through the bone of the head, not the air passages of the ear. They are uncomfortable and not very efficient, and are usually only used where some ear condition rules out an insert receiver.

Other devices and developments

Amplified telephone receivers, flashing lights (instead of telephones that ring and doorbells), remote receiver headphones for televisions, and teletypewriters have all been developed to improve circumstances for the deaf. New medical developments include cochlear implants (to help nerve conduction deafness), and temporal bone implants (for bone conduction deafness).

Cochlear implants, consisting of one or more electrodes implanted in or close to the cochlea, a receiver-stimulator implanted in the mastoid process of the temporal bone, and an external speech processor, were introduced in the late 1980s. They have been extensively reviewed and have been found to be highly successful in treating adults with profound deafness. Miniaturization, frequency manipulation techniques, and noise generation to mask tinnitus are likely to lead to great advances in hearing aid technology, so that people with hearing defects, including the increasing numbers of elderly people, can expect aids designed to match their exact spectrum of hearing loss, and the suppression of confusing background noise.

Sleep

Everyone has a natural rhythm of sleeping and waking, based on a daily rhythm cycle. About one-third of a person's life is spent in this state of near unconsciousness. However, a sleeper retains awareness of aspects of his surroundings, such as noises and lights, and some parts of his brain and body are less affected than others.

The part of the brain governing sleep is called the reticular formation in the central core of the brainstem. Neurons in this part of the brain have widespread networks of connections across the central nervous system. Three types of neuron dominate this part of the brain. They release the neurotransmitters norepinephrine, dopamine and serotonin. It is thought that serotonin might induce changes in the brain that bring about sleep. Other sleep-inducing chemicals are found in the blood, urine, cerebrospinal fluid and brain tissue, including the delta sleep-inducing peptide (DSIP) which induces delta-wave sleep, and a 'substance S', which may induce slow-wave sleep. The interrelationship between these substances is not yet understood.

Two systems in the brain interact: one that brings about sleep when stimulated, and an arousal system. The second can override the first.

5

Stages of Sleep

Slow-wave sleep

With drowsiness, the alpha rhythms – brainwaves characteristic of an adult who is awake with closed eyes – gradually gives way to a pattern of slow waves. As sleep deepens, the brainwaves show a progressively slower frequency and higher voltage. It takes 30 to 45 minutes to progress to deep sleep, then the process reverses, taking 30 to 45 minutes to return to a light sleep. During this phase the postural muscles retain tone and the heart and respiration rates fall only slightly.

REM (Rapid Eye Movement) sleep

During this phase of light sleep, electroencephalogram (EEG) readouts show a brainwave pattern similar to that when awake. During this phase, the eyes move rapidly behind closed lids. The postural muscles lose tone completely, but the limbs and facial muscles twitch in concert with bursts of rapid eye movement. Breathing, heartbeat and blood pressure go through irregular changes. Men experience an erection during REM sleep. Men who cannot normally achieve erection experience erection during REM dreaming, unless the penis is incapable of erection, because of nerve damage, for example. When awakened during this phase, subjects report they have been dreaming.

Through a night of 7 to 8 hours' sleep, the brain follows a cycle lasting an average 30 to 90 minutes of deep sleep followed by 10 to 15 minute REM episodes. Toward the end of an undisturbed night, slow-wave sleep diminishes and the numbers of REM episodes increase.

Patterns of Sleep

Consciousness

Shallow sleep
The dark shaded areas show dream periods

Deep sleep
Sleep is at its deepest early in the sleeping hours

Brain pattern
The electrical activity of the brain changes with different stages of sleep

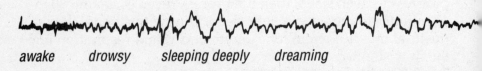

awake   drowsy   sleeping deeply   dreaming

The Need for Sleep

During deep sleep there is a rise in the output of the growth hormone in young people. This is also the time when repair processes are undertaken and dead cells replaced. During REM sleep, the postural muscles relax totally.

A person kept awake for long periods of time passes through periods of intense fatigue, but can recover from them and continue to function without sleep. Yet people deprived of sleep for long periods become increasingly disorientated, and both mentally and physically exhausted.

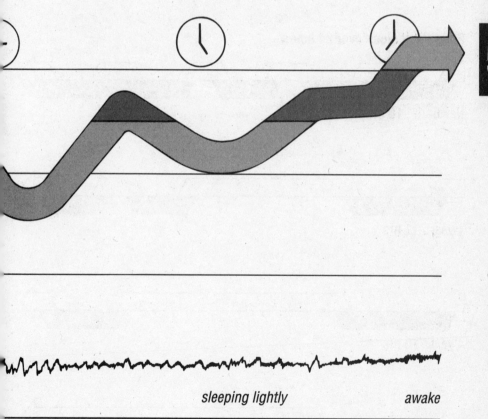

sleeping lightly   *awake*

After about 10 days of total sleep deprivation, death occurs. It seems that we do not sleep just because the body needs to rest. Lying down would be adequate for that. In fact, the body shifts regularly during sleep to prevent the muscles seizing up. If we go without sleep for several days, our automatic body processes can go on functioning in a fairly steady way.

It also seems that the brain can adapt to periods of perhaps two or three days without sleep. But eventually, lack of sleep brings irritability, irrationality, hallucinations and confusion. The brain does not rest during sleep. Some neurons are deactivated during sleep, but others are activated. The activity of the brain continues.

Patterns of sleep over 24 hours

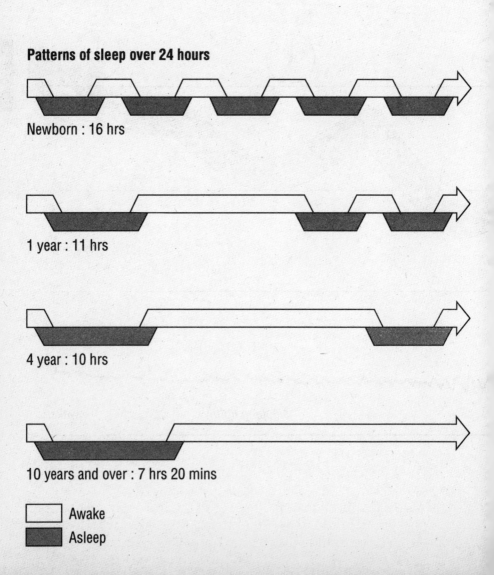

Newborn : 16 hrs

1 year : 11 hrs

4 year : 10 hrs

10 years and over : 7 hrs 20 mins

☐ Awake

■ Asleep

It is thought that one function of sleep is to allow changes to take place in the brain that enable learning to take place and memory to function. It seems that perhaps our feelings of physical exhaustion are produced by the brain, in its unwillingness to go on controling the body.

These ideas are, however, hypotheses. As research into the brain progresses, the function of sleep may be revealed.

Sleep requirements

Most of an unborn child's day is spent sleeping. After birth, the amount of sleep needed gradually declines with growth:
But there are wide variations around these figures. Some babies sleep 10½ hours, others 23 hours. Some adults sleep 14 hours, others 3 or less. There is a tradition that sleep requirements diminish with advancing age and that people over 65 need an average 5½ hours or less.

However, research shows that sleep needs are constant from adulthood.

The reasons for variations in sleep patterns are not understood. Time spent sleeping is not related to sex, exercise, diet or intelligence. It is highly personal, related, perhaps, to childhood training or psychology.

5

Dreaming

Dreaming takes up an average two hours of a night's sleep lasting 7½ hours. Everyone dreams, but many people do not remember their dreams. If a sleeper is woken in the middle of REM sleep, he will remember a vivid dream. If woken 5 minutes after REM he will have only a hazy recollection of a dream, and if woken 10 minutes afterwards he will remember nothing of it.

In tribal societies the world over, and in all civilizations, including the modern world, the significance of dreams has been sought and the content of dreams held to be significant in the interpretation of past and present events, and in the prediction of the future.

Throughout the 20th century psychologists have sought a scientific explanation for dreaming.

Freudian ideas

The Austrian founder of psychology, Sigmund Freud, suggested that dreams symbolize the unconscious needs and anxieties of the dreamer. He argued that society requires us to suppress many of our urges. We cannot act on them and we sometimes have to hide them from ourselves. This is unhealthy, and the subconscious, seeking to redress the balance, re-presents them to the conscious mind as dreams, which act as an outlet for repressed urges.

Jungian theories

Freud's Swiss colleague, Carl Gustav Jung, saw the diverse images in dreams as meaningful symbols, each of which may be variously interpreted according to its context in the dream. He believed that during the waking state the unconscious perceives, interprets and learns from events and experiences, and that during sleep it communicates this 'inner knowledge' to the conscious in a system of simple visual imagery. He attempted to classify the images in dreams in terms of their symbolic meaning. He believed that the symbols in dream imagery are common to all mankind – that they were formulated during the evolutionary development of the human brain and transmitted through generations by heredity.

Computer analogies

Since the development of computers, psychologists have compared the brain with a computer, carrying out tasks according to a set of instructions – a program. Reprogramming can take place only when the computer is not occupied with its daily tasks – that is, at night, when it is at rest. In sleep, the influx of new information into the brain falls considerably, so sleep may be the time when the brain reviews and organizes new information and reprograms itself accordingly.

New ideas

In the light of recent advances in knowledge about the brain, all of these theories are being increasingly dismissed as simplistic, and experiments are being carried out to try to determine scientifically the function – if any – of dreams and dreaming.

The respected theoretical biologist, Francis Crick, who is famous for having discovered, with James D. Watson, the double helix structure of DNA in 1953, has turned his attention to a study of the brain. He dismisses computer analogies, but suggests that in one respect the human brain and computers that organize information in parallel (in many locations at a time, as the brain does) may behave in a similar fashion. When overloaded with data, they react by throwing up 'pseudo-memories', which are composites of real ones. The brain may use pseudo-memories – dreams – as a way of reducing a memory overload.

Nevertheless, examples of the unconscious mind 'assisting' in the solving of some problem in a dream remain to be explained. The chemist, F.A. Kekule, who discovered the

chemical structure of benzene went to bed one night in a state
of anxiety because he could not see how to solve the problem
of the molecular structure of benzene. He dreamed of a snake
with its tail in its mouth – an ancient image, according to C.G.
Jung, found in mythologies the world over, and in ancient
Egyptian mythology. He subsequently proved the molecular
structure of benzene to be a ring.

Sleep Disorders

Somnambulism ('sleep walking') is sleep in which the parts of
the brain that control the muscles have stayed awake. The
person may speak, sit up, and even get out of bed and walk.
The senses are partly awake, for the walker avoids
obstructions, but does not remember the experience on
waking.
Paralyzed wakefulness is a condition in which a person wakes,
but cannot immediately move. The experience is frightening,
but harmless.

5

Insomnia
Perhaps for reasons of survival the body's waking systems are
easier to activate than those causing sleep. Perhaps this is one
reason why insomnia (sleeplessness) is such a common
problem. It is also thought that many people who find it
difficult to sleep do not have insomnia. In fact, many fail to
realize that they do not need so much sleep (pp 234-5), and
others in fact sleep while in bed, but very lightly and for such
short periods that they do not realize they have slept.
To know that the body is getting all the sleep it really needs
and is not deprived can be a source of comfort to a sleepless
person, removing one possible source of stress, can in itself
help to alleviate insomnia. Sometimes the best response to
insomnia is simply to get up, make a hot drink or eat a snack,
and calmly do something until you feel sleepy again. The
tension insomnia creates is most likely to prolong it. In fact, the
main cause of insomnia, whether occasional or regular, is
simply the fear that one is not going to sleep.

Causes
Causes of occasional insomnia include: feeling cold, or having
bedcoverings that are too light; indigestion; excessive fatigue;
excitement; nervousness; worry; pain or illness.
Causes of repeated insomnia include: difficulty in breathing
when lying down (as in heart and lung disorder); bad food
habits, especially eating a large meal, or drinking tea or coffee,

too late in the evening; needing to urinate during the night; a noisy, airless or overheated bedroom; lack of exercise during the day; trying to sleep more than you need; and psychological factors – anxiety, emotional upset, overwork and depression. In fact, insomnia is a common sign of psychological stress. People sleep badly because they cannot forget their problems at bed time. The insomnia aggravates feelings of tiredness and tension, which are a further cause of insomnia.

Treatment

It is better to try to cure insomnia naturally before resorting to sleeping pills. First, try to ensure that you are comfortable before you go to bed: wear comfortable bedclothing, open a window, and so on. Next, go for a short walk or do a few stretching and relaxing exercises before getting into bed, and have a warm bath. Have a hot milky drink (milk is thought to encourage serotonin production), and read, listen to the radio or watch television until you drift off. Developing a gentle routine is useful in re-educating the mind to the idea of a good night's sleep.

If you have to resort to sleeping pills, try 'natural' pills from a health food store. It is better to resort to pharmaceutical drugs only at times of serious and fairly short-lived outside emotional disturbances, such as acute grief at a death.

Psychosomatic Illness

Research into various disorders has often implicated the role of mental factors in their development and progression. Illnesses such as asthma and high blood pressure may be initiated or worsened by factors such as anxiety and overwork, although they have other causes. The contribution of emotional factors to other diseases, such as cancer, is less easy to quantify and is controversial.

Some physicians think that prolonged anxiety and depression caused by an accumulation of adverse life events, such as unemployment and family breakdown, have the effect of lowering the body's resistance to illness. Statistics indicate that this may well be the case, and animal experiments have shown that stress can affect the immune response. But the direct physiological effects of stress factors are hard to prove.

In extreme anxiety states, the psychological illness probably causes physical symptoms, such as breathlessness and rapid heartbeat, which disappear with successful treatment. The physical effects of life crises are not so clear, however. People

who suffer financial hardship or depression may be less
motivated to take an interest in a healthy diet or to take regular
physical exercise, for example.

Stress

Stress, broadly defined, is the response of the mind and body
to environmental changes which may be threatening to health
or life. In response to a rise in external temperature the body
will put into motion mechanisms to prevent dangerous
overheating. Similarly, in response to intense fright, the body
puts into operation physical processes that enable the
individual to run, fight or otherwise overcome the threat.
In recent years, the concept of stress has been widened to
include the effects of a vast range of experiences, from worry
over exam results to divorce or moving house. Most non-
medical people now believe that the 'stresses of modern life' –
domestic, social, or business stress – are a major factor in
causing ill-health.

5

Psychological stress

The acceptance of the idea of stress as a cause of physical
illness can be traced back to the work of Hans Selye, a
Canadian, who began investigating the effects of stress on the
body in the 1920s. He observed a three-stage response to stress:
alarm; resistance; and exhaustion. He proposed that long-term
stress leads to physical deterioration, shock, heart failure and
death.

During the major wars of the mid-1900s, post-traumatic stress
disorder was first accepted as a medical condition.

This is a severe personal anxiety disorder resulting from stress
caused not only by warfare experiences but also by other
terrifying events, such as assault, rape, involvement in a
disaster or personal injury. Symptoms such as nightmares,
insomnia, a sense of isolation, guilt, irritability, loss of
concentration, depression and loss of emotional feeling may
occur, immediately, or after a long delay. Support and
counseling are important in enabling the affected person to
recover.

The A-type personality

In the mid-1980s American heart specialists identified a
'coronary-prone' personality type and described it as the A-
type. This individual is ambitious, aggressive, restless and
obsessively concerned with time and deadlines. This type is
reported to be more than twice as likely to experience a severe

heart attack as the 'Type B' personality, who is less obsessive or aggressive, and achieves things in a more relaxed way. This book had immense influence during the late 1980s, and inspired a great deal of research into the effects of psychological stress on ilnesses such as atherosclerosis and heart attacks.

Subsequent investigation shows that certain personality types, most notably the 'A-type' personality and especially people who repress aggression, attract stress and suffer a higher than average incidence of heart attacks. However, people who abuse their bodies in any way – with drugs, alcohol or overeating – are more likely than average to develop illnesses. It is therefore suspected that there may be some confusion between cause and effect in the interpretation of these phenomena.

Stress tables

Thomas H. Holmes and Richard Rahe, two American psychiatrists, attempted to quantify the stress value of various life events in terms of their health-destructive effects. Their Social Readjustment Ratings Scale rates 43 stressful events in terms of their effects on the body. On a scale from 1 to 100, the death of a spouse ranks 100, divorce, 73; death of a close friend, 37; and a minor brush with the law, 11.

The facts

Research has shown that stressful life events affect physiology in many ways. The body increases production of epinephrine, also called adrenalin, a hormone produced by the adrenal glands on the kidneys. This hormone is released in response to frightening and threatening situations. It increases the heart and breathing rates, raises blood pressure and supplies more blood to the muscles to enable the body to respond by 'fight or flight'. The production of cortisol, a chemical also secreted by the adrenal glands which raises heart rate, blood pressure and blood sugar, also increases under stress.

Some physicians argue that recurrent or continuous stress results in continual overproduction of these hormones, resulting in raised blood pressure and other illnesses. Research shows that stressful events often perpetuate or aggravate long-standing or recurrent disorders such as eczema, hay fever and asthma.

The medical debate has turned to the extent to which these responses are harmful. Some physicians point out that some people are severely affected by states of stress, and claim that if these states are prolonged, the result is organic disease, such as

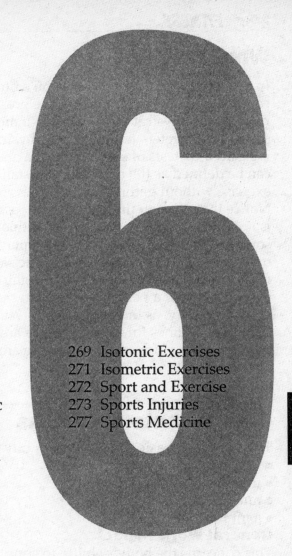

6

red blood cells into the blood, increasing its gas carrying capacity.

Skin

The skin's heat loss by sweat and radiation is determined not only by body mechanisms but also by external conditions. High environmental temperatures limit radiation loss; high humidity limits sweat loss.

The fit and unfit heart

The diagram shows the comparative amounts of work done by a fit heart (**A**) and an unfit heart (**B**) during different activities. The lower the heart rate, the more efficiently the heart is being used; the higher its beat rate, the harder the heart is working. An unfit heart has to work harder all the time, so is constantly under strain and in extreme stress will have to increase its work to a dangerously fast rate. A healthy heart works under a self-imposed maximum rate of about 190 beats per minute.

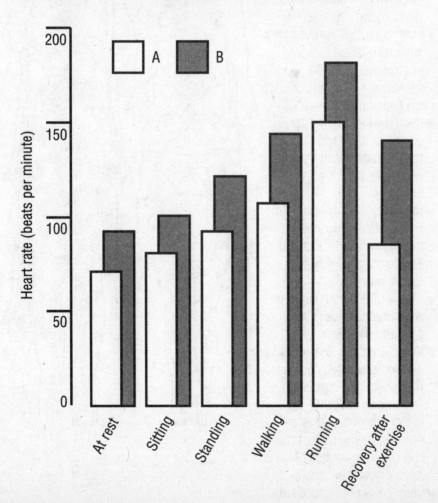

Heart rate (beats per minute)

At rest · Sitting · Standing · Walking · Running · Recovery after exercise

6

ulcers, high blood pressure, asthma, rheumatoid arthritis,
thyrotoxicosis, ulcerative colitis and dermatitis. However,
research into many of these illnesses shows other causes, and
has not proved that external stress is a major cause.
Moreover, the demonstrable physiological effects of stress are
temporary in most people, and have not been proved to result
in disease in large numbers of people.

The theory

In summary, there is no debate about the stressful nature of
many life events, or of the close inter-relationship between
body and mind, or of the fact that people burdened by
overwhelming troubles break down and develop severe
symptoms and disabilities.

On the other hand, there is no doubt that the idea that stress is
a major factor in determining ill-health has been so vigorously
promulgated in the popular medical press that a number of
myths have been disseminated and are widely believed.

At the other extreme of the debate, one body of thought is
probing the idea that stress is essential to well-being,
prompting the individual to confront and resolve problems
brought about by natural life changes.

There is no doubt that just as some people succumb to stress,
others sustain high levels of stress for long periods. The fact
that stress is experienced by everyone, but that individuals
react to it in widely different ways throws doubt on many of
the claims made about its harmful effects.

Stress management

Stress is, nevertheless, a daily reality, and most people find it
unpleasant. Learning and taking action to manage it, to control
its effects on the pattern of your life, is a sensible and positive
step which can only lead to greater self-knowledge. Good
stress management combines support and counseling with
personal reappraisal and some reorganization of one's life:

1. Find a confidant – a relative, a friend, perhaps a counseling
service – with whom to talk over problems and share worries.

2. Try to deal with your problems. Don't try to blot them out
with alcohol, drugs, smoking or overeating.

3. Try to accurately identify the real cause or causes of the
stressful feelings.

4. Seek professional advice for problems involving legal,
financial or medical problems.

5. Approach a counseling service or psychotherapy for any
problems that seem too burdensome to be relieved by talking
them over with a confidant.

6. Try to emphasize organization in your life, so that you have

5

time for the things you have to do and things you want to do.
7. Think about your physical health. Make a point of eating healthily – if minimally, and walk or get some other exercise every day, and resting, even if it is difficult to sleep.
8. Examine your attitudes and priorities. Are they the root cause of whatever is making you unhappy?
9. If your problem is frustrated relationships with friends or people at work, think about enroling on an assertiveness course. These courses help you evaluate and deal with relationships with other people, deal with aggression, and get what you want without upsetting people.
10. Try any stress-reducing strategy which can be learned: progressive relaxation, meditation, Alexander technique, yoga, a martial art, such as aikido or kendo, self-hypnosis, autosuggestion, biofeedback or coping in imagination.

Neuroses

This term describes relatively mild forms of mental illness which, nonetheless, are very distressing to the sufferer and may prevent him from leading a normal life. Neurosis generally represents a tendency to react excessively or abnormally to stress, and the level of anxiety felt appears inappropriate to the triggering factors. It may seem a part of the person's personality. Neurosis may take any of several forms, indicating severe underlying anxiety expressed in a characteristic but inappropriate way. Each type of reaction is described here, but neurosis can manifest itself in unusual behavior.

Anxiety states
The most common form of neurosis. Physical symptoms include trembling, sweating, breathlessness and nausea. Panic attacks are also sometimes associated with a particular situation; they are, therefore, also known as situational anxiety states or phobias. For example, agoraphobia is commonly defined as 'fear of open spaces' and is usually characterized by the onset of symptoms when the sufferer attempts to leave home, use public transport or enter crowded places.

Hysterical or conversion reactions
Sometimes anxiety is 'converted' into physical symptoms. Someone under severe stress may become blind or lose the use of a limb, apparently without any physiological reason. People with this form of neurosis appear relatively unconcerned by their disability, and symptoms disappear as the causes of

anxiety are removed. Other types of hysterical behavior, in which the person shuts himself off from unbearable anxiety, include sleepwalking, amnesia and (rarely) multiple personality.

Obsessional neuroses

It is not neurotic behavior to return quickly after leaving to make sure the door of your house is locked. It is simply reassuring. Obsessive neurosis is an extreme form of this behavior, characterized by continual feelings of unassuageable anxiety. These surface in persistent intrusive thoughts or repetitive patterns of behavior, which disrupt normal life.

Treatment

Treatments vary widely according to national practices and the treatments favored by the professionals consulted. If the behavior is very disturbed, specialist help will be needed. If the causes of anxiety are obvious, treatment will be directed at them. In the U.S. and parts of Europe, psychotherapy is extensively used. Deep-seated anxiety resulting from events in childhood may require lengthy psychoanalysis to help the patient recognize its causes and so come to terms with it. Behavior therapy, in which the patient is encouraged and supported in gradually confronting situations which cause anxiety, can be highly effective in dealing with anxiety states and phobias.

Obsessive compulsive behavior may also respond to re-educative forms of treatment. If relationships within the family are thought to be the principal cause of anxiety, family counseling with a doctor or a social worker may be most appropriate. Worries about health, money, or work may also require practical advice.

5

Psychoses

More severe forms of mental illness than neuroses, psychoses manifest themselves mainly as loss of contact with reality. Psychotic illness is thought to result from a chemical imbalance in the brain, or damage to a part of it. Drug treatment is often effective in controling symptoms; the underlying illness may be long-lasting, perhaps for life.

Schizophrenia

The cause or causes of schizophrenia have long been sought, and some factors have been identified. The tendency to develop it is at least partly inherited; pathological studies have demonstrated damage to the corpus callosum, the part of the brain linking the right and left hemispheres in some people. All people who are genetically at risk do not develop it. Factors like family problems may be triggers.

Faculties such as intelligence and memory are retained, but there are disturbances of emotional responsiveness and perception, resulting in apparent 'splitting' of the normally integrated processes of the mind. Some schizophrenics believe they are being persecuted. Others may hear voices telling them to behave in a certain way, or suggesting false ideas. Schizophrenics may also become withdrawn or, if overstimulated, very excitable.

Drug treatment can now 'damp down' symptoms sufficiently in most patients for psychological and social therapy to be beneficial. However, schizophrenia is usually a long-term problem.

Brain scans

PET scans have revealed abnormalities in the brain's glucose consumption. Scans of schizophrenics showed decreased glucose consumption in some areas. Scans of manic-depressives showed increased consumption during the manic phases.

Manic-depressive psychosis

Everyone experiences fluctuations of mood. One day we wake feeling full of energy and optimism, the next despondent and sluggish. Manic-depressive psychosis is an extreme disorder of mood swings. A phase of mania, with feelings of elation, restlessness and self-confidence in one's abilities – often misplaced and sometimes with disastrous consequences – alternates with deep depression during which suicide may be attempted. Imbalance of the brain chemistry which regulates mood is thought to be the main cause of the disorder, and closely monitored treatment with lithium carbonate is often effective in suppressing symptoms.

Depression

At some time in their lives, most people experience emotional lows of sadness or hopeless pessimism and seem to lose all interest in life. This may be as the result of loss of loved ones, the failure of a relationship, redundancy or job loss and many other causes. Usually after a period of mourning or coming to terms with things they recover; but when the symptoms develop into a state from which it seems impossible to emerge this can become clinical depression, when behaviour and physical health are affected. This occurs at some time in between 10% and 15% of lives. One in nine men seek help for depression at some time (compared with one in six women) but this may reflect a greater reticence to seek help rather than fewer effected. True depressive illness may be triggered by some physical diseases, such as hepatitis or stroke, it may also be due to hormonal changes and disorders. Depression which form part of a manic-depressive cycle may have an hereditary element.

Symptoms
A feeling of anxiety, even fits of crying for no apparent reason, tiredness, loss of appetite, difficulty in sleeping, inability to concentrate, loss of interest and pleasure in social life. Sometimes there may an agitated anxiousness, sometimes it may take the opposite form with thinking and physical activity slowed down. Feeling increasingly withdrawn, the sufferer may retire to bed and be loathe to get up, let alone face the world. Feelings of guilt, low self worth, thoughts of death and of suicide may even lead on to hallucinations of poisoning or persecution.

Treatment
Anti-depressant drugs are often effective in reducing symptoms, which may help the patient deal with their own problems, but the underlying emotional causes may require counseling and psychotherapy.

Aggression
In nature aggressive behaviour serves to deter competition for territory, food or mate, and to challenge dominance in a social hierarchy. In humans other factors often also seem to be involved, such as frustration and revenge, while some see it resulting from parental behaviour, or lack of affection, feelings of inadequacy or even as part of human creativity. The male sex hormones, androgens, appear to stimulate agressiveness, the female estrogen to suppress it, but social conditioning may also have a role in that aggressiveness has often been emphasised as an emblem of masculinity. Changing attitudes to gender stereotyping may help men to control aggression but alcohol and other drugs, dementia and some medical conditions can reduce or remove control of aggression which is also associated with such psychiatric conditions as schizophrenia.

5

FITNESS

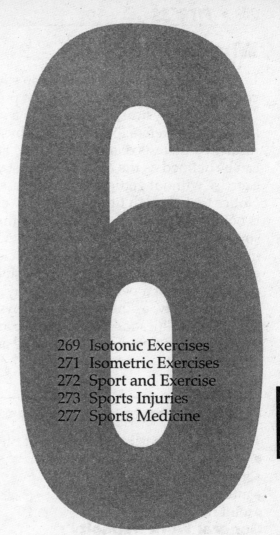

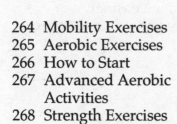

6

What is Fitness?

In the most general sense, a person's fitness is his ability to cope with his environment and the pressure it puts on his mental and physical system. But in a more usual, and useful, sense, fitness refers to the body's physical capabilities, as measured by tests of strength, speed and endurance. Fitness can be defined as the ability to withstand prolonged physical exercise without getting too breathless to continue.

Notice that, though fitness is usually associated with health, it is not the same thing. An Olympic athlete can be ill, and someone free of diagnosable illness may still be extremely unfit. In the absence of planned exercise, work and transport effort (such as walking or climbing stairs) are the main determinants of a person's actual physical capabilities. In modern society, as the element of physical activity in work and transport declines for most of us, we are increasingly dependent on planned exercise if we are to hold on to fitness and its benefits.

Components of Fitness

There are four basic components of physical fitness:
• general work capacity;
• muscular strength;
• muscular endurance; and
• joint flexibility.

General Work Capacity

This concerns the body's ability to supply itself with the oxygen and energy it needs to keep going during general physical activity. It depends on the efficiency of the cardio-vascular and respiratory systems. The limit of physical endurance is marked by labored breathing and a pounding heart, rather than by failure of a particular muscle group to respond any more.

Muscular Strength

This concerns the maximum force a particular muscle group can apply in one action. There are two types.
• Isometric strength is force applied against a fixed resistance.
• Isotonic strength is force applied through the full range of movement available to a certain muscle or muscle group (as set by the joint or joints acted upon).

An example involving both types of strength is arm-wrestling. The beginning, when the participants' arms first lock motionless against each other, involves isometric strength. The latter part, in which one participant's arm forces the other's down to the table, involves isotonic strength. The two types are at least partly independent of each other.

Muscular Endurance

This concerns the ability of particular muscle groups to go on functioning over a period of time. Again, there is both isometric and isotonic endurance. Isometric endurance involves the ability to maintain force as long as possible against a fixed resistance or in a fixed position (as when the opening lock of arm wrestling continues over a period of time). Isotonic endurance involves the ability to repeat a muscular movement against resistance as many times as possible (as with push-ups or repetitive weight-lifting). In both cases, the limit is marked by inability of the muscle group to respond anymore.

Flexibility

This concerns the range through which a joint will move. Except in the case of certain bone disorders, it depends more on the nearby muscles than on the structure of the joint itself.

Inter-relation

- Localization. Levels of muscular strength, muscular endurance, and joint flexibility are all localized, i.e. development of one part of the body does not necessarily imply the development of any other part.
- Inter-dependence. Muscular strength and endurance in any one muscle or muscle group are inter-related. For example (taking isotonic strength), a muscle capable of a maximum 200lb (90kg) force through its whole range of movement will be able to go on moving 50lb (22kg) through that range longer than one with an 80lb (36kg) maximum. Otherwise the components of fitness are fairly independent of each other.

Motor Abilities

An individual's physical capabilities are limited not only by his fitness, but also by his motor abilities: co-ordination, balance, agility, reaction time, speed, movement time (i.e. speed of moving a part of the body) and power (i.e. ability for explosive movement).

Human Efficiency

The efficiency of any system is measured by how much energy output (work) it gives, for a set amount of energy input (fuel). Its efficiency will vary, depending on how near to its limits it is working. The nearer it is to maximum energy output, the more units input are needed for each unit gain in output. But all systems are more or less inefficient over all their output range (i.e. all give less than 100% return). The average human body is between 16 and 27% efficient – which compares badly with several products of the human mind. But by regular exercise the body's efficiency can be raised to 56%, which is better than many machines.

Human efficiency

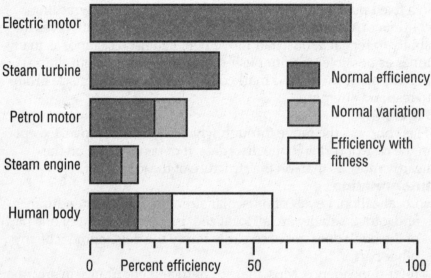

Factors Affecting Fitness

Potential Fitness
Even if everyone were as fit as possible, their physical abilities in terms of strength, speed and endurance would not be equal. Three main factors limit someone's potential fitness:

- age: different aspects of fitness reach peak potential at different times – speed is at its best at the beginning of adulthood, strength in the late 20s, and endurance in later life. The body's efficiency gradually declines with age, so the indices of fitness alter with age.
- sex: men have a greater potential for strength and speed than women; women are better able to withstand extremes of temperature, and have a longer life expectancy than men, so the indices of individual fitness differ between the two sexes.
- health: fitness and ill-health seem mutually exclusive, yet it is possible to be ill and unaware of it, so apparently fit. A man who is fit is not obviously ill, and his physical and mental

functions correspond to the averages within the individual's
age group.
- nutrition: a healthy diet is essential in order to attain and
  maintain fitness.
- weight: a man whose weight far exceeds the desirable weight
  for his height and body type is always functioning under the
  burden of an extra load. A man who is far below optimum
  weight lacks the capacity to function at maximum efficiency.
- regular physical activity: fitness can only be maintained by
  making regular demands on the body to perform physical
  exercise. With lack of activity, the body atrophies – muscular
  weakness follows confinement to bed.
- sleep: the body and mind need adequate rest in order to
  function at optimum efficiency.

Muscle strength: men and women compared

Skeletal muscle can generate around 3 to 8 kilograms (6½ to 17½ lbs) of
force per cm^2 (in^2) of muscle cross-section.

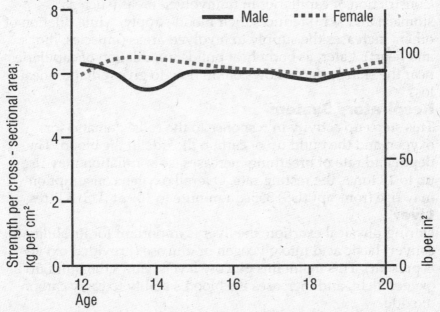

Men are usually 30-50% stronger than women when total muscle force is
compared on the basis of absolute force exerted. But the difference is
considerably reduced when strength is evaluated in relation to muscle
cross-sectional area. In an experiment comparing the strength of the arm
flexor muscle of men and women in relation to the cross-sectional area,
little difference was indicated. *(Ikai, M., and Fukunaga, T.: Calculation of
muscle strength per unit cross-sectional area of human muscle by means
of ultrasonic measurements. Arbeitsphysiologie, 26: 26, 1968.)*

Body during Activity

Any muscular effort requires some energy, and puts some demand on the rest of the body to supply that energy. When a large proportion of the body's muscles are involved over a period of time, the effects of this become noticeable.

Cardio-vascular System

The blood network supplies the cells of the body with the oxygen and other nutrients (glucose, fat, etc.) that they need for activity, and takes away the resulting waste products (carbon dioxide, lactic acid, etc). The heart is the pump that drives blood around the system. During exertion, more nutrient and product transportation is needed. This is mainly supplied by increased heart activity. The total rate of blood flow may rise by up to 600% due to increase both in the rate of heart beat and in the amount pumped at each stroke. Systolic blood pressure may rise up to 70%. At the same time, levels of nutrients build up in the blood, as physical need increases, and levels of waste products as usage exceeds disposal.
Constriction of capillaries in uninvolved areas (such as stomach and skin) reduces their blood supply, while dilation of others increases the supply to involved areas (muscles, lungs and heart). Later, as body heat builds up, dilation of capillaries near the skin surface allows blood flow to give radiation heat loss.

Respiratory System

This steps up activity in response to the cells' demand for oxygen and the build up of carbon dioxide in the blood. The depth and rate of breathing increases, so ventilation may rise up to 12 times the resting rate. Overall oxygen consumption may rise from ¾pt (US) 355cc a minute to 10½pt (US) 5 litres

Liver

During physical exertion, the liver is important for its ability to convert lactic acid into glycogen or glucose (provided oxygen is present). This maintains glucose levels, slows the build up of oxygen debt, and increases the blood's ability to carry carbon dioxide.

Endocrine system

The main short-term hormonal response to physical exertion is the release of adrenalin by the adrenal glands, stimulating the body to the 'fight or flight' response. Other hormonal activity controls, for example, body water, and aids increased energy mobilization.
It is possible that during exertion the spleen releases reserve

red blood cells into the blood, increasing its gas carrying capacity.

Skin

The skin's heat loss by sweat and radiation is determined not only by body mechanisms but also by external conditions. High environmental temperatures limit radiation loss; high humidity limits sweat loss.

The fit and unfit heart

The diagram shows the comparative amounts of work done by a fit heart (**A**) and an unfit heart (**B**) during different activities. The lower the heart rate, the more efficiently the heart is being used; the higher its beat rate, the harder the heart is working. An unfit heart has to work harder all the time, so is constantly under strain and in extreme stress will have to increase its work to a dangerously fast rate. A healthy heart works under a self-imposed maximum rate of about 190 beats per minute.

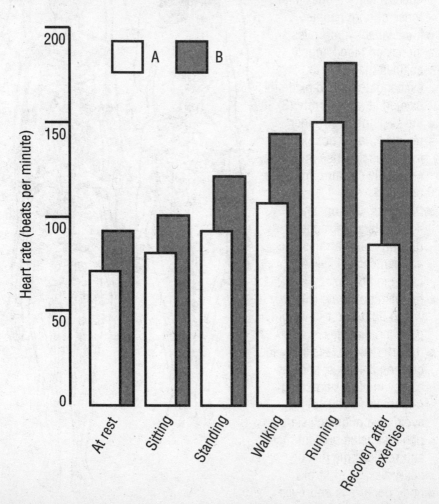

The Benefits of Fitness

Physically fit individuals differ from those who are unfit in many ways:

- they have a better tolerance of physical and mental stress, and cope better with illness and injury
- the coordination and responses of the nervous system improve (**1**)
- the heart (**2**) pumps more oxygen-carrying blood to the muscles, making them able to perform more effectively for longer than those of unfit people
- lung capacity improves and increased blood supply enables the lungs to exchange carbon dioxide for oxygen at a faster rate (**3**)
- the skeleton is stronger - people who do not exercise their muscles lose minerals, especially calcium, from the bones (**4**)
- the joints, tendon, and ligaments are stronger, making minor strains and accidents less likely to cause injury (**5**)
- the metabolic rate is higher, which fights excess weight gain and diabetes
- the arteries are less likely to develop diseases, such as narrowing and hardening (atherosclerosis) (**6**) avoidance of a cholesterol-rich diet helps prevent them and reduces the risk of heart disease or stroke.
- body posture is improved

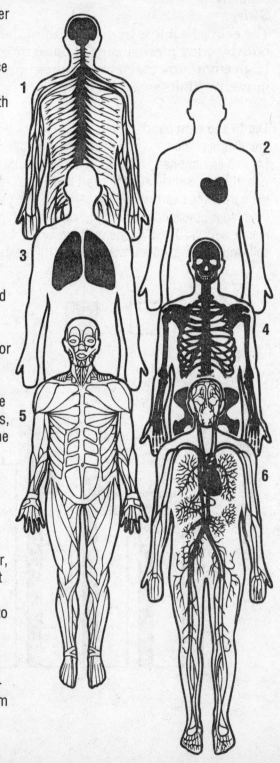

Tolerance of Exercise

In a mechanical system, use produces wear and deterioration. In the human body, the changes during strenuous activity are drastic. Despite the beneficial effects of exercise, some harmful effects can occur from ill-judged exercise:

Sudden, fast or violent exertion after a period of inactivity can cause injury to the muscles, tendons, ligaments and joints. In people with high blood pressure or heart disease it can cause overload and death. This is true of people of any age – severely inappropriate exercise can damage even a healthy heart.

Exercise increases the pressure of blood through the aorta, the main artery leading from the heart. If the blood flow through the heart is blocked by narrowed arteries or a blood clot, a heart attack may occur.

Anyone who has or may have high blood pressure, angina pectoris, or any other form of heart disease should see a physician before beginning any exercise or training, and should follow a carefully planned exercise program that is specially formulated for people with your condition. A well-structured exercise program that permits gradual, monitored build-up of activity can improve these conditions. It will also prevent undue strain on the joints, muscles, ligaments and tendons.

6

Warming up

Muscles, tendons, ligaments, and joints are susceptible to injuries and accidents if exercise is begun without warming-up exercises. They stimulate the blood flow to the muscles and

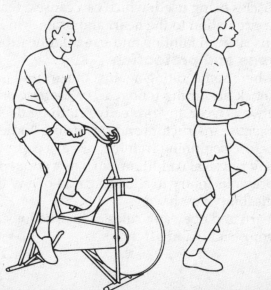

Warming up involves exercising the large muscles groups by stretching, jogging gently in place, skipping rope, or cycling on a stationary bicycle for a few minutes. The warm-up activity should be carried out slowly but rhythmically and continuously.

cause the body temperature to rise, which increases the release of energy by the body. Warming up improves the function of muscles, tendons and ligaments. People with high blood pressure and heart disease should never exercise without first warming up, and should be especially careful to warm up thoroughly if exercising in cold weather. Sudden activity in a few muscles when the rest of the body is cold can send the blood pressure soaring.

Pacing yourself

A physician or your exercise supervisor can assess your upper exercise limits by monitoring you as you work a treadmill, ride a stationary bicycle, or step on and off a low bench. However, the body signals its own tolerance. If you feel exhausted, if your heart pounds intolerably, if you feel pain, especially in the chest or in a joint, if you feel you cannot breathe fast or deeply enough to continue – STOP. Exercise is only beneficial if it enables you to adapt gradually to greater physical stress. Notice pain and strain, and ease off. Sudden unaccustomed movements can wrench muscles and joints. You should get accustomed to new movements gradually, so your body can learn what positions and efforts it can safely allow. When exercising, work up gradually from gentle movements to forceful.

Cooling down

At the end of an exercise session, slow down over 5 to 10 minutes, never stop dead. Slowing allows the metabolism and blood circulation to drop to low-activity levels. Stopping suddenly can cause blood to pool in the veins leading from the muscles being used, which can cause a temporary lowering of the circulation to the heart and brain. This can cause dizziness, nausea, even fainting and irregular heartbeat.

Dress and protection

- where some jolting against the ground is inevitable, use shock-absorbing footwear, or exercise on a suitable surface
- always wear any protective clothing deemed necessary by exercise instructors and governing bodies of sport
- before beginning training, always warn your instructor of any physical condition, such as a slipped vertebral disk or a previous injury to a tendon, and of any illness, disease or disability you have
- learn and obey any rules or instructions designed to protect your health and safety.

The Overload Principle

Regular exercise gives an individual a sense of well-being and relaxation. Many people find physical activity enjoyable, and keep practicing sports and games they enjoy right into old age. This keeps them fitter and healthier longer than someone who leads a sedentary life, or who stops exercising at some stage. People who did stop exercising and want to start again should bear in mind that their body is weak and unadapted for physical activity. The capacity of the heart and lungs is insufficient to supply the muscles with sufficient energy for very powerful or prolonged use.

The capacity for exercise must be built up over a long period of regular exercise that makes gradually increasing demands on the body. This concept of achieving fitness through progressively more demanding exercise is called the 'overload principle'. It must be followed by anyone beginning a new exercise regime, from teenager to octogenarian, and competing athlete to convalescent heart patient.

Anyone starting exercising after a period of inactivity must follow an individualized training program that combines activities to exercise different muscle groups, and exercises of different frequencies, intensity, and duration.

6

Exercise and age

Exercise is essential for the middle aged and elderly – so much so that the United States Public Health Service includes as one of its most important 'Healthy People 2000' objectives getting more people involved in slow to moderate levels of physical activity, with emphasis on the development of muscular strength and flexibility. Research shows that physical training renewed at any age reverses the decline in exercise capacity brought about by a sedentary lifestyle. It also:

● prevents a decrease in muscle strength. In one experiment, strength conditioning improved muscle strength, tone, and function of healthy men aged 60 to 72 within a 12-week period;
● improves joint flexibility. Exercises designed to move joints through their full range of movement can improve flexibility by 20 to 50% in people of every age;
● through life, slows the loss of neurons from the brain and spinal cord;
● can slow the reduction in lung function that tends to be a sign of aging;
● arrests the reduction in the heartbeat and the hardening of the arteries, and increases the blood flow to the tissues.

Nine men aged 87 to 96 years underwent 8 weeks of high intensity resistance training to improve the action of the quadriceps and hamstring muscles while seated. The training took place 3 days per week and consisted of 3 sets of 8 repetitions (6 to 9 seconds per repetition), with a 2-minute rest between sets. Improvement averaged 174%. This experiment showed that disuse, lack of exercise and inadequate nutrition account for declining muscular strength in elderly people. (*From Fiatarone, M.A., et al.: High-intensity strength training in nonagenarians. J.A.M.A. 263:3029, 1990.*)

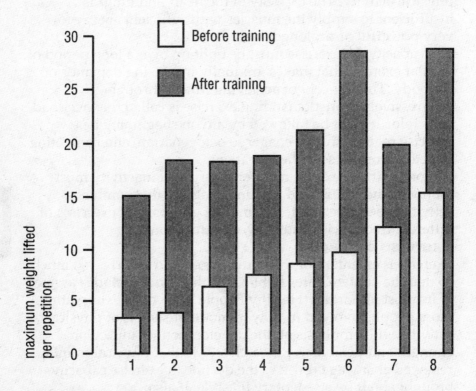

Note: emphasis on the 'sudden death syndrome' of older people taking up exercise after a long period of sedentary living is now known to have been exaggerated. Research has shown that sudden death rates have declined over the past 20 years, while there has been an increase in the numbers of people exercising. In one study of nearly 3000 exercisers there were only two (nonfatal) cardiovascular medical complications, and only three per 100,000 hours of exercise for men. However, older people who are unused to exercise should, where possible, exercise under the supervision of a qualified instructor. They must always begin slowly and progress gradually, and always warm up before sessions and cool down afterwards.

Inactive Man

It is chiefly disuse that causes deterioration. Once growth has ceased, there is no physical improvement without increased physical demand. This is true not only of muscular strength and cardio-vascular and respiratory response, but also of motor abilities such as co-ordination and reaction time. Inactivity fails to develop latent capacity and results in a general deterioration of body systems through disuse.

The effects on the muscular system are the most obvious. There are 639 muscles in the body, accounting on average for 45% of body weight. Loss of muscle tone results, for example, in:

● general physical weakness and tiredness;

● a weak and sagging abdomen;

● back pain due to weak back muscles; and

● a weak and lethargic heart.

Degeneration of the abdomen and heart have, in particular, general effects throughout the system. Abdominal weakness favors digestive trouble, while sluggish blood flow encourages blockage of arteries and capillaries.

In general terms, the effects of inactivity show themselves in reduced vitality, lowered resistance to infection, and perhaps in such mental conditions as lack of enthusiasm, inability to concentrate, nervousness, irritability and insomnia. Physical inactivity also increases food intake, often producing excess weight with all its harmful consequences.

When inactive man does have to undergo physical stress, his heart cannot greatly increase its stroke volume. A pounding heart results, as it tries to keep up with demand just by beatmg faster.

6

Tests of Fitness

Fitness for all types of training can be tested, e.g. isotonic strength by the weight of barbell that can be lifted, isometric strength using strain gauges and dynamometers. But only cardiovascular testing gives a good guide to general fitness. Muscular endurance tests may also be interesting for following progress.

Aerobic training

The step test given here is safe for most age groups. It measures heart rate response after aerobic activity and, thus, the body's capability for aerobic metabolism. It involves stepping up and down at a given rate between the ground and a single step, bench or stool. Afterwards the pulse rate is taken. General rules for any step test are:

- face the same way all the time and always step back to the ground on the same side;
- 'one step' is one complete ascent and descent;
- keep the correct step rate;
- take the pulse at wrist or throat (but if at the throat do not press too hard as this can alter the rate);
- do stop before the time limit if the test is too hard (count this as putting you in the lowest fitness category); and
- to compare performances over time try to repeat under similar conditions (e.g. time of day, and time and size of last meal); recent physical activity, health and sleep; and step rate). Do not be discouraged by apparent lack of progress: temporary factors may be involved.

Muscular Endurance

Isometric endurance tests judge the duration for which a certain contraction can be held (e.g. how long a known weight can be held at arm's length). More relevant for general fitness are isotonic endurance tests which judge the number of times a given movement can be repeated. Typical tests (with average performances of male college students in brackets) include pull-ups (8 completed) push-ups (25) sit-ups (40) and bar dips (9).

Step Test

For ages 10 to 69 (unless in poor health). Use 8in bench. Step at rate of 24 steps a minute for 3 minutes. Wait for exactly 1 minute after exercise. Then count heartbeats for 15 seconds. Multiply that count by 4.

Heartbeat counts for men of all ages

Excellent	under 68
Good	68-79
Above average	80-89
Below average	90-99
Very poor	100 plus

Adapted from Montoye, Willis and Cunningham
Journal of Gerontology, 1968.

Heart-rate and Exercise

The step test gives you a guide to your general physical condition. You can use this to judge how high you should allow your heart-rate to go during exercise.

Someone in the lowest ('very poor') category on the test (100 beats a minute or more) should begin exercising very gradually.

- At the start of the first month he should exercise for 5 minutes a day at not more than 100 beats per minute. During that month he can gradually increase the time up to 10 minutes, but must keep the same heart-rate limit.
- During the second month the time allowed again increases from 5 to 10 minutes, but the heart-rate limit is now 110 beats.
- During the third month the same happens, but the limit is now 120.
- Thereafter the person may allow his heart-rate to rise to the desirable limit for his age.

Someone in the 'below average' step test category should follow the same routine, but can begin at 'b' and go on to 'c' in the second month. Someone in the 'above average' category can begin at 'c'.

Age limit

As the resting heart-rate declines with age, the maximum possible and desirable rates also fall.

The estimated maximum possible heart-rate for a healthy fit young adult is about 220 beats per minute. For a rough estimate of the maximum rate for anyone aged 30 years or older, the age should be subtracted from this figure. For example, the maximum heart rate of a man aged 40 is 220 – 40=180 beats a minute. To find the maximum heart rate that should be allowed in a fit person during exercise, the figure of 20 should be subtracted. For example, the maximum desirable rate for a fit man aged 40 is 180 – 20=160 beats a minute.

Using heart-rate guides

- Count the number of pulse beats in 15 seconds and multiply by 4. Unlike the step test, count while still exercising if possible (e.g. if walking).
- With a little practice, it is easy to make a rough judgement of the speed of one's heartbeat at any moment, and when it is getting a bit too high. This then becomes the most practical method.

6

The table gives some idea of levels of heartbeat in different common activities for fit young adults.

Intensity	Heart rate	Walk/run (mph/kmph)	Cycling (mph/kmph)	Climbing (Grades)	Sports	Occupation
Maximum	200	13.0/20	20/32	12	running	digging
Very heavy	150	6.0/9.6	14/22	6	mountain-eering	chopping wood
Heavy	140	5.5/8.8	12/19	5	tennis	pick and shovel
Fairly heavy	130	5.0/8	10/16	4	volleyball	gardening
Moderate	120	4.5/7	9/14	3	golf	house painting
Light	110	4.0/6.4	8/12.8	2	table tennis	auto repair
Very light	100	3.5/5.6	7/11.2	level	bowling	shopping

Need for exercise

Work and travel are increasingly sedentary – and leisure equally usually a matter of sitting. (It has been estimated that on average 75 hours are spent by people in spectating – films, tv, sport, etc – for every 1 spent in physical participation.) So we have to plan and work to achieve enough activity to keep us physically fit. But a high level of physical fitness can often be reached in just a couple of months' daily physical training – and maintained after that by exercising vigorously 3 days a week. In theory, adequate fitness might perhaps be maintained every day by: walking briskly a mile or two to and from work; standing doing something for a couple of hours; using vigorous toweling movements after washing; stretching occasionally, and hurrying up a hill or stairs carrying a fairly heavy load. But in practice few have the time or taste or consistent discipline to organize even this; and most of us are well below desirable levels of fitness. So formal exercise, over and above the normal daily demands, becomes essential for the achievement of an efficient, strong and durable body. There are very many different approaches to physical fitness. The remaining pages of this chapter are concerned not with setting you a particular routine of exercise, but with telling you what kinds of exercise are available, what each can and cannot do, and how you should approach the general problem of keeping fit.

Types of Exercise

There are many different ways of exercising, ranging from intense bursts of activity to motionless exercise. On the following pages one or two examples of exercises from each different category are illustrated and explained. A full training program will, however, include many different exercises.

Anaerobic exercise

There are two main types of exercise: aerobic and anaerobic. Anaerobic exercise is 'all-out', maximum performance exercise, which can last for a short time only. It is fueled by energy made available by the anaerobic (literally 'without oxygen') breakdown of high-energy phosphates called ATP and CP, which are stored in the body's cells, and from lactic acid, the by-product of the breakdown of glucose by the muscles. Fast-action sports like sprinting, high jump, cycle-racing and long jump use anaerobic energy. The training involves strenuous physical activity.

It is thought that genetically, some people are highly adapted to anaerobic activity. However, a person who is unfit would be better to begin exercising with mobility and aerobic exercises.

Aerobic exercise

This is long-term exercise. If vigorous exercise is sustained for more than 2-3 minutes, the cells of the body start to utilize oxygen to produce enough ATP and CP for energy needs. This is aerobic (literally 'with oxygen') exercise. During the first 2 to 3 minutes, the amount of oxygen utilized by the cells is high; between the third and fourth minute a plateau, or 'steady state' is reached, from which point the use of oxygen remains fairly constant throughout the exercise period. With regular exercise, this steady state is reached more quickly than at the beginning of an exercise program. The advantage of aerobic exercise is that it causes relatively little lactic acid to be produced by the muscles, which means that the person exercising does not tire so quickly.

Aerobic exercise includes using cycling, rowing and other exercise machines, brisk walking, jogging, running, cycling, swimming, jumping rope and running in place.

6

Mobility exercices

If you have not exercised regularly for some time, begin with mobility exercises, which strengthen the muscles and improve the efficiency and range of movement of the joints. Start very gently, with one or two repetitions each day, and work up slowly to a maximum 30 repetitions. Go on to other mobility activities – swimming, golf, racket sports, and track and field events.

Arms and shoulders

Stand with your arms loosely at your sides; bend forward, then backward (**1**). Raise your arms and cross them in front of your face, then behind your sides; lower your arms and cross them first in front of your body, then behind your back (**2**). Stand with your feet together about 18in (0.46m) from a wall, lean forward with your arms outstretched until your hands rest against the wall; bend your arms until your chest touches the wall, then straighten your arms (**3**).

1

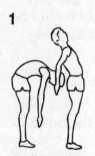

2

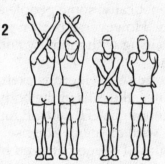

3

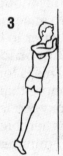

Waist and trunk

Stand with your arms loosely crossed, then twist your trunk as far as possible to one side, then the other, keeping your feet flat on the floor (**4**). Stand with your legs apart and your arms loosely at your sides, then keeping your trunk facing forward, bend as far as your can to one side, then the other (**5**). Lie on your front, raise your head and your feet, then try to grasp an ankle in each hand and to raise your knees and thighs off the ground (**6**).

4

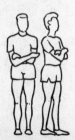

5

6

Legs and hips

Support yourself with your left hand against a wall or a table, stand on your left leg, lift your right leg as high as you can to the side, and lower it to the floor (**7**); then swing it forward as far as possible, then back as far as possible (**8**). Turn to support yourself with your right hand and repeat the exercise with your left leg. Stand with your feet together, keep them flat on the ground, and bend your knees while twisting them to the left. Straighten, then repeat the exercise, twisting to the right (**9**). Keeping your feet together jump as high as you can to one side, then to the other (**10**).

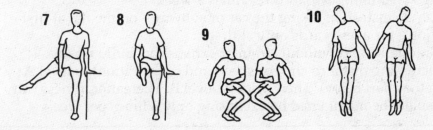

Aerobic exercises

Aerobic exercises improve endurance and promote fitness. They are especially important in improving the performance of the heart and blood circulation, and increasing lung capacity and efficiency. To bring about these improvements, however, it is necessary to impose heavy demands on the body by
● the duration of the exercise.
● its intensity as shown by the heart-rate response.
The demand needed for improvement depends on age and level of fitness, but in a fit young adult, for example, exertion at 140 to 150 beats a minute would be needed for 8 to 10 minutes several times a week. After a time, however, a rate as low as 120 beats gives improvement.
Intensity depends on
● the proportion of muscle involved (for example, jogging is more intense than sit-ups).
● the pace of exercise (for example, running is more intense than jogging).
Very low intensity exercise, such as slow walking, may not give improvement, whatever the duration. If the permissible heart rate is limited by a formerly sedentary lifestyle, it is important to improve fitness before increasing pace, then plan a program that exercises but does not overtax the system.
Step aerobics is a form of low-impact exercise providing a good cardiovascular workout. It is suitable for most men and involves stepping on and off of a low step for periods of up to an hour.

6

How to Start

If you are very unfit, ease your body gradually into aerobic exercise. Never go above your maximum recommended pulse rate, and have a thorough physical examination before beginning. Begin by joining an aerobic exercise or aerobic dance class, where your fitness and progress will be properly measured and monitored, or try some simple aerobic activities:
- walk instead driving to the station, the supermarket, etc.
- go swimming two or three times a week
- cycle instead of taking the car or subway – on the flat at first
- jog – for a few yards only at first

Gradually, and without strain or exhaustion, build up (by increasing distance and/or speed and/or duration) to level A in the chart below. Then work to level B. Thereafter, fitness can usually be maintained by exercising only 3 times per week.

	Distance	Rate	Time per day	Days per week
STATIONARY RUNNING				
A		70 to 80 steps per min.	1 minute	5
B		80 to 90 steps per min.	20 mins.	3 or 4
RUNNING				
A:	**1:** 1 mile/1.6km	1 mile in 13 minutes (walk)	13 mins.	3 to 5
	2: 1 mile/1.6km	1 mile in 11 minutes	11 mins.	5
	(walk and run alternately)			
	3: 1 mile/1.6km	1 mile in 9½ minutes	9½ mins.	5
B:	2 miles/3.2km	1 mile in 8½ minutes	17 mins.	3
COMBINATION				
A	*Walking*			
	1: ½ mile/.8km	120 steps per minute	5	
	2: 1 mile/1.6km	120 steps per minute	5	
B	*Alternate jogging and running*			
	1: 1 mile/1.6km	120 steps per minute	5	
	2: 3 miles/4.8km	120 steps per minute	5	
SWIMMING				
A	**1:** 25 yds, 4 times*	25 yds in 35 seconds	2½ mins.	3 to 5
	2: 100 yds (91m)	100 yds in 2½ mins	2½ mins.	5
	3: 100 yd increases	100 yds in 2½ mins	5 mins., 7½ mins.etc	
B	1000 yds (910m)	100 yds in 2 mins.	20 mins	3 or 4

* 4 separate occasions, with rests between

Advanced Aerobic Activities

When you have built up fitness through walking, jogging or cycling, the following activities will provide more strenuous aerobic exercise:
- racket sports entail a great deal of running;
- ball games such as football, soccer, hockey, basketball and volleyball involve running and jumping;
- competitive sports such as canoeing, rowing, skiing, swimming, hurdling, skating and cycling provide aerobic exercise at competition speed, but are not recommended for anyone unfit, or with heart or circulatory problems. Performed non-competitively they give less aerobic benefit;
- hill-walking, orienteering and cross-country skiing give good aerobic activity if you keep up a brisk walking pace and cover several miles or more.

Distance	Rate	Time per day	Days per week
CYCLING			
A 1 mile	12 mph	5 mins.	5
B 8 miles	20 mph	25 mins.	3 or 4
BENCH STEPPING			
A 8in (20cm)bench	30 steps per minute	3 mins.	3 to 5
B 15-18in (37-45cm) bench		30 steps per minute	
5 mins.	3 to 4		

'One step' is one complete ascent and descent, involving four leg movement counts: first foot up, second foot up, first foot down, second foot down. At the rate specified above, this gives 120 counts per minute i.e. 2 per second.

TENNIS			
Also squash, badminton, basketball,		**A** 10 mins.	3 to 5
handball (singles)		**B** 60 mins.	3
		or 45 mins.	4
ROPE SKIPPING			
A **1:** ½ minute skip, 1 min rest, ½ minute skip		2	3 to 5
2: ½ minute skip, 1 min rest, ½ minute skip, 1 min rest, ½ min skip.		3	5
etc. building to gradually to:			
3: 2 minute skip, ½ minute rest, 2 min skip,		2	5
4: 2 minute skip, ½ minute rest, 2 min skip, ½ minute rest, 2 minute skip		3	5
5: 4-5 minute skip		1	3 to 4
B 6 minute skip		1	3 or 4

6

Strength Exercises

These exercises, some involving the use of weights, give the muscles shape and tone, and build up their size and power. They are extremely beneficial because strong muscles help the body cope with activities that require more strenuous physical effort than usual. They are therefore essential to success in many sports. They have been shown to improve the strength of individual muscles or groups of muscles even in people aged over 90. Begin gently and with one or two repetitions each day, and build up gradually to a maximum of 20 repetitions.

Arms and shoulders

Throw and catch a large heavy ball, such as a medicine ball, until your arms are tired (**1**). Holding Indian clubs or heavy books, raise your arms above your head, then keeping them straight, lower your arms, stretching them out to the sides and then down (**2**).

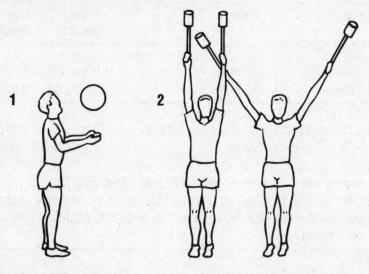

Abdomen

Lie face down with your hands under your chin and lift one leg as high as possible, then the other (**3**). Sit on the floor, raise your legs and try to clasp your ankles with both hands (**4**).

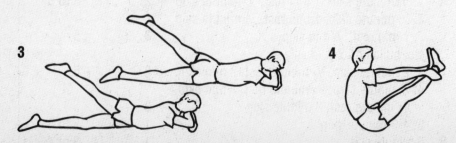

Legs

Run up and down stairs quickly, as often as your can until you begin to feel out of breath (**5**). Sit on the bottom step of a staircase with your feet on the floor. Raise your legs until they are horizontal, extending your arms until they are parallel, and balance in this position (**6**). Lie face down with your arms at your sides and your legs straight, then lift both legs as high as you can off the floor (**7**).

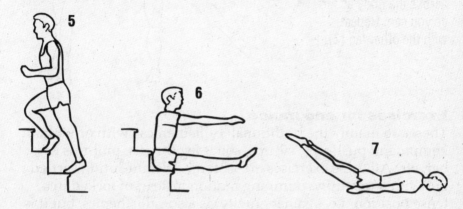

Isotonic Exercises

These consist almost entirely of weight-lifting. This gives the progressive resistance necessary to test, and increase, the maximum strength of a single joint movement. They use all potential muscle strength, whereas other forms of exercise use 20-30%. Isotonic exercises are important because they help build muscular strength and endurance. Develop isotonic exercises gradually, under expert guidance, starting with a low weight.

Exercises for strength

Arms and shoulders

Crouch with a dumbbell in each hand, knuckles uppermost, keeping your back straight. stand up, bending your arms and lifting the dumbbells to shoulder height, then thrust the dumbbells to arm's length above the head (1).

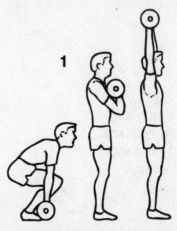

Thighs and calves

Using foot weights, stand with your hands on your hips, stretch your right leg to the side as far as you can, then swing the leg across the body as far as you can. Repeat with the other leg (**2**).

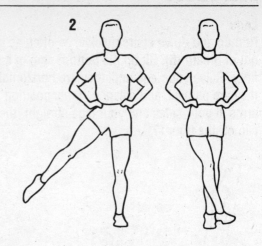

Exercises for endurance

These are mainly the traditional 'callisthenics', with or without equipment: push-ups, sit-ups, squat leg thrusts, pull-ups to a bar, etc. All these exercises are isotonic. Weight-lifting carried out with a repetitive pumping motion instead of locked in a tense position (i.e. against gravity) is also callisthenics, but it is usually used to increase muscle size instead of strength.

Arms and shoulders

Balance on your toes and your hands, then, keeping your back straight, bend your elbows to lower your body to the floor; then straighten your arms (**3**).

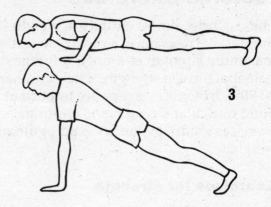

Abdomen

Lie on your back with your knees bent, your feet flat on the floor and your hands behind your head. Sit up without using your hands to help you (**4**).

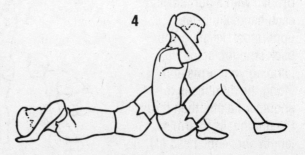

Isometric Exercises

These are exercises without motion, which use the force of one body muscle or muscle group against another or against a fixed point such as a wall or a bar. Towels, ropes, and door frames provide simple accessories, but health studios are equipped with complex machines that provide variable resistance according to strength. It has been shown that a single muscle can be strengthened by an isometric exercise lasting as little as 6 sec a day. Hold these exercises for a maximum of 6 sec, and repeat them only once a day.

Legs
Sit with your legs apart and your hands on your knees, and try to push your knees together while resisting the pressure with your legs; repeat the exercise with your hands crossed (**1,2**). Sit well back on a chair with your legs raised and your hands on your shins, press down with your hands and upward with your legs (**3**).

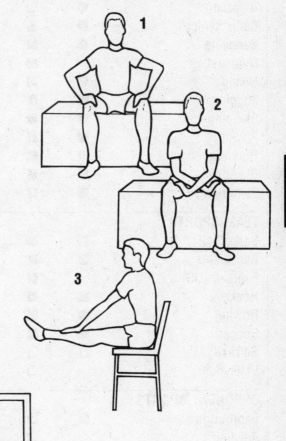

Arms
Push with your hands against the inside of a door frame as hard as you can (**4**).

6

Sport and Exercise

Here we show the effect of different sports on fitness; eg, running has a high effect on heart and lung capacity, but little on strength.

	CR Capacity	Muscular endurance	Strength	Power	Agility
❑ some effect ■ considerable effect					
SOLO ACTIVITIES					
Archery		■	❑		
Bicycling	■	❑	❑		
Callisthenics	■	■	❑		
Canoeing	■	■	❑		
Gymnastics		■	■		■
Hiking	■	■			
Jogging	■	■			
Skipping	■	■			
Rowing	■	■	❑		
Running	■	■			
Skiing	■	■	❑		■
Swimming	■	■	❑	■	■
TEAM SPORTS					
Basketball	■	■		■	
Baseball	❑	■		■	
Football (US)	❑	■	❑	■	■
Hockey	■	■	❑		■
Rowing	■	■	❑		
Soccer	■	■	❑		■
Softball	❑	❑			■
Volleyball		❑		■	■
OPPONENT SPORTS					
Badminton	■	❑			■
Bowling		❑			
Canoeing	■	■	■		
Golf	❑			■	
Handball	■	❑		■	■
Tennis	■	❑		■	■
Skating	■	■	❑		■
Skiing	■	■	❑		■
Swimming	■	■	■		

Sports Injuries

The term 'sports injuries' refers to injuries which occur during sport and may even be named after specific sports – such as 'golfer's elbow' and 'jumpers knee' – but in fact, such injuries can result from other, often quite common, activities. These injuries may be caused by accident or overuse and include broken bones, stress fractures, dislocations, joint and ligament injuries; muscle strains, tears, and inflammations (including injury to muscle tendons) as well as muscle cramps and muscle soreness after training; inflammation of bursae (fluid-filled sacs which normally prevent friciton between bones, muscles and ligaments); open wounds such as cuts and blisters; friction burns; having a 'stitch'.

Injuries are to be expected in combat and contact sports which are relatively violent but all sports carry risk of injury. Players, and coaches especially, should be trained in the recognition of injury and its first-aid treatment. No one should indulge in physical sports or exercise without an appropriate warm-up and sudden pain should always be taken as a sign to stop and find out what it is. Many strains, sprains, tears and pulled muscles could have been prevented by keeping fit and always warming-up before exertion. Repeated overuse of particular muscles can lead to repetitive strain injuries, such as 'tennis elbow' or inflammation of the Achilles tendon.

- Always wear protective clothing as appropriate: shields and pads, gloves, helmets and goggles — and bouyancy aids and wetsuits for water sports. Men should always wear a 'box' to protect the genitals in vigorous and contact sports.
- Wear comfortable clothing. Ill-fitting shoes are a common cause of bursitis and some trainers with a high back can cause Achilles tendinitis.
- Always warm-up before a game or exercise session.
- When taking up or resuming a sport, work on your general fitness first. Take the early sessions easy, building up gradually to more strenuous and demanding activity over a number of sessions.

These are the most common injuries in different types of sport:

Gym sports

Remember, going for 'burn' can mean going for injury.
In weightlifting/weight training, bad technique can lead to injury: keep the back straight — a belt can help to transfer more force to the abdominals. Excessive pressure in the abdomen can lead to rupture or to fainting if not enough blood returns to heart and brain. Overdoing bench presses can lead

6

to strained biceps, shoulder separation and chest wall pain. Gymnasts can easily overstretch flexible joints. Back injuries caused by frequent overextension and sway back elbow (lax ligaments which make a joint unstable) are common. Overstrenuous aerobics without proper preparation has led to heart attacks, especially in older participants.

Combat sports

Boxing injuries are mainly to face and head, with concussion and brain damage a constant danger (which enforced rest after a knock out may help to minimize). Blow to the eye can detach the retina.

Wrestling and judo have a good safety record, probably because they are rigorously supervised, but shoulder dislocations and, in judo, rib, collarbone, finger and toe fractures ,do occur. Repetition of arm positions can also lead to tennis elbow and ligament injuries.

Fencing injuries can be caused by faulty equipment.

Contact sports

In American, Australian rules and rugby football broken bones, spinal injuries, shoulder separation, damage where the ribs joint the sternum and quads haematoma (bleeding within muscles caused by a blow) are all common injuries - though the protection worn by American footballers makes it much safer than it used to be.

Injuries from twisting in a scrum can be minimized by conditioning the muscles. Collapsing a rugby scrum is now illegal - it had led to the paralysis of players.

Wearing a sweat band on the head can minimize cauliflower ears.

Association football

Hamstring sprains are common among weekend players.

A kick with the inner side of the foot can produce adductor strain.

Knee ligament and cartilege are vulnerable, shinbone fractures and sprained ankles. Repeated minor injuries will also stretched ligaments producing 'footballer's ankle'.

Sidestepping and backing movements can loosen the symphasis ligament producing inflammation ('footballer's groin').

Basketball

Basketball, netball and volleyball can lead to foot injuries and ankle injuries when played on hard surfaces.

Mistimed catches can disclocate and fracture fingers or sprain thumbs, a blow to the tip produce 'mallet finger' (a swollen end joint).

'Jumper's knee' (patella tendinitis) groin and shoulder problems can result from jumping, backing and overhead throwing.

Hard and softball field sports

Baseball, softball and cricket can produce 'pitcher's elbow' and other joint injury from round-arm throwing; bowling pitching and sliding shoulder and back injuries.

Hard ball catching can result in fractured or dislocated fingers and mallet finger (see above).

Athletics

Runners risk hamstring sprains and adductor strain, especially from one-sided running and sudden and explosive movements. Long-distance work on hard surfaces can make runners prone to stress fractures and shin splints.

Hurdlers and discus throwers can suffer from 'footballer's groin'.

Javeline-thrower's elbow is caused by round-arm throws.

Shot-putter's finger is a sprain on the three fingers used for final acceleration.

Kick movements aggravate quads and mechanism injuries.

High-jumpers can twist the lower leg on take-off (Fosbury flop ankle).

Golf and hockey

These are played with a bias to one side which can lead to similar back and hamstring injuries .

Gripping clubs too tightly or frequently hitting turf can produce 'golfer's/tennis' elbow.

Running and bending make hockey players liable to high knee and hip pain, and they can suffer from 'footballer's groin'.

Target sports

Wear earmuffs when shooting with firearms to avoid damage to the middle ear.

To avoid accidents , never point a gun at a person, always assume the gun is loaded, always break the gun before putting it in a car or climbing over an obstacle.

Faulty archery technique can lead to 'tennis elbow'.

Racquet games

'Tennis elbow' can come from an over-tight grip on the racquet, or from faulty backhand in tennis. Tight grip can also produce 'squash-player's finger'.

Twisting, turning and lunging in squash, raquetball and badminton, especially at speed and in badly fitting shoes, can cause foot, ankle, knee and toe injuries. Frequent overhead shots in badminton can produce shoulder injuries.

6

Snow and ice sports

Accidents cause most skiing injuries. Loose ski-bindings may allow your skis to come off but reduce the risk of a broken leg or twisted ankle; modern bootsprotect against ankle fracture but put more strain on the knee, where twisting and turning may stress ligaments. Skiers should wear filtered goggles to protect the eyes from glare.

Skaters with ill-fitting boots risk bursitis ('skater's heel') but fractures are more of a risk than ligament damage. Jumps in figure skating can stress the tibia to fracture, falling onto an outstretched hand can produce radius and scaphoid fractures.

Horseriding

Falls are the greatest hazard. Always wear a proper helmet which will minimize the risk to the head, but any neck pain, or numbness or weakness in the limbs calls for urgent medical attention. Fractures to shin, thigh and collarbone, shoulder separation and strained and ruptured knee ligaments are common fall injuries.

Cycling

Falls are the main cause of injury. Always wear a safety helmet and goggles to keep out grit and insects and prevent watering.

Roller sports

Falls and collisions are the main cause of injury. As well as safety helmets, roller skaters, skateboarders and rollerbladers should wear knee and elbow protection

Water sports

Swimming within 90 minutes of eating a meal can lead to cramp, because there is less blood around the muscles.

Diving into very cold water produces shock with immediate hyperventilation and increased pulse and blood pressure. It can be fatal, especially in the elderly and unfit. Impact velocity on diving can cause wrist, thumb and shoulder injuries and badly executed dives can also risk fatal neck injuries. Accidents can occur from diving from too great a height into shallow water. Always check depth and that there is no obstruction before attempting a dive - and with a springboard ensure that you dive beyond the board!

The strains of long-distance swimming can cause shoulder and knee problems, otherwise swimming rarely causes injury.

Heavily chlorinated water can sometimes lead to conjunctivitis (so wear goggles), but untreated water increases the risk of picking up fungal and bacterial infections from other swimmers.

Waterskiers, surfers, windsurfers and sailors should wear life-jackets, even if good swimmers, a blow on the head from a ski, board or boom could render them unconscious. Wet suits, if properly fitting, protect both from hypothermia and the risk of high-pressure edema.

Sailing often demands muscular work by static limbs which can produce quad and abdominal strain. Dehydration and hypothermia are other risks for sailors: proper clothing and drinking water are essentials, eye protection and a sunscreen desirable.

Rowers and canoeists need to develop abdominal muscles to avoid backpain. Gripping oars and paddles too hard can produce 'paddler's wrist' and 'tennis elbow'. Blisters are a common problem, lessened by wearing gloves or toughening the skin with surgical spirit) and piles are sometimes an affliction.

Sports Medicine

Sports medicine is a branch of medicine concerned with the treatment and prevention of sports-related medical disorders. Physicians working within this field may:

- supervise fitness testing
- give advice about training methods
- give advice about the correct clothing, footwear and protective equipment needed to reduce the likelihood of injury
- provide nutritional advice to improve performance, including advice about fluid requirements to prevent dehydration
- give advice about the negative effects of drugs
- provide on-site treatment at sporting events
- give details about immunization required before competition abroad, as well as providing information about the effects of jet lag and how to cope with changes in altitude and climate.
- give advice about the psychological preparation needed before sporting events.
- carry out the diagnosis and treatment of injury and illness
- supervise the rehabilitation of an athlete after injury or illness

As not all sporting injuries occur as a result of sporting activity, not all those treated by sports physicians are sportspeople.

6

FOOD

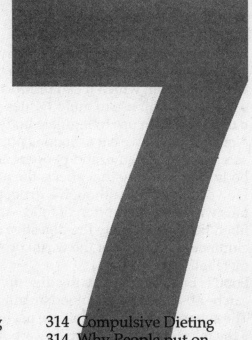

7

Food and Nutrition

Food is anything taken into the body with a chemical composition which can provide the body with:
● material from which it can produce energy
● material it can use to build tissues
● material it can use to regulate body processes.
Not everything we eat as food is nutritious. Flavorings such as saccharin, aspartame, and pepper cannot be utilized by the body. Tea is a drug that affects the nervous system, not a food. However, alcohol, although a drug, provides energy and so falls within the definition of food. And bran, which contains fiber, helps to regulate the digestive system, facilitating the elimination of some of the waste products produced by metabolism.
Food is broken down by the digestive system into forms that can be absorbed by the bloodstream and lymphatic systems. The substances in food that are useful to the body are:
● the micronutrients: proteins, carbohydrates and lipids (fats);
● vitamins and minerals;
● water.

Food Efficiency

At every step in the food chain, only 10% of the energy within the food is passed on. For example, to produce 1lb (0.45kg) of human requires 10lbs (4.54kg) of bass, which requires 100lbs (45.36kg) of minnows, which requires 1,000lbs (453.59kg) of water flies, which requires 10,000lbs (4540kg) of algae. Meat and animal products are usually a much more concentrated source of human dietary needs than plant products. But their production involves more steps in the food chain, so they are far less efficient. The diagram opposite compares energy loss in a potato crop and in beef cattle.

Potato
a Plant metabolic loss 37%
b Farming loss 24%
c Available for processing 39%
  Available after processing 30%

Cattle
d Plant metabolic loss 34%
e Farming and feeding loss 25%
f Animal metabolic loss 35%
g Available for processing 6%
  Available after processing 4%

Energy loss in the food chain

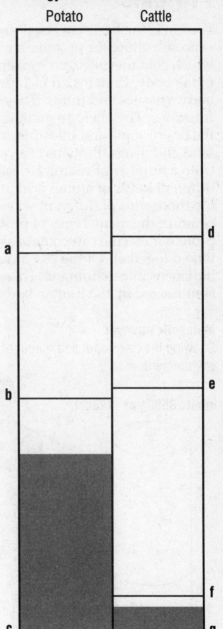

Potato   Cattle

Available after
processing

7

Proteins

Protein is the basic chemical unit of the living organism. There is no substitute for protein, for it is the only constituent of food which contains nitrogen – essential for the growth and repair of the body. Proteins, in fact, provide the raw materials for the body's tissues and fluids. They also have certain specialized functions. They help to maintain the chemical fluid balance in the brain, spine and intestine, and they aid the transport of food and drugs. Proteins are very complex substances made from a number of chemicals called amino acids. About 20 different kinds of amino acid are found in protein food, and the thousands of different ways these can be linked up produce the many types of protein that exist in food. A single protein molecule can contain as many as 500 amino acid units linked together. Of the 20+ amino acids in protein food, 9 are indispensable to humans. These proteins cannot be synthesized by the human body. Of the remaining amino

Metabolic turnover
Showing the daily input and output of a 154lb (69.91kg) man in a closed environment.

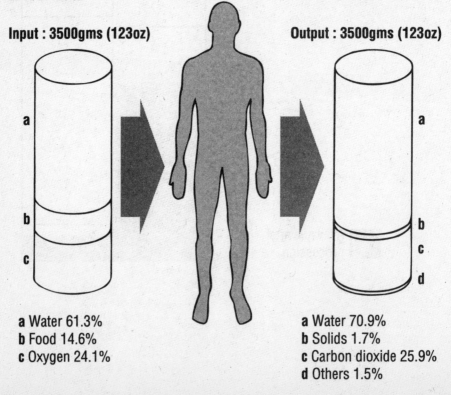

Input : 3500gms (123oz)

Output : 3500gms (123oz)

a Water 61.3%
b Food 14.6%
c Oxygen 24.1%

a Water 70.9%
b Solids 1.7%
c Carbon dioxide 25.9%
d Others 1.5%

acids, 9 or 10 are needed in the diet, but can be synthesized by
the body under certain circumstances. These are called
'conditionally essential' amino acids. The remaining 3 are
readily synthesized by the body, and are called 'inessential'.
The two main sources of protein are from animals, in the form
of meat, fish, eggs and dairy produce, and from plants in the
form of nuts, peas and beans, grains and grain products (such
as wholemeal bread), and in small quantities in many tubers
and vegetables.
Most animal proteins contain all the 8 essential amino acids
that humans need, and so are called complete proteins. But
although all vegetable proteins contain some of the essential
amino acids, none contains the full complement. Vegetarians
must therefore take care to mix vegetable groups in their meals
to ensure that their diet contains all the essential amino acids.

Calories

The nutrients in food that enable the body to grow and repair
its tissues cannot all be measured on one scale. But the
nutrients that provide energy can all be measured on a single
scale and added together, for in the end all of them can be
measured in terms of the amount of heat they produce in the
body.
The basic unit for measuring any energy, including heat
output, is the scientist's calorie. This is defined as the amount
of energy needed to raise the temperature of 1 cubic centimeter
of water by $1°$ Centigrade. The measure used in talking about
food and human energy needs is 1000 times larger than this:
the kilocalorie, which is sometimes written as 'Calorie' (i.e.
with a capital 'C'), but is now more usually expressed as 'kcal',
or simply as 'calorie'.

7

Nutrient energy yields

Nutrient	Energy yield: kcal. per gram
Carbohydrates	4
Lipids (fats)	9
Proteins	4
Vitamins	0
Minerals	0
Water	0
Fiber	0

Carbohydrates

Organic compounds of carbon, hydrogen and oxygen are abundant in nature and easily converted into energy by the body. They provide our main source of energy for immediate use, so they are essential in sustaining the functioning of the internal organs and the central nervous system, and in heart and muscle contraction.

The human body cannot manufacture carbohydrates, so we get them from plants or from animals that feed on plants. Carbohydrates are synthesized in the green leaves of plants out of the reaction of sunlight on water and carbon dioxide. The end product of this process is first sugar, then starch, which is stored in the plants for future use.

There are several different kinds of carbohydrate:

Monosaccharides

These are the simple sugars, soluble in water:

- **glucose** circulates in the blood as glucose, and it is oxidized to give energy.
- **fructose** (from honey and fruit) and **galactose** (a sugar in milk) are converted into glucose before they can be used by the body.

Disaccharides

These are more complex sugars, including **sucrose** (cane sugar), **lactose** (milk sugar) and **maltose** (a sugar produced during digestion from starches and glycogen). During digestion they are split by the body into two monosaccharides.

Polysaccharides

These are complex sugars, not soluble in water. They are:

- **plant starches and cellulose** – the form in which plants store energy manufactured from sunlight. Starch is found in many plant seeds, especially grains, cereals and potatoes. It is intended for use in maintaining the growing plant until it is able to feed itself by photosynthesis. Unripe fruit also contains starch, which converts to sugar as the fruit ripens. Starch is composed of complex chains, linked by glucose units. It is indigestible unless it is cooked, when the granules swell and burst. Cellulose is fibrous and indigestible, but, as fiber, it is an important component of the diet.
- **glycogen** – the form in which glucose is stored in the liver and in the muscles. It is broken down into glucose molecules when the body needs energy.

Oligosaccharides

These are sugars found in legumes (beans and peas). They are broken down in the digestive system not by the action of

enzymes, but by fermentation in the large intestine.
Starch forms the largest part of the carbohydrate in our food.

Fats

Lipids, or fats, are organic compounds composed, like
carbohydrates, of carbon, hydrogen and oxygen, but they
contain more hydrogen than do carbohydrates. The body
absorbs the main constituents of lipids: fatty acids – its main
fuel substances – and glycerol. Lipids differ according to the
different fatty acids they contain.
Fat is stored by the body in fat cells, which form a thick layer
beneath the dermis. It provides heat insulation and padding,
giving the body shape and protecting it against injury. It is also
the body's most concentrated source of energy.
Fats are of two main types:

- **Saturated fats** are animal fats and they contain a high
  proportion of hydrogen. They include butter, milk and other
  dairy products. They tend to solidify at fairly high
  temperatures. Saturated fats are believed to be harmful to
  health, particularly in encouraging the development of
  atherosclerosis (see p 76).
- **Unsaturated fats** are found in vegetable and fish oils and
  they contain a lower proportion of hydrogen. They are
  thought to inhibit the development of atherosclerosis and to
  be more beneficial to health than saturated fats (see p 304).

Fats are not soluble in water, although they are soluble in
alcohol, ether and chloroform. But by chemical treatment with
alkalis, fats can be broken down into their separate units, and
then can be mixed with water. Soap is made by this process,
and it also occurs during the digestion of fats.
Mineral oils such as Paraffin or Vaseline cannot be saponified.
They are therefore no value as food.

7

Vitamins

Vitamins are organic compounds that occur in minute
quantities in food. They function as co-enzymes: chemicals that
work with enzymes to effect chemical processes in the body,
and thus influence growth and development, and protect
against illness and disease. Vitamins are essential in the diet, as
most cannot be manufactured by the body.
The role of vitamins in nutrition was only discovered in the
20th century, but there are now known to be about 40, of which

about 12 are essential in the diet. Because of their haphazard discovery, they were originally identified by letters and numbers, but since their chemical structures have been identified, chemical names are often used for many of them. Analysis has also enabled them to be synthesized.

Vitamins are essential to the manufacture of tissue-building materials, hormones and other regulators; for nerve and muscle function; for the production of energy and for the breakdown of waste products and toxic compounds.

The vitamins are chemically very different. The body can manufacture only vitamin D (from sunlight) and pyridoxine, a B vitamin (from bacteria in the intestine); the rest come from food. Vitamins in the diet can be divided into those soluble in fat (A, D, E and K), and those soluble in water (C and the B vitamins). All are needed by the body in only tiny amounts. For example, the body needs only 1 ounce (28.3g) of thiamine (vitamin B1) in its lifetime, although that 1 ounce (28.3g) is vital. However, whereas excessive quantities of water-soluble vitamins can be diluted and excreted in the urine, unused quantities of fat-soluble vitamins remain in the body and, if they are present in large quantities, become poisonous.

Vitamins and free radicals

Vitamins E and C are antioxidants – substances capable of combating the chemically very active atoms called free radicals, which are capable of causing immense damage to the system. To protect the body from attack by free radicals, these vitamins need to be taken regularly in doses much larger than the body's minimum daily requirement.

Minerals

Minerals are chemical elements that are needed in the diet in tiny amounts. Their roles in the body include:
- regulating the water balance of the body cells;
- regulating the acid-base balance – the acidity level – of the body fluids;
- regulating the reactability of nerve and muscle tissue;
- they are components of many compounds synthesized by the body, such as hormones and enzymes;
- they are important to many reactions that take place in the body, acting as catalysts ;
- they are important to growth and repair.

More than 20 minerals are needed by the body. They are grouped as major minerals, needed by the body in relatively large amounts; and trace minerals which are needed by the

body in minute amounts and which have known functions.
However, these groupings do not reflect the importance of
their member minerals – many trace elements carry out vital
functions in the body.

Water

Water is essential to the functioning of all body cells – the body
is about two-thirds water. It is the body's main transport
system. The blood, which is made up mainly of water, carries
dissolved nutrients and oxygens to the tissues and carries
away dissolved waste products, including carbon dioxide, to
be filtered by the kidneys and lungs, and excreted.

Body water content				
Body weight	Total water content	Cells	Tissue spaces between cells	Blood
143 pounds	70 pints	38+ pints	25+ pints	8-9 pints
64.92kg	39.77 liters	21.59liters	14.20 liters	4.83 liters

Water is a simple compound of oxygen and hydrogen and
always contains dissolved minerals and other solids, and
gases. The nature and amount of these depends on the rocks
and soil the water passed through before being channelled for
drinking. Water is also found in most solid food.

Clean water

More than half the world's population does not have access to
clean water. In industrialized Western countries, where public
water systems are readily available to all, the water is often
contaminated with lead from old piping, and nitrates and
other chemicals used in agriculture, which seep into rivers and
reservoirs. It may also contain aluminum, chlorine, fluoride,
and other substances added with the intention of improving
the health of the population.

To ensure clean water, it is advisable to see that cold water
tanks are cleaned regularly, that old lead piping is removed and
replaced, and that the water you use for drinking is filtered. In
addition to jug filters, it is possible to fit filtering devices to the
mains supply. These are advisable, since jug filters remove only
a limited number of chemicals and pollutants with larger
particles. To prevent bacterial contamination it is essential to
replace the cartridges of all filters regularly and to keep filtered
water cool to prevent bacteria from multiplying.

7

Vitamins Chart: WATER-SOLUBLE VITAMINS

Name	Function	Found in
B1 (thiamine)	role in the removal of carbon dioxide	whole grains, pulses, pork, milk, fruit
B2 (riboflavin)	role in carbohydrate and protein metabolism	milk, eggs, liver, fish, spinach, broccoli, asparagus
Niacin (nicotinamide)	role in cellular respiration, fatty acid metabolism	liver, lean meat, oatmeal, pulses, rice, wheat
B6 (pyridoxine)	essential to synthesis of neurotransmitters hormones (e.g. insulin), and to protein metabolism	meat, vegetables, wholegrain cereals
Pantothenic acid	important in fat and carbohydrate metabolism	wholegrains, legumes, animal products
Folic acid (folate)	essential to synthesis of DNA and red blood cells and amino acid metabolism	green leaf vegetables, liver, legumes, bacteria in bowel
B12 (cobalamin)	essential to fatty acid metabolism	muscle meats, eggs, diary products (not present in plant foods)
Biotin	important to the synthesis of essential fatty acids and in amino acid metabolism	liver, egg yolk, cooked egg white, cereals, yeast, soy flour
Choline (vitamin-like substance)	used in the metabolism of fats and formation of neurotransmitter acetylcholine	lecithin, found in egg yolk
C (ascorbic acid)	formation of collagen	fruit juices, citrus fruits, green vegetables, tomatoes, strawberries, potatoes

NB: All the B vitamins are co-enzymes: they enable enzymes to function.

Figures given here for recommended daily intake for men

Deficiency causes	Excess	Destroyed by	Recommended daily intake
beriberi and polyneuritis (nervous system damage)	excreted	overcooking food	1.2 mg
blurred vision, cataracts, corneal ulcerations, dermatitis	mainly excreted, some stored in liver, kidney and heart	overcooking food	1.7 mg
pellagra (dermatitis, diarrhea, nervous and mental disorders)	flushing, peptic ulcers	overcooking food	19 mg
lesions of lips and mouth, nousea, retarded growth	100-1000 mg daily causes impaired memory	heat and overcooking; some drugs; some molds and fungi	2 mg
deficiency symptoms reported only in starvation	excreted	overcooking	4-7 mg
megaloblastic anemia (abnormal red blood cell production)	no known ill effects	antibiotic treatment	0.2 mg
pernicious anemia, nervous and mental disorders	excreted, some is conserved	overcooking meat	0.002 mg
fatigue, nausia, loss of appetite, muscle pains, dry skin, anemia, high blood cholesterol	no ill effects reported in up to 10 mg per day intake		0.1 mg
memory loss	not known		500-900 mg in normal diet. RDA not established
scurvy, poor healing of wounds, internal bleeding	excreted	exposure to air and cooking, especially in presence of copper and alkalis	60 mg RDA 1000 mg+

7

continued on next page

Vitamins Chart (continued):

FAT-SOLUBLE VITAMINS

Name	Function	Found in
A (retinol)	antioxidant; health of bones, lining tissues, immune system; protects against cancer; normal vision; protects skin	whole milk, butter, cheese, egg yolk, liver, yellow and green vegetables, fish liver oils
D (ergocalciferol)	increases absorption of calcium; promotes growth	cod-liver oil, eggs, dairy produce, fortified milk and margarine
E (tocopherol)	antioxidant; protects all cell structures	wheat germ oils, alfalfa, lettuce
K (phylloquinone)	important in formation of blood factors	green leafy vegetables; some in cereals, fruits, meats

Deficiency causes	Excess	Recommended daily intake
night blindness, dry eyes, hair and skin, slow and faulty development of bones and teeth	causes skin irritability, nausea, headache, loss of appetite, intense sleepiness, enlarged liver and spleen	1 mg RDA
rickets (bone deformities) in children; osteomalacia (bone softening) in adults	deposition of calcium in the tissues, including kidneys, arteries; vomiting, diarrhea, kidney failure	0.005 mg
degenerative changes in brain, nervous system; impaired vision; anemia; fluid retention; skin disorders	abdominal pain, nausea, vomiting, diarrhea	10 mg
hemorrhaging;	not known	0.06-0.08 mg

7

Minerals Chart

Name	Function	Found in
Calcium	essential to strong bones and teeth; role in nerve impulse transmission, muscle contraction and blood clotting	dairy products, meat, milk, eggs, fish, legumes, dark green vegetables
Chloride	acid-base balance, formation of gastric juices	salt
Chromium	glucose and fat metabolism	fats, meats, vegetable oils, brewers yeast, legumes, whole grain, nuts
Cobalt	constituent of vitamin B12	muscle meats, eggs, dairy products (not present in plant foods)
Copper	important in iron metabolism, energy release and protein synthesis	meat, drinking water
Fluoride	role in maintaining healthy bones and teeth	drinking water, tea, milk, seafoods
Iodine	constituent of thyroid hormones	fish and shellfish, dairy produce, vegetables
Iron	essential to the formation of haemoglobin and in synthesising certain enzymes	green leaf vegetables, lean meat, liver, whole grains, legumes
Magnesium	essential to protien synthesis	green leafy vegetables, whole grains, lean meat, fish, milk
Manganese	activates enzymes involved in fat synthesis	green leafy vegetables, tea
Molybdenum	constituent of some enzymes	legumes, cereals, organ meats, vegetables
Nickel	activates some enzymes	in many foods

Deficiency causes	Excess	Recommended daily intake
stunted growth, osteoporosis, rickets	vomiting, diarrhea, kidney damage	800 mg
muscle cramps, loss of appetite, mental apathy	vomiting, dehydration	750 mg
raised blood sugar	skin and kidney damage – an occupational hazard	not known; 0.05-0.10 mg in normal diet
not known	inhibits enzyme function	0.003 mg
stunted growth, anemia in children	nausea, vomiting, diarrhea, cirrhosis, brain damage	1.5-3 mg
dental caries	discoloration of teeth, densening of bone tissue	0.5-1 mg
enlarged thyroid gland (goiter), inhibition of proper mental development in young	inhibits thyroid function	0.12-0.15 mg
anemia	cirrhosis of the liver	10-12 mg
muscular tremors, anxiety, depression	diarrhea, nausea, vomiting and muscle weakness	350 mg
not known	nervous and mental disorders	not known (3-8 mg in normal diet)
not known	not known	not known (0.4 mg in normal diet)
not known	acute pneumonia	not known

7

continued on next page

Minerals Chart (continued)

Name	Function	Found in
Phosphorus	bone and teeth formation, acid-base balance, role in muscle contraction and nerve impulse transmission, component of DNA, RNA and many enzymes	dairy produce, white meat, cereals, fish, nuts
Potassium	essential to water and acid-base balance, nerve and muscle function, heart rate	in many foods
Selenium	essential to synthesis of specific enzymes	meat, whole grains, seafood, milk
Silicon	not known	in many foods
Sodium	essential to water and acid-base balance, nerve function	salt
Sulfur	constituent of hormones and vitamins, cartilage, tendons, and other tissues	protein in diet provides sulfur containing amino acids. Also fish, dairy produce and beans
Tin	not known	in many foods
Vanadium	not known	occurs in many foods
Zinc	major constituent of many enzymes; protects against free radical damage; essential to immune system; important in synthesis and metabolism of proteins	lean beef, pork, dairy produce, whole wheat, maize, rice, yams

Deficiency causes	Excess	Recommended daily intake
osteoporosis, weakness	erosion of jaw	800 mg
muscular weakness, paralysis, fatigue, abnormal heart rhythm	kidney damage, and, in severe cases, heart failure	2000 mg
heart muscle damage	dermitits and nervous disorders	0.05-0.07 mg
not known	silicosis	not known
muscular cramps, loss of appetite, apathy, fainting	high blood pressure increasing the likelihood of heart and circulatory diseases, and kidney damage	500 mg
not known	not known	bodily needs extracted from proteins and certain B vitimins
not known	vomiting	not known
not known	lung irritation	not known
loss of appetite, hair loss, diarrhea, slow healing of wounds; in children, impairs growth and delays sexual development	fever, vomiting, diarrhea; absorption can be reduced by tin	15 mg

7

The Digestive System

The digestive tract, also called the alimentary canal, forms a tube more than 30ft (9.1m) long, beginning in the mouth and ending at the anus. Between these, it includes the esophagus (gullet), stomach, small intestine and large intestine.

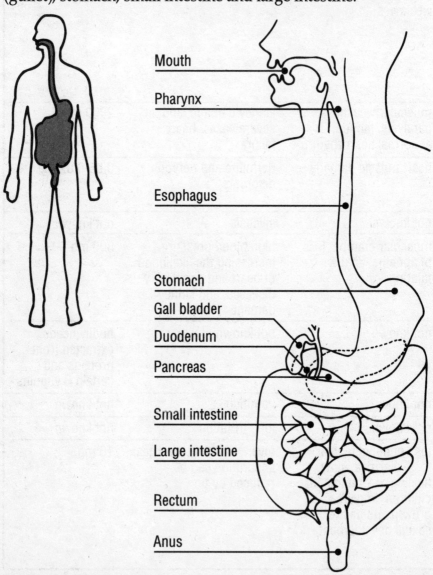

Mouth

Pharynx

Esophagus

Stomach

Gall bladder

Duodenum

Pancreas

Small intestine

Large intestine

Rectum

Anus

Digestion timescale:

Mouth and esophagus (chewing and swallowing):	about 1 minute
Stomach (churning and mixing with digestive juices):	about 4 hours
Small intestine:	about 5 hours
Large intestine:	5-24 hours

Digestion and Absorption

Digestion begins in the mouth as a mechanical process in which food is chopped and ground by the teeth into smaller and smaller particles, liquefied by saliva, and formed into a rounded mass, a 'bolus', to facilitate swallowing. Saliva is a digestive juice secreted by the parotid and several other salivary glands in the mouth, which begins the digestion of starch.

The bolus passes through the pharynx and down the oesophagus aided by peristalsis – regular contractions of the muscular wall, which move food along the digestive tract at a controlled speed – into the stomach.

The stomach varies in shape and size according to its contents. Its maximum capacity is about 3 U.S. pints. Its movements churn food into smaller particles and mix it with the gastric juices. The stomach produces gastric juices, principally hydrochloric acid, and thick mucus, which protects the stomach lining from erosion by hydrochloric acid. The **pyloric valve** opens to allow the liquefied food, called 'chyle' to pass into the small intestine.

In the **duodenum**, the first 12in (30cm) of the small intestine, the food is mixed with digestive juices produced by the duodenum, the **pancreas**, a gland located just behind the stomach, and with bile from the **gall bladder**, a substance produced by the liver, which aids in the digestion of fats. Here, and in the remaining 21ft (6.4m) of the small intestine, nutrients are broken down into simple chemical forms that can be absorbed through the walls of the intestine into the blood and lymph streams. (The lymphatic system circulates tissue fluid to the cells of the body).

The **large intestine**, or colon, is a continuous tube about 5ft (1.5m) long. Its main function is to absorb water and electrolytes (potassium, magnesium, sulphate and phosphate) from the digested food, while transporting it to the rectum and anus. It also encourages the growth of bacteria capable of synthesizing certain vitamins.

The waste products of digestion reach the **rectum** as feces, a soft, solid mixture of indigestible remains and unabsorbed water. The feces are expelled from the body via the **anus**.

7

Carbohydrate digestion (1)
The enzyme amylase in the salivary glands of the mouth begins the breakdown of polysaccharides (complex sugars), into disaccharides. This is continued in the small intestine by amylase secreted by the pancreas. The pancreas also produces insulin, which stimulates the storage by the liver of glucose as glycogen. The enzymes maltase, sucrase, and lactase break down disaccharides into simple sugars in the duodenum, which are absorbed through the intestinal walls. Some forms of carbohydrate (e.g. cellulose and fiber), cannot be digested and pass through the digestive system as bulk, or roughage.

Protein digestion (2)
Pepsin in the stomach begins the chemical breakdown of proteins into peptides. Rennin coagulates milk protein. The pancreas produces trypsin, an enzyme which completes the digestion of proteins. In the duodenum, the enzyme erepsin converts any partially digested proteins into amino acids. These are absorbed into the bloodstream through the walls of the small intestine.

Fat digestion (3)
Lipase, a digestive juice in the stomach, begins the chemical digestion of emulsified fats (fats that are finely dispersed in water, as in homogenized milk). In the duodenum, bile emulsifies fats, and pancreatic juices convert them into fatty acids and glycerol. These are absorbed into the lymph vessels (70%) and the bloodstream (30%). Fat-soluble vitamins are absorbed at the same time.

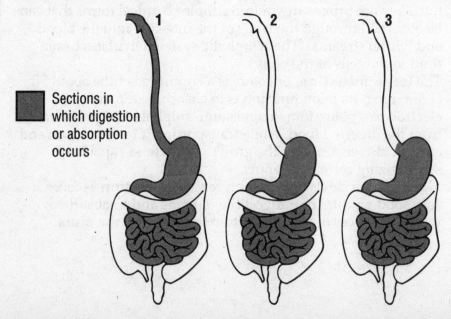

Sections in which digestion or absorption occurs

The Liver

The liver is a chemical factory connected to the digestive
system, and has many digestive functions. Among the most
important are:
- the conversion of monosaccharides (simple sugars) into
  glucose, and its conversion into and storage as glycogen;
- neutralizing hydrochloric acid from the stomach;
- inactivating unneeded insulin, a substance that is important
  in the regulation of blood sugar levels;
- the production of bile, using cholesterol to produce bile
  salts, which convert non-soluble fats into fats that can be
  absorbed into the blood and lymph streams;
- regulating the concentration of amino acids in the blood,
  converting unused amino acids into glucose;
- destroying old red blood cells, extracting and storing the
  iron content;
- synthesizing cholesterol and lipoproteins from fatty acids.

Cholesterol and Lipoproteins

Cholesterol is an important component of the body – it is, for
example, an essential part of the structure of cell membranes
and of the sex hormones, as well as bile. It is a fatty substance,
synthesized by the liver from fatty acids. Large quantities of
cholesterol are released into the large intestine through the bile
duct every day, and most is reabsorbed into the blood and
lymph steams.
Cholesterol is carried in the blood as part of complex
substances called lipoproteins. Lipoproteins are, as their name
suggests, combinations of fats and proteins. There are many
types. Those that circulate in the bloodstream are classified by
the density of protein they contain in three principal ways:
- as HDL or high density lipoprotein (high protein, low
  cholesterol content).
- as LDL or low density lipoprotein (low protein, high
  cholesterol content)
- as VLDL or very low density lipoprotein.

LDLs and atherosclerosis
The role of LDLs, which contain high levels of cholesterol, is to
transport lipids to muscles and to fat stores. Cells needing
cholesterol to manufacture membranes synthesize receptors
which bind an LDL circulating in the blood. They then imbibe

the LDL and utilize its cholesterol.

LDLs are, however, associated with the accumulation of atheroma (fatty plaques) in the walls of arteries, leading to atherosclerosis and stroke (see pp 76-7).

HDLs, on the other hand, appear to have an important role in protecting against these diseases. HDLs circulating in the bloodstream absorb cholesterol unused by cells and return it to the liver, where it is processed.

Food Intake

What people eat varies enormously. For many people in tropical countries, a typical day's food is two small bowls of rice and a little vegetable – totaling perhaps 160 kcals, and containing only tiny amounts of necessary proteins, vitamins, and minerals. Yet in industrial countries, the daily diet of a food lover may total over 3500 kcals and supply in all respects about twice the body's needs. Even taking national averages, great differences remain. In Ghana, on a diet mainly of roots, cereals, and vegetables the average total daily intake is perhaps 90% of daily needs, including 47gm of protein of which only 11 are of animal origin. In Denmark, on a diet of meat, dairy produce, cereal products, vegetables, and fruits, the average intake is on average 130% of daily needs, including 95gm of protein (62 of animal origin). Diets also vary greatly in their variety, their range of geographical source, and their handling and processing before consumption. Perhaps 75% of the world lives on a basic diet of one food, usually a cereal (typically rice), usually grown by themselves, and usually eaten in a simple boiled form. Average individual grain intake on such a diet in a poor country totals perhaps 400lb (181.4 kg) a year. In contrast, about 1700lb (771.8 kg) of grain enters the food chain of a North American each year – but only 30% is ever eaten as cereal products. The rest goes to feed livestock for meat and dairy produce. Industrial man buys widely from restaurants, carry outs, and vending machines, as well as from an average supermarket stock of 7000 different food items that have been stored, transported (perhaps imported), usually processed and preserved, and wrapped for sale. As a result of this overabundance, in the US, where the daily kilocalorie supply is on average 130% of daily need, 12% of men and 15% of women are obese, according to World Health Organization statistics for the late 1980s.

Energy Needs

A person's need for energy from food is measured in calories (kilocalories, see p 283). Needs vary from person to person, depending on a variety of different factors. Age, sex, size, physical activity and climate all affect the amount of energy you need. An increase in weight results if a person takes in as food more calories than are needed. If the intake is below requirements, fat stored in the body is converted to energy and weight is lost.

Daily Calorie Needs

The chart gives daily calorie requirements for men by age and is based on USA National Research Council statistics for the late 1980s. For men aged under 50 they are based on an average daily level of physical activity; for men aged over 50 they are based on a desirable daily level of physical activity .

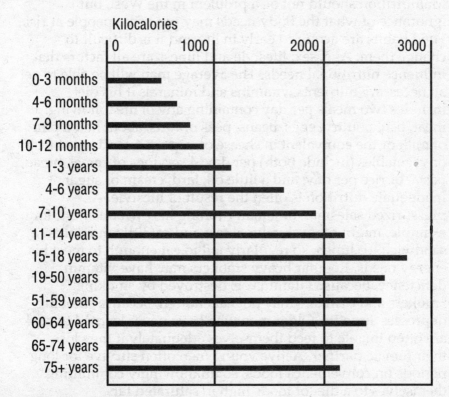

Calories and exercise
People use up calories whatever they are doing, even when asleep, when the calorie expenditure is used to maintain body functions.

The following table gives average calorie expenditure on different activities:

Activity	Energy kcal/h
Basic metabolic rate (lying still while awake)	77
Sitting still	100
Operating keyboard rapidly	140
Walking, 2.6mi/h (3.8km/h)	200
Sexual intercourse	280
Jogging	570
Running at top speed	1440

Inadequate Nutrition

Malnutrition should not be a problem in the West, but ignorance of what the body needs may put some people at risk. Food habits are acquired early in life and it is difficult to change them. Age, sex, lifestyle and illness are all factors that influence nutritional needs. The average man will be able to get all necessary nutrients, vitamins and minerals if his diet includes two meals per day containing any of the following: meat, fish, poultry, eggs, beans, peas or nuts; about half a pint of milk or the equivalent in cheese or yogurt; 4 servings of fruit or vegetables (include both) per day; 4 servings of cereal, bread, pasta, or rice per day; and a little oil, lard, cream or sugar. Inadequate nutrition is often the result of lifestyle. A pressurized salesman or a man running his own business, for example, might often skip breakfast and eat little more than a sandwich for lunch, so regularly fail to eat enough to meet his energy needs. Regular heavy smokers may have vitamin deficiency, because vitamin C is destroyed by smoking. Smokers and drinkers may not eat enough, because smoking depresses appetite. Older men who have never learned to cook are often unable to feed themselves adequately if they lose their female partner. Active young men often survive for long periods on convenience foods, so unknowingly committing themselves to a diet of foods high in saturated fats.

Nutrition and disease

The West offers the most varied, cleanest, and most readily available supply of food in the history of the world. But this brings its own problems, including heart disease, obesity, diabetes (associated in some cases with excessive carbohydrate intake) and digestive diseases associated with lack of fiber. Known links between diet and disease include:

- **Atherosclerosis**, associated with a high intake of saturated fats.
- **Night blindness** which may be caused by a lack of vitamin A.
- **Inflamed tongue** may be a result of B-vitamin deficiencies.
- **Bleeding gums** may be a sign of scurvy — lack of vitamin C (which is destroyed by smoking).
- **Rashes**, itching, soreness scaliness, and cracking of the skin may indicate a number of vitamin deficiencies.
- **Obesity** is the result of eating too much food. It can cause breathing difficulties, backache and heart disease.
- **Soft bones** may indicate rickets, caused by lack of vitamin D).
- **Loss of motor function** in the legs may be a sign of beri beri (lack of vitamin B1 or thiamine).
- **Kidney stones** may form as a result of insufficient fluid intake.
- **Gallstones** are associated with a fatty diet.
- **Cirrhosis of the liver** is caused by too much alcohol.
- **Constipation and piles** (hemorrhoids) often result from a lack of fiber in the diet.
- **Painful feet** may be a sign of vitamin B12 deficiency.

7

Healthy Eating – The Facts

The concept of a balanced diet has altered considerably over the last 20 years, as research has revolutionized knowledge about food and nutrition. The principles of healthy eating are set out below – but see also the Vitamin and Mineral charts (pp 288-95). New facts will, however, undoubtedly continue to change the picture over the next few years.

Carbohydrates Intake

Carbohydrate intake in the American diet ranges from 250 to 800 grams (8.82 to 28.24 oz) per day. Some two-thirds of this comes from starch and the remainder from sugars – sucrose used as a sweetener – and lactose from milk.

Slow-release carbohydrates

It is now widely accepted that the bulk of the diet – half to two-thirds – should consist of carbohydrates containing a high proportion of fiber. These are called slow-release carbohydrates because, by contrast with sucrose, they release energy slowly. They include pasta (made from durum flour, which is high in protein), brown rice, high-fiber wholemeal bread, muesli, and breakfast cereals with no added sugar or fat. These foods tend to lose their energy content if overcooked. Government health departments in the US and Great Britain have emphasized the importance of cereal foods (which include pasta) in replacing foods rich in fats and sugars as the main source of energy in the diet. In the past, and still in many of the poorer countries, cereals, very simply cooked, were the major food. Their widespread replacement by refined and sweetened carbohydrate products has serious implications. Pastries, cakes, chocolate and ice cream have little nutritional value, and they tend to be high in saturated fats.

Fats Intake

Fats are an essential part of a balanced diet. They provide energy in concentrated form; they enable the fat-soluble vitamins, A, D, E and K, to be absorbed from the intestines; and they stimulate the production of bile by the gall bladder, which aids digestion. They also make food more palatable, by making its texture and smell more appealing.

The body can synthesize some of the 9 essential fatty acids (pp 282-3) from other foods, but three are made only from fats. The amount of fat in the diet varies enormously from culture to culture. Textbooks cite the Indian Ho tribe, which consumes less than 4 grams (0.14oz) of fat per day; and the East African Maasai, who live on a diet of cattle blood and milk.

The average amount of fat in the Western diet can only be estimated. In Great Britain, for example, people eat an average 100 grams (3.53oz) of fat per day, which provides about 42% of their daily energy needs. However, these figures are based on foods consumed at home. The amount of fat consumed may be different when a proportion of daily food intake is consumed in restaurants.

Saturated and unsaturated fats

Fats fall into two major categories: saturated fats (containing a high proportion of hydrogen); and unsaturated fats (with a low hydrogen content); fats with minimum hydrogen content are called polyunsaturated. Saturated fats, which harden at room temperature, are in meat and dairy produce, solid shortening products, coconut oil, cocoa butter, and palm oil (used in bought cookies and pastry). Research has shown a relationship between consumption of saturated fats and high levels of cholesterol in the blood, and heart disease see (see p 75 and p 300). A high level of saturated fats in the diet is also associated with intestinal cancers.

Many vegetable fats are unsaturated. Polyunsaturated fats are found in vegetable oils, especially safflower, soybean and corn oil. Some authorities believe that consuming polyunsaturated fats can counteract the effects of foods high in saturated fats. It is difficult to lower blood cholesterol levels (see p 283) simply by reducing cholesterol in the diet, because whenever the level of cholesterol in the blood falls, the liver starts to synthesize cholesterol to replace it. Cutting cholesterol out of the diet completely would reduce blood cholesterol levels by 5 to 10%. However, it is now known that the saturated fatty acids, of which saturated fats are mainly composed, tend to stimulate the liver to produce more cholesterol instead of converting blood cholesterol to bile. But the polyunsaturated fatty acids which predominate in vegetable oils cause cholesterol and bile acids from the liver to be excreted.

Fish oils, such as halibut and cod liver oil, are known to be especially effective in reducing LDLs (see p 76), and so protecting against atherosclerosis.

Until recently, animals fats constituted a very high proportion of daily fat intake in the average diet. The U.S authorities recommend reducing the total intake of saturated fat to less than 10% of the daily diet, substituting fats high in polyunsaturates, which should ideally provide about 7% of daily energy needs. Fats in total should make up no more than 30% of total food intake.

7

Protein Intake

The American diet typically contains about 125 grams (4.41oz) of protein, making up 10-15% of the diet. In fact, only about 50 grams (1.76oz) is needed every day to supply the amino acids the body needs.

Daily protein requirements

The following table gives US government recommendations for the daily amount of protein in the diet for men of all ages:

Protein requirements grams/day

Age	0	10	20	30	40	50	60	
0-3 months								13.0
4-6 months								13.0
7-9 months								14.0
10-12 months								14.0
1-3 years								16.0
4-6 years								24.0
7-10 years								28.0
11-14 years								45.0
15-18 years								59.0
19-50 years								55.5
50+ years								55.0

The discrepancy between the typical and the recommended intake reflects a major change in thinking about diet over the last two decades. Until recently, protein was considered the most important constituent of the diet, since it has a vital role in growth and repair, as well as energy provision. However, given that protein needs vary according to age and other factors, reassessment of the amount of protein needed to maintain health has tended to reduce recommended daily amounts of pure protein in the diet and substitute slow-release (high-protein) carbohydrates, which should form the bulk of the diet. US government recommendations estimate that 50% or more of the body's total food energy of an adults should be supplied by carbohydrates.

Dietary Fiber Intake

Cellulose and other plant tissues that humans cannot digest are collectively called dietary fiber. Bran – the outer husks of cereal grains, which are removed during processing – is dietary fiber. Carrots and cabbage have a high fiber content. Fiber is simply a natural laxative. The urge to defecate depends on distension of the rectum. Fiber absorbs a large amount of water, creating bulk and causing distension. Constipation – difficulty in expelling feces – affects approximately 10-12% of the population of UK, yet the condition is unknown in people on high-fiber vegetarian diets. Wholegrain cereal foods are most effective in preventing constipation.

However, recent research has shown that dietary fiber has other important roles. Studies in 1990 showed evidence that a high intake of vegetable fibre protects against the formation of gallstones – crystals of cholesterol in the bile duct. Evidence from studies in the 1980s and early 1990s suggests that soluble fiber binds bile cholesterol so preventing its reabsorbtion into the body. The effect is to lower the level of cholesterol circulating in blood.

Fiber is most often eaten in the form of wholemeal bread, muesli, brown rice, pulses, fruit and vegetables.

Water Intake

Water in the diet is derived from food, and the breakdown of food during digestion, as well as from fluids drunk. The average need for water for an adult is 7 to 10 glasses per day, but individuals should be guided by instinct. The thirst center in the brain provides an excellent warning of dehydration and the need to take in fluids, and the desire to drink is severely inhibited if too much fluid is taken in.

7

Assessing Your Eating Habits

Although there are many different views on healthy eating, one point on which all experts agree is that you need to follow a varied diet that includes all the different food types. They recommend that you cut down on sugar, other refined foods and animal fats, replacing them as far as possible with more fresh fruit and vegetables, wholegrain cereals and unsaturated fats.

To change your eating habits, you first need to know exactly what they are. Make a chart using the suggestions below as guidelines. Fill in the chart honestly for two weeks, and see if a pattern emerges. Each time you eat, ask yourself why you are eating: are you hungry, or is it just because it is the time when most people have a meal? Do you really dislike vegetarian meals, or are you just used to having red meat at every meal? Use the information you have collected to help yourself plan a healthier eating pattern.

Keeping a Food Diary

FREQUENCY OF EATING
Time started
Time finished

WHAT EATEN
List what you eat
every time you eat

TYPE OF FOOD
Convenience
Fresh

COOKING METHOD
List how food was
cooked (raw, fried,
steamed, etc.)

**POSITION IN WHICH
YOU EAT**
Sitting
Standing
Walking
Running
Lying

EFFECTS OF EATING
Fullness
Hunger
Physical discomfort

```
FREQUENCY  OF  EATING
                       TIME
                  STARTED FINISHED  KING
Monday  BREAKFAST  8:20    8:35    HOD
        LUNCH     12:05   12:20    AW
        SUPPER     7:10    7:30    ILED
Tuesday BREAKFAST  8:15    8:30    EAMED
   ○    LUNCH     12:10   12:25    IEO
                                   SAMED
Wednesday BREAKFAST 8:20   8:35
        LUNCH     12:05   12:20
        SUPPER     7:10    7:30
```

Buying and Preparing Food

Choose ingredients that look and smell fresh. Fruit and
vegetables should not be wilted or discolored. Cracked or
wilted vegetable leaves indicate a mineral deficiency in the
plant, so they may not provide you with the minerals you
need. White meat and fish contain less saturated fat than red
meat. Brown rice, wholewheat bread, wholewheat flour, and
wholewheat pasta contain more fiber, minerals and vitamins
than their white equivalents. The vitamin content of raw fruit
and vegetables is reduced by boiling, but some vitamins will
pass into the cooking liquid, which may be used as stock. It is
sensible to eat at least one salad a day and to cook foods
without adding fat – steaming fish instead of deep frying,
boiling, baking, and grilling (broiling) instead of frying.

Replace foods high in fat with a low-fat alternative; for instance, use plain yogurt instead of cream to top a fruit salad. Statistics show that men tend to eat more red meat than white meat or fish because they see it as macho, but the fat content of some red meats is higher than that of chicken or fish. If you must eat red meat, choose game, such as venison, which is a low-fat red meat. Grill meat, instead of frying it. Try substituting white meat or shellfish once or twice a week. Then try an occasional vegetarian meal. You may find that, gradually, your tastes change.

Know Your Food

This list shows the calorific changes that take place in a potato when it is cooked by different methods or processed commercially.

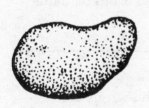

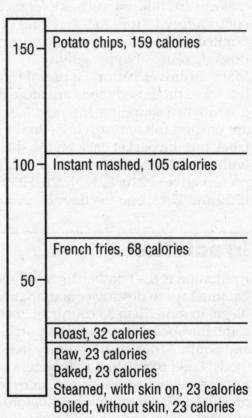

150 —	Potato chips, 159 calories
100 —	Instant mashed, 105 calories
	French fries, 68 calories
50 —	
	Roast, 32 calories
	Raw, 23 calories
	Baked, 23 calories
	Steamed, with skin on, 23 calories
	Boiled, without skin, 23 calories

7

Food Additives

A food additive is any substance not normally consumed as food, which is added to food to preserve it, or to enhance its flavor, color or texture. Most packed foods contain additives. About 3500 additives are currently in use worldwide. Some occur naturally, such as pectin, used to set jams, which comes from plants. Others are made by food manufacturers, for instance azodicarbonamide, which is added to flour to improve the consistency of bread dough.

Growing public concern has led governments in several countries to pass legislation obliging food manufacturers to list all the ingredients in their products; they are now listed in descending order of weight; additives usually have to be listed by type and chemical name or by number, or both.

Improved labeling helps people avoid additives that might provoke an allergic reaction; most people do not have an obvious reaction to additives, but a significant minority does. Symptoms of additive intolerance are wide-ranging. They may include asthma, rashes, headaches and a general feeling of malaise. In children, such intolerance may also be an important contributory factory to behavioral problems. Research has pointed to the artificial azo dyes, such as Tartrazine, as a possible cause of hyperactivity.

Many additives perform a useful function in preserving food, but some processed foods are more additive than food. Be on guard when shopping and read labels before you buy. Many are purposefully mystifying – so if you cannot understand a label, put the packet back on the shelf and choose something with few additives. Do not buy foods that contain the azo dyes, preservatives E210, E211, E220, E250 and E251; anti-oxidants E320 and E321; and the flavor enhancer 621.

Irradiation

Irradiation is the bombardment of food with high-intensity gamma rays to destroy contaminating microorganisms. It is illegal in more than 30 countries, including the US the UK, and some European countries, but potatoes are widely irradiated, and South Africa is one country that irradiates a wide range of foods. Food irradiation kills beneficial bacteria, prevents food from smelling bad when 'off', does not destroy toxins produced by microorganisms before radiation, lowers the nutrient content of the food (which may then lose more nutrients through cooking), and, most importantly, produces damaging free radicals.

Vegetarianism

A vegetarian is a person who does not eat the meat of any animal, bird or fish. There are two main types of vegetarian.

a vegans, who eat nothing at all of animal origin; and
b lacto-ovo-vegetarians, who do allow themselves animal
products such as milk, cheese, eggs and honey.
Some people call themselves vegetarians but eat fish. Reasons
for vegetarianism vary from society to society and individual
to individual. It has been advocated for religious,
philosophical, moral, economic and health reasons. It has also
been adopted as a necessity. Many people have lived on a diet
of fruit, nuts and berries, with meat only when it could be
obtained. Powerful arguments for vegetarianism in modern
society are:
● the inefficiency of the animal food production chain in an
  overpopulated and underfed world;
● the relative cheapness of the ingredients of vegetarian diet;
and
● the possible unhealthiness of eating meat that contains crop
  pesticides, antibiotics and hormones given to the animals and
  that has been processed in many ways that are not
  necessarily hygienic or beneficial.
● the slaughter of animals is cruel and debasing, and that
  vegetarianism is part of a more peaceful and harmonious life.
A person who chooses to give up meat must be careful that his
diet still provides enough of the right nutrients. Protein,
vitamins D and B12, iron and calcium must be planned for but
there is no problem with:
● healthy carbohydrates (grains, cereal products, potatoes,
  fruits);
● fats (vegetable oils, dairy products, nuts, margarine); and
● minerals and most vitamins (vegetables and fruits).

7

Diet Planning

Protein is readily available from eggs and dairy produce, nuts,
soybeans, raisins, grains and pulses. But a vegetarian should
be sure to get a good selection of essential amino acids at each
meal. This is not difficult where eggs or dairy produce are
eaten: cereal and milk, bread and milk, and bread and eggs are
all good amino acid combinations. But vegans must depend on
soyabeans, or on carefully planned vegetable combinations.
These include: lentil soup and hard wholewheat bread; and
beans and rice -1½ cups of beans to 4 of rice have protien
equivalent to ¾lb (340 g) steak.

Vitamins requiring particular attention in a vegetarian diet are:

- cobalamin (vitamin B12) – available from dairy produce and yeast and particularly useful for vegans, in synthetic form;
- vitamin D – also needed in synthetic form by vegans where sunlight is insufficient.

Iron and calcium are also worth mentioning, as they are sometimes lacking even in diets of meat-eaters. In fact, there are many excellent vegetarian sources.

Iron is found in raisins, lentils, wheat germ, prunes, spinach and other leafy vegetables, and in bread, eggs and yeast.

Calcium occurs in dairy produce, dried fruit, soybeans, sesame seeds and in leafy vegetables.

Eating Disorders

Anorexia nervosa

True anorexia nervosa has been described as the 'willful pursuit of thinness through self-starvation'.

Symptoms and behavior

Dieting begins because the anorexic either is or believes himself to be overweight. It develops into a morbid fear of fatness and continues to the point of extreme emaciation (rarely recognized by the anorexic).

Background and causes

Anorexia nervosa and its causes are highly complex. It is often associated with preexisting stresses, such as tensions within the family, academic pressures, or sexual abuse in childhood. The anorexic may feel that he lacks control over anything except his body.

Many anorexics suffer from an overwhelming sense of ineffectiveness. Continuous starvation and refusal of food represents a gesture of independence, possibly from an overdominant parent, while slimness is seen as desirable.

Self Image

All people have a distorted view of their own body proportions, but whereas the normal person underestimates face, chest and hip size, while slightly overestimating waist size, the anorexic grossly overestimates each of these sizes when severely emaciated.

Bulimia Nervosa

This illness is characterized by bouts of grossly excessive eating ('bingeing'), usually of any food available, followed by self-induced purging through vomiting or laxatives. (In a related form, known as 'exercise bulimia', excessive exercise is used instead of purging to burn off calories.)
Bulimia may coexist with anorexia nervosa and can endanger long-term health, although it is not likely to be fatal. The root causes and treatment are similar for both bulimia and anorexia.

Treatment

Treatment for anorexia and bulimia has moved away from techniques such as enforced bedrest and drug therapy. Most treatments involve pressure to eat until a specific weight is reached, or strong encouragement to reach weight-gain targets, but these are accompanied by counseling or psychotherapy.

Compulsive Eating

The obesity that results from compulsive eating can cause considerable distress. Many people indulge in occasional bouts of 'stuffing', but these are rarely significant. The compulsive eater, however, is addicted to food. He may use it to relieve feelings of stress, loneliness, isolation, frustration, dissatisfaction or boredom. He may use it to comfort himself if he feels guilty, depressed or unattractive. Overeating – a secret and solitary activity – needs handling with sensitivity and understanding. To help overcome the problem, avoid being alone for longer than necessary, ensure that only low-calorie snacks are kept in the house, and seek diversion in physical activity when the craving for food starts. Severe cases often need clinical help. Reasons for compulsive eating vary, but the vicious circle illustrated here is common to many. In self-help groups and 12-step groups such as Overeaters Anonymous, participants explore their self-image and attitudes to food and their bodies, and many find their own way to recovery. Compulsive eaters should keep a food diary to pinpoint when binges are likely to occur, so that avoidance measures can be taken.

7

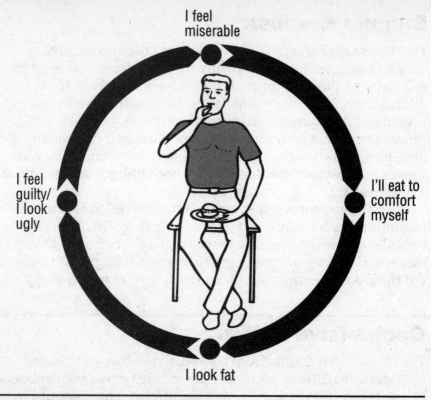

I feel
miserable

I feel
guilty/
I look
ugly

I'll eat to
comfort
myself

I look fat

Compulsive Dieting

Compulsive dieting, like anorexia and compulsive eating, is a disorder related to self-image. Often the image is distorted, as in anorexia. Sometimes the act of dieting itself becomes a crutch or a reaction to stress or disappointment. Although it is unlikely to be fatal, compulsive dieting can be harmful. Evidence is growing to show that prolonged or repeated low-calorie dieting merely alters the body's metabolism, slowing it down and making it more energy efficient. When dieting stops, the body has a greater tendency to store fat than it did before. Worse, in a very low calorie-restricted diet or fast, weight loss will consist largely of lean tissue such as muscle. Hunger pangs may lead to bingeing on fatty, unhealthy foods and to eating disorders.

Why People Put on Weight

Overweight is always caused by taking in more food energy than the body uses up. The bulk of food energy is taken in in the form of carbohydrates and fats. Both these supply calories (the measure of energy); and both are converted to fat deposits if the calories they supply are more than the body uses. The diagram shows what happens to the food energy input.

- Most of it is used to supply body energy needs – to maintain basic life processes and for all physical activity (see pp 300-1).
- It is still the subject of scientific controversy, but it does seem that some people get rid of surplus input because their bodies automatically speed up their metabolism and burn up the surplus rather than store it. This burning up process is called 'thermogenesis'. Also, there is a rise in the body's metabolism after every meal. So two people may eat exactly the same, but one will burn up more than the other if the food is taken in several small meals rather than two or three large ones.
- Food energy that is neither needed nor burned up is stored by the body in the form of fat. In overweight people the store far exceeds any normal future demand.

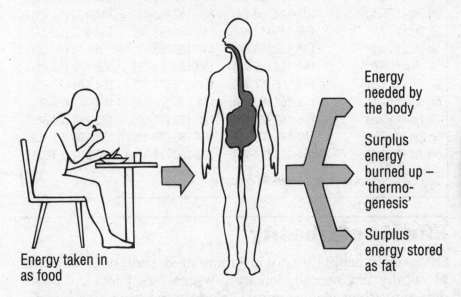

Energy taken in as food

Energy needed by the body

Surplus energy burned up – 'thermo-genesis'

Surplus energy stored as fat

7

Are You Overweight?

It is not always easy to say whether a person is overweight. But there is no doubt that weight problems are on the increase in modern industrial society.

One way of learning whether you are among the overweight is to check your weight against a desirable weight table – such as the one given in p 316. (Note that 'desirable' weight tables give lower figures than 'average' weight tables – in a society where more people are overweight than underweight, the average will be higher than is healthy.)

Even without weighing yourself, it is possible to do a quick check for overweight. Start by asking yourself the following questions. Do you have any telltale bulges? Do you look much fatter than you used to? Have your measurements increased appreciably? If you pinch your upper arm, thigh or midriff, is there more than 1in (2.5cm) of flesh between your thumb and forefinger?

Desirable weights (in lbs/kg for men 25 and over, in indoor clothing

Height in bare feet	Small frame	Medium frame	Large frame
5ft 1in (1.54m)	112-120 (51-54)	118-129 (54-59)	126-141 (57-64)
5ft 2in (1.57m)	115-123 (52-56)	121-133 (55-60)	129-144 (59-59)
5ft 3in (1.60m)	118-126 (54-57)	124-136 (56-62)	132-148 (60-67)
5ft 4in (1.62m)	121-129 (55-59)	127-139 (58-63)	135-152 (61-69)
5ft 5in (1.65m)	124-133 (56-60)	130-143 (59-65)	138-156 (63-71)
5ft 6in (1.67m)	128-137 (58-62)	134-147 (61-67)	142-161 (65-73)
5ft 7in (1.70m)	132-141 (60-64)	138-152 (63-69)	147-166 (67-75)
5ft 8in (1.72m)	136-145 (62-66)	142-156 (65-71)	151-170 (69-77)
5ft 9in (1.75m)	140-150 (64-68)	146-160 (66-73)	155-174 (70-79)
5ft 10in (1.77m)	144-154 (65-70)	150-165 (68-75)	159-179 (72-81)
5ft 11in (1.80m)	148-158 (67-72)	154-170 (70-77)	164-184 (74-83)
6ft 0in (1.82m)	152-162 (69-73)	158-175 (72-79)	168-189 (76-86)
6ft 1in (1.85m)	156-167 (71-76)	162-180 (73-82)	173-194 (78-88)
6ft 2in (1.87m)	160-171 (73-78)	167-185 (76-84)	178-199 (81-90)
6ft 3in (1.90m)	164-175 (74-79)	172-190 (78-86)	182-204 (83-93)

Source: Metropolitan Life Insurance Company.

Effects of Obesity

Overweight people are not just more tired, short of breath, and physically and mentally lethargic, with aching joints and poor digestion. They are also more likely to suffer from high blood pressure, heart disease, diabetes, kidney disorders, cirrhosis of the liver, pneumonia, inflammation of the gall bladder, arthritis, hernias and varicose veins. They have more accidents, are more likely to die during operations, and have higher rates of mortality in general (including three times the mortality from heart and circulatory disease). Someone who weighs 185lb (84kg) when he should weigh 140lb (63.5 kg) has his life expectancy shortened by 4 years. Some of these effects arise from mechanical causes: the burden of extra weight and its particular location as fat deposits. Others arise chemically, from the need to supply more body tissue than normal.

Appetite

Most people have an effective appetite control, or 'appestat', which prevents them from putting on too much weight. The appestat is remarkably precise. For example, eating an extra half slice of bread a day (30 calories) above energy output would bring a weight gain of 110lbs (50kg) over a 40-year period. The appestat normally protects people against this type of weight gain.

However, some people ignore the messages from their appestats, for a number of reasons:

● social habit or custom;
● excessive love of food in general or of certain foods ;
● habits of overeating acquired during childhood;
● lack of exercise;
● eating for psychological support.

Some people put on weight because their appestat is put out of action by an excessively sedentary existence. When physical activity falls below moderate levels, research has shown that appetite may increase – even though the body has no need for the extra food. Increasing the amount of exercise increases calorie output and puts the appestat back into good working order. However, exercise above moderate levels increases the appetite.

Losing Weight

7

Losing weight involves permanently changing lifestyle by learning how to control eating habits and change exercise patterns. Many people find this very difficult, and it demands discipline, patience and a change in attitudes.

Before you start:

● discuss your intentions with your physician, who will help you plan your diet and support you in your efforts.
● do not be tempted by any promise of easy weight loss. There is none.
● aim to lose weight steadily over a period at a rate of no more than 2lbs (1kg) per week, until you reach your target.
● make an exercise plan along with your diet plan.

Weight loss plan

Your physician will give you a meal-by-meal diet planner if you feel you need one, but following general guidelines is equally effective:

1 Cut down on fat in your diet:
- substitute skimmed milk for whole milk; buy margarine that is high in polyunsaturates and low in saturates.
- buy lean meat, especially white meat, or fish instead of pork or red meat. Cut any skin or fat off the meat you buy,
- steam or grill your food. Do not fry it.
- substitute dressings for rich sauces.

2 Cut down on sugars:
- have sweeteners in hot drinks instead of sugar. Try cooking using sweeteners instead of sugars.
- eat fruit and nuts instead of sweets, cakes and chocolates.
- buy wholewheat bread, brown rice, wholewheat pastas, to cut down on refined carbohydrates.

3 Enjoy your mealtimes:
- eat small meals frequently. Allow yourself time to relax and enjoy your food, with a rest afterwards.
- build small snacks into your diet. Stop and enjoy them.

4 Dealing sensibly with cravings:
- if you find yourself craving for cream or chocolate, allow yourself a small ration at an appropriate time
- if possible, try to distract yourself from a craving by going out, getting some exercise, or doing something different from what you usually do at that time.

5 Work at changing your eating and exercise habits, and your lifestyle, instead of becoming obsessed with your diet. Joining a slimming club gives many dieters support and a valuable social boost.

Slimming Aids

There is always a great variety of slimming aids on the market, not all effective or recommended:
- substitute meals (wafers, chocolate bars, packaged foods, etc.) have a stated calorie content and sometimes contain cellulose to give a full feeling. Some slimmers find them useful, but they do nothing to encourage the eating habits needed to stay slim.
- low-calorie, low fat substitute foods and drinks, such as skim milk, slimmers' bread, and crispbread, can help slimmers reduce total calorie intake.
- proprietary slimming pills are often suspect. Some claim to suppress appetite, but the amounts are so small that their effectiveness is questionable.

- saunas, Turkish baths, and reducing garments cause loss of body water through sweating. This can reduce measurements and weight, but the effect is rapidly cancelled out by the drinking needed to replace the fluid loss.
- vibrator belts and other massagers are meant to break down fat deposits, but there is little evidence to support their claims.

Exercise

Regular, progressively more difficult exercise will tone muscles, make you generally fitter, and help to keep your willpower strong. Exercise is an important accompaniment to slimming, but may not on its own enable you to lose weight.

Diets

Never fall for the claims of fad diets. Many are dangerous. A number of readily available diets can be useful: but always bear in mind that fats, not carbohydrates, provide the most energy, and that cutting down on fats is more efficient than cutting down on carbohydrates:

- Low-calorie plans set a numerical limit to daily calorie intake (usually 1000 to 1500 calories). Calorie tables make it easy to calculate the energy content of a meal.
- No-count plans, simplified versions of the low-carbohydrate system, divide food into three categories: high-carbohydrate food that must be avoided; high-calorie, non carbohydrate food that can be eaten in moderation; and unrestricted food.
- Liquid diets have been developed that provide approximately 330 calories per day. As calorie intake is under 1000 calories per day, these diets should only be followed for brief or intermittent periods, and under medical supervision.
- Machines using electric impulses to relax and contract muscles are recommended by some slimmers.
- Liposuction is an option; many plastic surgeons now practice this technique of removing unwanted body fat.
- Exercise will not on its own make much difference to your weight. It would, for example, take 12 hours of tennis to lose 1lb of fat. Exercise does, however, increase the sense of well-being that dieting brings.
- Attending a support group such as Overeaters' Anonymous can be an effective, though expensive, way of getting slim, and can give an invaluable psychological boost.

7

Excluding Meat

A vegetarian is a person who does not eat the meat of any mammal, bird, or fish. There are two main types of vegetarian:
● vegans, who eat nothing at all of animal origins, and
● lacto-ovo-vegetarians, who do allow themselves animal products such as milk, cheese, eggs and honey.
There are also people who call themselves vegetarians but do eat fish.

Reasons for vegetarianism

Reasons for vegetarianism vary from society to society and individual to individual. It has been advocated for religious, philosophical, moral, economic and health reasons. It has also been adopted as a necessity. Many peoples have lived on a diet of fruit, nuts and berries, with meat only when it could be obtained.

Perhaps the most powerful arguments for vegetarianism in modern society are:
● the inefficiency of the animal food production chain (see p 281) in a largely underfed world;
● the relative cheapness of the ingredients of vegetarian diet; and
● the possible unhealthiness of eating meat that contains crop pesticides and antibiotics and hormones given to the animals, and that has been processed in many ways that are not necessarily hygienic or beneficial.

Also, many people feel that the slaughter of animals is cruel and debasing, and that vegetarianism is part of a more peaceful and harmonious way of life.

Vegetarian diet

Despite the claims of some vegetarians, there is no established evidence that eating meat is unhealthy in itself. But it is certainly as possible for a vegetarian to be healthy, strong and long-lived as it is for a meat-eater.

A person who chooses to give up meat must be careful that his diet still provides enough of the right nutrients.
There are no problems with:
● healthy carbohydrates (grains, cereal products, potatoes, fruits);
● fats (vegetable oils, dairy products, nuts, margarine); and
● minerals and most vitamins (vegetables and fruits).
Obtaining an adequate supply of protein and certain vitamins can, however, be more problematic for vegetarians than for meat-eaters (see below).
Vegetarians must take particular care that their diet provides

them with adequate supplies of the following nutrients.
Protein is readily available from eggs and dairy produce,
nuts, soybeans, raisins, grains and pulses. But a vegetarian
should be sure to get a good selection of essential amino acids
at each meal.
This is not difficult where eggs or dairy produce are eaten:
cereal and milk, bread and milk, and bread and eggs are all
good amino acid combinations. But vegans must depend on
soybeans, or on carefully planned vegetable combinations.
These include: lentil soup and hard wholewheat bread; and
beans and rice.
Vitamins requiring particular attention in a vegetarian diet
are:
● cobalamin (vitamin B12) – available from dairy produce and
   yeast and, particularly useful for vegans, in synthetic form;
● vitamin D – also needed in synthetic form by vegans where
   sunlight is insufficient.
Iron and calcium are also worth mentioning, as they are
sometimes lacking even in the diets of meat-eaters. In fact,
there are many excellent vegetarian sources.
Iron is found in raisins, lentils, wheat germ, prunes, spinach
and other leafy vegetables, and in bread, eggs and yeast.
Calcium occurs in dairy produce, dried fruit, soybeans, sesame
seeds, and in leafy vegetables.

Nutritional Medicine

7

Nutritional medicine, also called nutrition therapy, is in some
ways related to naturopathic healing techniques. Naturopathy
aims to help the body assert its own powers of healing in the
face of disease; nutritional medicine emphasizes the role of
healthy eating habits as an essential part of this process. Many
of the dietary principles propounded by naturopaths agree
with traditional medical thinking: both agree on the
harmfulness of eating large amounts of fats and refined
carbohydrates. However, nutritional therapists think that
many ailments are provoked by poisonous or allergy-
producing substances in a normal diet; they may recommend
supplements of vitamins, minerals and other substances,
calculated on individual requirements. Treatment with
supplements should always be under the guidance of a trained
practitioner. Attention to diet has proved beneficial for all
manner of ailments.

DRUGS

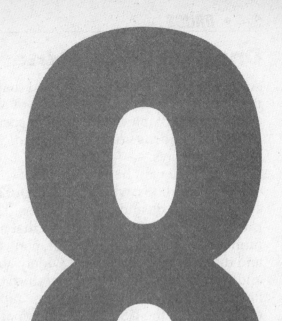

8

Drugs and Drug Abuse

A drug is any chemical compound that can affect the body's functioning. Drug abuse is the use of any drug for any purpose that is unacceptable for medical or social reasons. This includes the misuse of drugs obtained in medically or socially acceptable ways.

Especially relevant here are psychoactive drugs: those having effects on the body which bring about behavioral changes, such as euphoria and hallucinations. The use and often the production of many of the drugs that are abused by large numbers of people are illegal in many countries, but alcohol and tobacco, two of the most widely abused drugs, are legally and widely available. However, since the dangers of smoking have been proved, the habit is now rapidly becoming socially unaccepted in the US, the UK, and many Western countries.

Reasons for Drug Abuse

There are many reasons for drug abuse, including:

Social conformity If the use of a drug is accepted in a group to which a person belongs or with which he identifies, he will feel a need to use the drug to show that he belongs to the group. This is true of all drugs, from nicotine and alcohol to heroin.

Pleasure One of the main reasons people take drugs is to induce pleasant feelings, ranging from well-being and relaxation to mystical euphoria.

Availability Illegal use is highest where there is a ready supply – such as large cities. Legal drug use also increases with availability: for example, alcoholism is common in the liquor trade.

Curiosity about drugs and why people take them can start people taking drugs.

Alienation Drug use may seem a valid symbol of opposition to the values of society. When a person rejects society and all alternatives, including himself, his hopes and his goals, the resulting feelings of meaninglessness, isolation, and inadequacy will predispose him to chronic drug abuse.

Affluence and leisure can result in boredom and loss of interest in life, so that drugs can seem to supply stimulation and escape.

Escape from psychic stress Most people manage to get along without letting life's more stressful events overwhelm them, but others react by seeking refuge in a form of dependence. Drugs often become a false center around which their lives revolve.

Men and Drugs

The traditional male roles of competitor and breadwinner, and the qualities expected of men – strength, self-reliance, dependability, control over personal emotions – necessitate suppressing personal feelings and human qualities, and so cause stress. Add to this life's flashpoints: puberty, examinations, cohabitation, loss of partner, work, threatened job or business, marriage, parenthood, and so on, and the tendency of some people to develop dependence on drugs – legal or illegal – becomes very understandable.

Now, more relaxed attitudes to sexual roles, and closer relationships between men and women are giving more and more men the opportunity to explore their emotional sensitivities. The ideas of modern writers, such as the American poet Robert Bly, have encouraged men in the US to form groups, in which they explore their roles, behavior, and relationships. Men's groups are now becoming common in Great Britain and other European countries. They can give positive support which, during stressful periods of life, can help to provide an alternative to dependence on harmful drugs.

What is Addiction?

'Addiction' has become a general term, covering several forms of dependence:

Tolerance of a drug increases as the body gets used to it. The quantity of the drug the body needs to produce the original effects increases as tolerance increases.

Dependence is the term used to describe the state in which the body has become used to functioning under the influence of a drug. When the drug is withdrawn, the user experiences extreme discomfort, called withdrawal symptoms.

Psychological dependence is popularly thought to be the need or compulsive desire to continue using a drug, whether or not there is physical dependence. However, it is unsafe to say that any drug does not cause physical addiction. A person may become addicted to an apparently non-addictive drug after very long-term use, or use under a specific set of circumstances. For example, there are reports of mild addiction

8

to marijuana after regular use in the evenings for a number of years, resulting in chronic insomnia after withdrawal. The physiology of addiction is not understood, but there have been important breakthroughs in understanding how the body may become tolerant to psychoactive drugs (drugs that affect the brain and perception).

The Mechanism of Drug Tolerance

Many psychoactive drugs are chemically similar to neurotransmitters – the substances released by nerve endings when stimulated by an impulse. Neurotransmitters interact

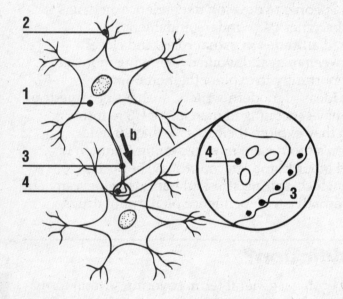

1 Neuron
2 Dendrite
3 Axon
4 Synapse
5 Receptor
b Direction of impulse

1 Before drug: natural neurotransmitter activates 50% of receptors
2 Drug is taken:
All receptors activated Drug-taker experiences euphoric state

3 Drug wears off
Feedback of natural neurotransmitter-releasing neurons is inhibited 50% of receptors activated Euphoria decreases

4 Increased drug dose
All receptors activated Drug taker experiences euphoric state
Inhibition of natural neurotransmitter-releasing neurons

 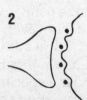 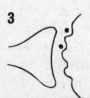 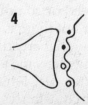

with receptors – sensory nerve endings which can receive impulses and respond to them. Serotonin and the endorphins are neurotransmitters. They control mood, emotion and hormone function, and inhibit pain.

It is thought that psychoactive drugs enhance the effects of these natural neurotransmitters, producing an increased response from their receptors (the 'high'). Feedback then causes less of the natural neurotransmitter to be released. If a drug is taken repeatedly, release of the neurotransmitter is inhibited, so the drug no longer enhances its effect. More and more of the drug is then needed to achieve the same 'high'. Withdrawal of the drug results in unpleasant physical effects, since the natural neurotransmitter does not begin to be released again for some days, during which the body is without either the drug or the neurotransmitter.

What Psychoactive Drugs Do

Some drugs inhibit and other drugs stimulate nervous activity in the brain, which is the reason for their different mental effects. Other reasons include the amount of the drug taken, its purity and concentration, and how it enters the body. The mental and physical state of the consumer, his expectations and reaction to his environment are other factors: a drug may heighten an existing psychic state or release a suppressed one. The effects are likely to be enhanced if the consumer is tired or has an empty stomach.

The Depressants

Psychoactive drugs fall into four main categories, according to their effects: depressants; stimulants; hallucinogens; and marijuana. Alcohol is one of the depressants.

Alcohol: The Chemical and the Drink

Alcohols are volatile, colorless, pungent liquids, composed of three chemical elements: carbon, hydrogen, and oxygen.

Ethyl alcohol (ethanol) is the type taken in alcoholic drinks. It may also be prescribed medically, to stimulate the appetite, or form a medicinal base in which other ingredients are dissolved.

Methyl alcohol (methanol, or 'wood alcohol') is used

commercially as a fuel and solvent. It is poisonous, and
drinking it causes blindness and death.

Alcoholic drinks

In the domestic and industrial production of alcoholic drinks,
ethyl alcohol is produced by 'fermentation', that is, the
degencration of a starch (such as maize, barley, rice, potatoes,
grapes) by bacterial action. The drink that results depends on
the starch used (e.g. malt and barley give beer and grapes give
wine). Beers and wines are produced by fermentation alone.
Only about a 15% level of alcohol is possible by this method.
'Spirits', with their higher alcoholic level (whisky, gin, vodka
liqueurs, etc) also require 'distillation'. That is, the alcohol is
evaporated off, leaving water behind, and resulting in a higher
alcoholic concentration in the eventual liquid. Distilled alcohol
may also be added to wines (sherry, port, etc) and beers to
strengthen them.

Men and Alcohol

Moderate drinking of alcohol is not harmful to health.
Statistics show that drinking moderate amounts of alcohol can
have a beneficial effect on the heart, and appears to prolong
life. However, alcohol affects the brain so never drink and
drive.

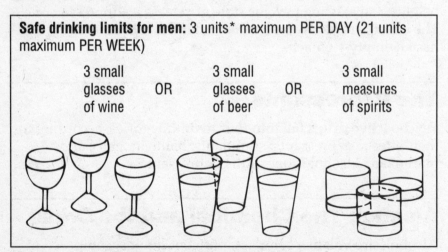

Safe drinking limits for men: 3 units* maximum PER DAY (21 units maximum PER WEEK)

| 3 small glasses of wine | OR | 3 small glasses of beer | OR | 3 small measures of spirits |

Excessive drinking causes social embarrassment,
hangovers, and inefficiency at work in the short term; in the
long term it causes irreversible liver damage, loss of memory
and a decline in mental functioning, insomnia, slowed reflexes
with a consequent increased danger of accidents, and
impairment of judgement and emotional control. Although

men's physical tolerance of alcohol is greater than that of
women, male alcoholics have a higher risk than normal of liver
damage, of developing many cancers, and of malfunctions in
the immune system.

Alcohol in the Body

About 20% of any alcohol drunk is absorbed in the stomach,
and 80% in the intestines. It is then carried around the body by
the bloodstream. The liver breaks down (oxidizes) the alcohol
at an almost constant rate: usually about $2^1/_2$ bottles (1 pint) of
beer or 1oz (29.6cc) of whisky per hour. This process
eventually disposes of about 90% of the alcohol, forming
carbon dioxide and water as end products. The remaining 10%
is eliminated through the lungs and in the sweat. Alcohol in
the body has four main effects:

1 It provides energy (alcohol has high calorific value, but
contains no nutrients).
2 It acts as an anesthetic on the central nervous system,
slowing it down and impairing its efficiency.
3 It stimulates urine production. With heavy alcohol intake, the
body loses more water than is taken in, and the body cells
become dehydrated.
4 It puts part of the liver temporarily out of action. After heavy
drinking, as much as two-thirds of the liver can be
nonfunctioning – but it is usually fully recovered within a
few days.

Blood Alcohol Level

8

The effect of alcohol on behavior depends on the amount
reaching the brain via the bloodstream. This 'blood alcohol
level' is determined by several factors, apart from the quantity
of alcohol drunk.

● The size of the liver decides the rate of oxidation and
elimination.
● The size of the person decides the amount of blood in the
system because blood volume is proportionate to size. The
larger the person the greater the diluting effect of the blood
on the alcohol consumed and the more it takes to produce the
same effect.
● The speed and manner which the alcohol is consumed is
important. The longer one takes to drink a given quantity,
the less effect it has.

● Alcohol consumed on an empty stomach will have a greater and more immediate effect than that consumed during or after eating. Food acts as a buffer to absorption.

What's Your Poison?

Commercially, the strength of an alcoholic beverage is expressed as so many 'degrees proof'. This describes the liquid's specific gravity, not the percentage of alcohol it contains. National proof measurement regulations vary. In the US., the percentage of alcohol is half the specific gravity. For example, a spirit that is 100 proof (written '100°') contains 50% alcohol. Most aperitifs contain 25% alcohol. The bottles in the chart are arranged in order of increasing percentage alcohol.

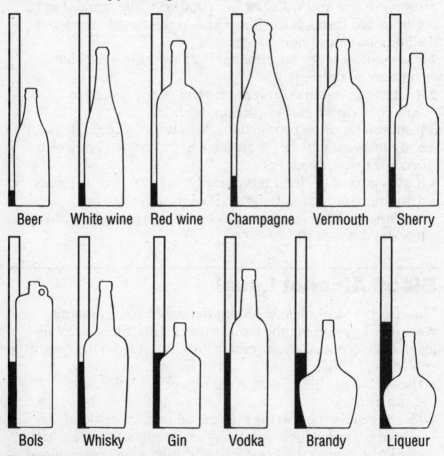

| Beer | White wine | Red wine | Champagne | Vermouth | Sherry |

| Bols | Whisky | Gin | Vodka | Brandy | Liqueur |

Typical alcohol contents

Beer and lager	up to 8%
White wine, Red wine, Champagne	9-15%
Vermouth, Sherry	20%
Whisky, Gin, Vodka, Bols, Brandy, Liqueurs	40-50%

Drinking and Driving

The behavioral effects of alcohol make drinking and driving
very dangerous, both to the drinker and to others. Tests have
shown that errors of judgement and control increase as soon as
there is any alcohol in the bloodstream. Many countries
prescribe a legal limit to the blood alcohol level of anyone in
charge of a vehicle. In the US this varies from 10 to 15mg/dl; in
Utah it is 8mg/dl; Iowa, New Mexico and Texas have no
restrictions. European countries vary from 5mg/dl
(Scandinavia) to 8 mg/dl (UK). In Australia it is 150mg/dl.

Drink Equivalents

If we assume a person of average size (150lbs or about 10
stone/68kg), drinking at an average rate on an empty stomach,
any of the following would give a blood alcohol level of 30
milligrams per deciliter:

1 24 oz or 2 bottles
US beer
2 ¾ pint UK beer
3 5½ oz or just
under 1 glass
table wine
4 3½ oz or just over
½ glass sherry
or fortified wine
5 1½ oz or about 1
measure spirits

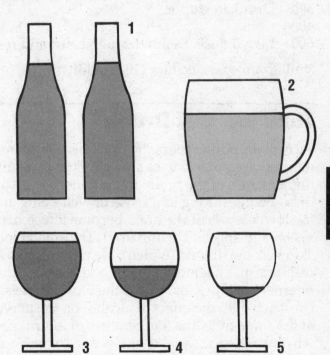

8

Behavioral Effects

As the level of alcohol in the blood rises, the drinker's brain and nervous system are increasingly affected, and his behavior changes:

mg/dl*

20	Sense of warmth, friendliness. Visual reaction time slows.
40	Impaired driving ability at speed.
60	Sense of mental relaxation and general well-being. Further slight decrease in skills.
90	Exaggerated emotions and behavior. Tendency to be loud and talkative. Loss of inhibitory control. Sensory and motor nerves increasingly dulled.
120	Staggering. Fumbling with words.
150	Intoxication.
200	Incapacitation, depression, nausea, loss of sphincter control.
300	Drunken stupor.
400	Coma.
600+	Lethal dose. Death through heart and respiratory failure.

*milligrams per deciliter (100 milliliters)

How We Get Drunk

As consumption occurs the transmission of impulses in the nervous system becomes slowed. First to be affected are the higher levels of the brain: inhibitions, worry and anxiety are dissolved, resulting in a sense of well-being and euphoria. As the lower levels of the brain become affected, co-ordination, vision and speech are impaired. The small blood vessels of the skin become dilated (widen). Heat is radiated and the drinker feels warm. This means that blood has been diverted from the internal body organs, where the blood vessels are already constricted by the effect of alcohol on the nervous system. So, at the same time, the temperature of internal body organs falls. Any increase in sexual desire is due to the depression of the usual inhibitions. Physical sexuality is more and more impaired as blood alcohol level rises. Eventually, the poisoning effect of excess alcohol causes nausea and possible vomiting.

Hangover

A hangover is the physical discomfort that follows the consumption of too much alcohol. Symptoms can include headache, upset stomach, thirst, dizziness and irritability. Three processes produce the hangover. First, the stomach lining is irritated by the excessive alcohol, and its functioning is disrupted. Second, cell dehydration occurs because the quantity of alcohol consumed exceeds the liver's ability to process it, leaving a prolonged level of alcohol in the blood. Third, the level of alcohol has a 'shock' effect on the nervous system, from which it needs time to recover.

Avoidance

The best way to avoid a hangover is not to drink too much. But there is less likelihood of a hangover if the alcohol is taken with meals: consumption and absorption are spread over a greater period of time, and the food acts as a barrier. Non-alcoholic drinks taken at the same time or afterwards, dilute the alcohol; and there is usually less of an after-effect when alcohol is consumed in relaxed surroundings, and when cigarette smoking is cut to a minimum.

Treatment

The stomach is relieved by a fresh lining: milk, raw eggs, or simply a good breakfast! Only then should aspirin or other pain relievers be taken to help the headache. The danger of stomach irritation from pain-relieving drugs is always much worse when the stomach is empty. Citrus fruit juices, honey, and vitamin C are all known to contain an 'anti-hangover factor'. Fizzy drinks may have a soothing effect upon the stomach. Liquids of any sort help the dehydrated cells recover their fluid content. Coffee or tea can be used to clear the head (the caffeine content stimulates the nervous system) and sugar can be taken to provide energy; but both these may leave the sufferer feeling worse when the immediate effects wear off. Similarly, for temporary relief, another alcoholic drink (in moderation) invigorates the sluggish nervous system and seems to dispel the unpleasant after-effects. But this is only a postponement: the original hangover and that of the extra alcohol, still await!

8

Alcohol and the Law

Chemically, alcohol is one of the most dangerous drugs known to man. But, over centuries of experience, society has managed to develop cultural attitudes which allow alcohol to be available without it causing too great disruption or harm. Most countries have a minimum age for its purchase, restrict the number of hours of the day during which it can be sold, control the number, ownership, and location of bars and liquor stores, and keep up strict observation of their orderliness. Liquor laws vary by state, county, municipality, and even town. In most cases, the minimum age for purchasing alcohol, or drinking it in bars, is 21. 'Open container' laws prohibit the consumption of any alcoholic beverage in the street or in a vehicle. In some Midwest states 'blue laws' restrict the sale of alcohol on Sundays. Local laws against driving while intoxicated are becoming markedly stricter throughout the US.

Alcoholism

Alcoholism is the regular, compulsive drinking of large quantities of alcohol over a long period. It is the most serious drug addiction today, involving between 1% and 5% of the population of most countries. An alcoholic's drinking is compulsive, in response to psychological or physical dependence.
Anyone can become an alcoholic. However, studies have shown that the children of alcoholics run 4 to 6 times the risk of becoming addicted to alcohol as the children of non-alcoholics.
It is estimated that more than two-thirds of alcoholics are men. Case studies show that alcoholism is often part of a general picture of depressive illness. Many alcoholics have emotional problems stemming from disturbed childhoods, often typified by the loss, absence or inadequacy of one or both parents.

Stages in alcoholism

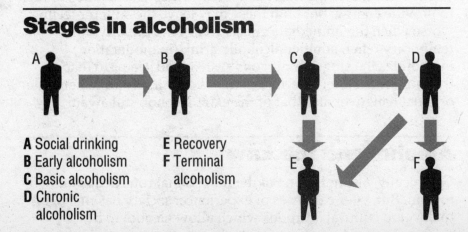

A Social drinking
B Early alcoholism
C Basic alcoholism
D Chronic
   alcoholism
E Recovery
F Terminal
   alcoholism

- **Social drinking** can lead to alcoholism: because a drinker begins to turn to alcohol for relief from stress ('symptomatic drinking'), or because his social drinking is so heavy that the beginnings of dependence are not noticed ('inveterate drinking').
- **Early alcoholism** is marked by the beginning of memory blackouts. Surreptitious drinking and the urgency of first drinks indicates increasing dependence. The drinker feels guilty, but cannot discuss the problem.
- **Basic alcoholism** The drinker can no longer stop unless forced by intoxication. He bolsters himself with excuses and grandiose behavior, but his promises and resolutions fail. He starts avoiding family and friends, and neglects food, interests, work and money. Physical deterioration sets in. Finally, tolerance for alcohol decreases.
- **Chronic alcoholism** is marked by further moral deterioration, irrational thought, vague fears, fantasies and psychotic behavior. Physical damage continues. The drinker has no alibis left and can no longer take any step to recovery for himself. Reaching this point may take from 5 to 25 years.
- **Recovery** usually depends on the alcoholic undergoing a treatment program. Psychologically, he regains the desire to be helped and thinks more rationally as a result. Ideally, he also develops hope, moral commitment, outside interests, self-respect and contentment in abstinence.
- **Terminal alcoholism** is the result if the alcoholic refuses treatment, or relapses after treatment. Irreversible mental and physical deterioration usually ends in death.

Physiological Effects of Alcoholism

8

The effects of alcoholism on the body include:
- **constant inflammation** of the stomach and later the intestines, with severe risk of ulceration.
- **malnutrition** and vitamin deficiency diseases, such as scurvy, pellagra and beriberi, caused by neglecting diet for drink.
- **cirrhosis of the liver:** the liver shrivels, its cells are largely replaced by fibrous tissues, and its function is impaired. Ten percent of chronic alcoholics have cirrhosis of the liver, and 75% of people with cirrhosis have an alcoholic history. There are few symptoms until the cirrhosis is fairly advanced, then the alcoholic complains of general ill health, loss of appetite, nausea, vomiting and digestive trouble. The toxic effects of alcohol are the cause of the condition.

- **alcoholic myopathy:** muscular degeneration resulting from alcoholism. Causes are disuse of the muscles, poor diet, and alcoholic damage to the nervous system. In **alcoholic cardiomyopathy**, the heart muscle is affected.
- **destruction of brain cells** and degeneration of the nervous system, sometimes resulting in pneumonia, heart or kidney failure, or organic psychosis.
- **delirium tremens** (the 'DTs') a condition of extreme excitement, mental confusion, anxiety, fever, trembling, rapid and irregular pulse, and hallucinations, which often occurs when a bout of heavy drinking is followed by a few day's abstention.

Tranquilizers

Depressants ('downers') reduce nervous activity. They include tranquilizers and the opiates. Taken in small doses, they have a sedative effect; in larger doses they bring on sleep. An overdose can kill: nervous activity is so reduced that vital functions, such as respiration are impaired and may cease.

Barbiturates

Drugs made from barbituric acid (nicknamed 'barbs' plus many other short-lived names) reduce the nervous impulses reaching the brain, and so have been provided to relieve anxiety and tension and induce sleep. Some have been used as anesthetics. Barbiturates vary in the immediacy and duration of their effect according to the rate at which they are metabolized and eliminated; e.g. Seconal is short-acting, Phenobarbital long-lasting. The barbiturates cause tolerance and physical dependence.

Symptoms of barbiturate use include drowsiness, restlessness, irritability, belligerence, irrational behavior, mental confusion, and impaired coordination and reflexes with staggering and slurred speech. The pupils constrict and sweating increases. The user experiences euphoria at first, then depression.

Withdrawal symptoms can be more severe than those of alcohol or heroin, and include irritability, restlessness, anxiety, insomnia, abdominal cramp, nausea and vomiting, tremors, hallucinations, severe convulsions and sometimes death.

An overdose (excessive amount) depresses the nervous system so much that unconsciousness results, followed in extreme cases by death from respiratory failure.

Types of abuse
Addicts are attracted by:
- the possibility of escaping from emotional stress through sedation.
- the feelings of euphoria on initial ingestion, when large amounts of the drug are tolerated.
- the ability of barbiturates to counteract the effects of stimulants. This cyclical use of 'uppers' and 'downers' can lead to dependence on both.

The common use of barbiturates to induce relaxation and sleep has resulted in the largest group of dependent people being the middle-aged, especially women who do not work outside the home. The same ready availability also makes the drug a common suicide weapon, while the combination of barbiturates' depressive effects with those of alcohol has brought many accidental deaths through taking barbiturates after heavy drinking.

Barbiturates

Drug	Description		Nickname
Amobarbital		Green/blue	'Blues', 'Blue devils'
Pentobarbital		Yellow	'Yellows', 'Nembies'
Secobarbital		Red	'Reds', 'Red devils', 'Red bird'
Tuinal		Red/blue	'Rainbows', 'Tooeys'
Thorazine		Orange	
Miltown		White	
Librium		Green/white	
Valium		Various	'Goofers'

8

Benzodiazepines
Because of their addictive effects, barbiturates have been largely replaced by benzodiazepine drugs, such as Valium (Diazepam) and Librium for the treatment of anxiety, tension and insomnia. They cause drowsiness, dizziness, and confusion, but an overdose is rarely fatal. They are habit-forming and should not be taken regularly for more than two weeks. Withdrawal should be gradual to avoid symptoms that may include extreme anxiety, sweating and sometimes seizures.

The Opiates

The opiates, opium and its derivative, heroin, are the archetypal 'hard' drugs – the drugs of addiction, but codeine and morphine, which are also derived from opium, are better known for their medical uses.

All depressants inhibit the central nervous system, impairing coordination, reflexes, etc. Opiates, particularly morphine, prevent pain signals being transmitted from sites called opiate receptors in the brain to the rest of the body. This action may cause initial excitement, as inhibitions are removed. In large doses, the opiates act on the pleasure centers of the hypothalamus, producing feelings of peace, contentment, safety and euphoria.

General symptoms of opiate use include loss of appetite, constipation, and constriction of the pupils of the eye. An overdose of an opiate is likely to cause convulsions, unconsciousness and death.

All opiates create tolerance and physical dependence. The symptoms of withdrawal from abusive use begin with stomach cramps, followed by diarrhea, nausea and vomiting, running eyes and nose, sweating, and trembling. These are accompanied by irritability and restlessness, insomnia, anxiety and panic, depression, confusion and an all-consuming desire for the drug.

Opium

Opium is the dried juice of the unripe seed capsules of the Indian poppy. The plant is cultivated in India, Persia, China and Turkey, and opium is prepared in either powder or liquid form. The poppy possesses its psychoactive powers only when grown in favorable conditions of climate and soil. Poppies produced in temperate climates have only a negligible effect. Opium is traditionally smoked, using pipes, but it can also be injected or taken orally.

Codeine

Codeine (methyl morphine) is the least effective of the opiates. It is white and crystalline in form and is often used with aspirin for treating headaches. Because of the inhibiting effect on nervous reflexes it shares with all opiates, it is used in many cough medicines, and sometimes in the treatment of diarrhea, since it reduces peristalsis (the automatic rhythmic contractions of the intestine). The risk of tolerance and abusive use are very small because of the large amounts necessary to produce pleasant effects.

Morphine

Morphine is the basis of all opiate action – it is opium's main active constituent. It was isolated from opium in 1805 and since then has been medically important as a painkiller. It is 10 times as strong as opium, and must be administered with great care to avoid tolerance and physical dependence.

Heroin

Heroin (diamorphine) was isolated in 1898. It is 3 times as strong as morphine, and has a quicker and more intense effect, though a shorter duration. Among drug takers it is often known as 'H', or 'smack'. In the USA it is not used medically. Its production, possession and use are all connected with drug abuse. A grayish-brown powder in its pure form, for retail purposes it is mixed with milk or baking powder. This results in a white coloring. The high cost of the drug, and its necessity to those who are dependent on it, account for the high crime rate associated with its users.

The powder may be sniffed but is usually injected – normally into a muscle when use begins, but then into a major vein ('mainlining') as tolerance develops. Mainlining gives more immediate and powerful effects. Constant injection into the same vein causes hardening and scarring of the tissue and eventual collapse of the vein. Unhygienic conditions and use of unsterilized needles can also cause infection, often resulting in sores, abscesses, hepatitis, jaundice, thrombosis and transmission of the HIV virus.

Almost immediately upon injection, intense feelings of euphoria and contentment envelop the user. The strength of these depends on the purity and strength of the heroin, and the psychological state of the user – the higher the previous tension and anxiety, the more powerful the subsequent feelings of pleasure and peace. It is the force of the initial pleasure that makes heroin more popular than morphine. Physical dependence on heroin is reached if one grain (60mg) of heroin is used in a period of up to two weeks. Withdrawal effects will then begin four to six hours after the effect of the last shot has worn off. These include intense abdominal cramps, diarrhea, vomiting, shivering, insomnia and restlessness. Heroin addicts also suffer from malnutrition and weight loss due to inadequate diet, impotence, infections such as hepatitis B and AIDS transmitted by sharing infected needles, and death from overdose.

8

Glue-sniffing

The fumes of adhesives, gasoline, nail varnish, lighter fuel, and paint-thinners are used to get a 'high'. Effects are very much like the effects of alcohol abuse: slurred speech, confusion, dizziness, hallucinations, and afterwards, a headache.
Sniffing glue is not illegal, but in several countries it is now an offense to sell solvents to anyone under 18 if the vendor believes they will be misused. School students are those most likely to abuse solvents 'for kicks' or out of boredom.
No evidence shows that solvent abuse causes direct permanent damage, but inhaling similar fumes daily in a factory sometimes results in damage to the liver and kidneys. A very real danger is the occurrence of an accident during intoxication.

Stimulants

These stimulate nervous activity, especially in the sympathetic nervous system, which mobilizes the body for action. So these drugs prolong activity and suppress the desire for sleep. They include nicotine, caffeine, the amphetamines and cocaine and its derivatives.

Nicotine

Nicotine is a poison extracted from the leaves of the tobacco plant, *Nicotiana*. An injection of 70mg (0.002oz) is enough to be fatal, but in the very small doses obtained by smoking cigarettes, it is a mild stimulant which acts on the sympathetic nervous system to increase the amount of adrenaline released into the blood. It is the substance in cigarette smoke responsible for causing addiction. It also increases the heart rate and raises the blood pressure by narrowing the small arteries.

Tobacco Consumption

Cigarettes account for the bulk of tobacco consumption. The tobacco they use is usually flue-cured. This gives a neutral cigarette smoke which is easily inhaled (i.e. taken down into the lungs).
Cigars are generally made of air-cured tobacco. The smoke is

more pungent and seldom inhaled (i.e. it only enters the mouth and perhaps the throat) but much of the nicotine content is absorbed through the linings of the mouth.

Pipe tobacco is generally air, sun, or fire-cured. It, too, is seldom inhaled, and there is only a small amount of nicotine absorption through the mouth.

Snuff is a powdered tobacco that is sniffed into the nostrils. Nicotine is absorbed through the linings of the nose, and some snuff probably passes down into the lungs.

Chewing Tobacco is a mixture of tobacco and molasses. Nicotine is absorbed through the mouth. With the spread of cigarette smoking after World War I, other forms of consumption declined, especially the taking of snuff and chewing tobacco. But recently, as the dangers of cigarette smoking have been recognized, there has been some slight rise in the relative proportion of cigar and pipe smokers.

Percentage of men smoking cigarettes in the US weight in lbs (kgs)

1965	51.9	**1987**	31.2
1974	43.1	**1990**	28.4
1979	37.5	**1991**	28.1
1983	36.1	**1992**	28.6
1985	32.6	**1993**	26.2

The Plant and Production

Tobacco comes from the plant *Nicotiana tabacum*, and is produced in about 80 different countries, giving a world total of 8000 million lb (3628 million kg) a year. Half this is from the US and China. After cultivation, tobacco is 'cured' (dried) in one of four ways. Air curing takes place in a barn provided with a steady circulation of air, and takes about six weeks. Sun-cured leaves are first exposed to the sun, and then undergo a similar process.

Fire-cured leaves are hung over wood fires, and come into direct contact with the smoke.

Flue-cured leaves are also cured by the heat of a fire, but do not come into contact with the smoke. The method of curing affects the finished product. For example, flue-cured tobacco has a lower nicotine content than other kinds, and instead contains 15 to 20% more sugar. It also affects the leaf color. Air-cured leaves are reddish brown, sun-cured rather darker, fire-cured simply dark brown, and flue-cured light brown to yellow.

8

Up to 90% of tobacco is flue-cured. After curing, the tobacco is left to mature, and then graded ready for manufacture. Grading is done by the size, color and texture of the leaf. Different grades are used for different products.

Smoking

Smoking has many ill-effects due to more than 3000 substances other than nicotine that are found in cigarettes. These substances and not nicotine are the cause of smoking-related cancers. However, its effects on the circulatory system encourage the build-up of fatty plaques inside blood vessels, which can result in heart disease and stroke. Inhaling nicotine in tobacco smoke irritates the bronchial passages in the lungs, causing breathlessness, bronchitis, emphysema (destruction of the alveoli, the sacs in the lungs through which oxygen passes into the bloodstream). Nicotine together with carcegenic products inhaled from cigarette smoke can combine to lower the quantity and quality of sperm a man produces. A man who smokes tends to produce fewer sperm and has larger numbers of damaged sperm. This can impair his fertility and increases the chances of conceiving a child with congenital abnormalities.

Tobacco Smoke

Tobacco smoke contains at least 300 different chemical compounds. These enter the lungs in the form of gases or solid particles. The solid particles condense to form a thick brown tar. (The inhaled smoke of 10,000 cigarettes, i.e. under 2 years' smoking at 15 cigarettes a day, yields about $^3/_8$lb of this tar.) It lines the passages down which the smoke travels, and collects in the lungs. The contents of tobacco smoke fall into five main categories.

Carcinogenic substances (i.e. those that induce the growth of cancer). There are at least 15 carcinogens in tobacco smoke, including certain hydrocarbons, benzpyrene, and perhaps a radioactive isotope of polonium.

Co-carcinogens, or cancer promoters, do not cause cancer themselves, but accelerate its production by the carcinogens. They include phenols and fatty acids.

Irritant substances disturb the bronchial passages, increasing mucus secretion but damaging the processes for expelling this mucus from the lungs. Many are also co-carcinogens.

Gases occur at dangerous levels in tobacco smoke. They include carbon monoxide at 400 times the level considered safe in industry, and hydrogen cyanide at 160 times the safe level.

Nicotine One cigarette contains 0.5 to 2.0mg, depending on how the tobacco was cured. How much of this is absorbed depends on the method of smoking. Inhalation can absorb as much as 90%, non-inhalation as little as 10%.

Filter-tip and low tar cigarettes 90% of all cigarettes sold are now filter-tipped. The filter removes many of the harmful substances from cigarette smoke. Low tar, low nicotine cigarettes with a good filter reduces the risk of mortality by some 16%. However, some filter-tipped cigarettes allow more of the poisonous gas, carbon monoxide, into the lungs.

Who Smokes Cigarettes

The chart below compares male and female smokers over various age groups.

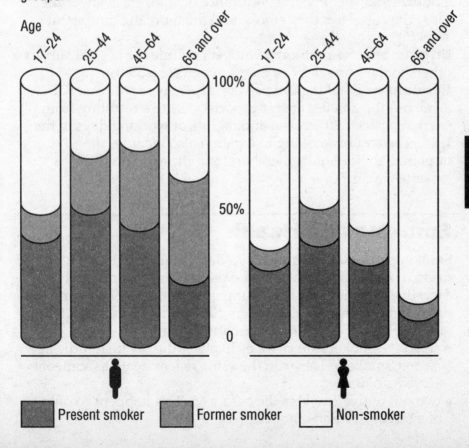

Present smoker   Former smoker   Non-smoker

Some Effects of Smoking

Dependence Smoking gives many smokers a comforting habit that helps them relax and avoid stress. For others, it is just a meaningless activity that cannot be stopped. Both cases result from the dependence that cigarettes create. Withdrawal symptoms on stopping smoking may include intense craving, depression, anxiety, instability, restlessness, sleep disturbance, difficulty in concentrating, altered time perception, sweating, drop in blood pressure and heart rate and gastro-intestinal changes. These symptoms seldom occur with any intensity, however: most people experience only very mild discomfort or none at all.

Accidents Smokers have four times more accidents than non-smokers. This may be due to a slowing of the reflex actions, lasting about 20 minutes, that follow smoking a cigarette. (It may also be linked with differences between the kind of people who become smokers and those who do not.) Smokers also run a higher risk of death or injury by fire – the most common cause being smoking in bed.

Endurance The physical endurance of smokers is lower the more the cigarettes they smoke and the more the time spent smoking.

Effects on non-smokers Smokers pollute the air and subject others to the same risks as themselves. (see p 350).

Economics Smoking can be very expensive on a personal level, but the greatest cost is to society. Illness resulting from smoking causes 20% of the annual loss of working days in the USA. The cost of smoking to a nation also includes the impaired abilities of its members, and the extra medical expenses incurred.

Smoking and Health

Smoking is the largest single avoidable cause of ill-health and death. It can damage the cardio-vascular, respiratory and digestive systems, and it encourages the growth of cancer in many parts of the body. Smokers run a much higher risk than non-smokers of illness and premature death:

- cigarette smokers are twice as likely to die before middle age as non-smokers. They run the same risk of death as someone 10 years older.
- two out of five smokers die before 65. This happens to only one out of five non-smokers.

● the average smoker aged 35 has a life expectancy 5½ years shorter than a non-smoker.

How much damage smoking does depends on several things: the type of tobacco; the form it is smoked in; the temperature at which it is burned, the effectiveness of any filtration; whether inhalation occurs; the length of time the individual has been smoking; the amount he smokes; and the general state of his health. Smoking of all sorts is harmful, but usually cigarette smoking is the most deadly. The nicotine content of cigarette tobacco is often smaller, but the higher burning temperature and the greater tendency to inhale make up for this. Also the tendency to inhale favors lung damage and especially lung cancer, which is often not diagnosed till too late. Pipe and cigar smokers are more likely to develop the more noticeable – and so more curable – cancers of the mouth, pharynx, and larynx. The convenience of cigarettes may also encourage more smoking than pipes or cigars.

Your Odds on Surviving

Your odds on surviving into the next age group.
Smoker A: 25 or more cigarettes a day
Smoker B: 15-24 cigarettes a day
Smoker C: 1-14 cigarettes a day

Age 45–54

Person	Odds
Smoker A	10–1
Smoker B	13–1
Smoker C	19–1
Non-Smoker	27–1

Age 35–44

Person	Odds
Smoker A	22–1
Smoker B	50–1
Smoker C	47–1
Non-Smoker	75–1

Age 65–74

Person	Odds
Smoker A	2–1
Smoker B	2–1
Smoker C	2–1
Non-Smoker	3–1

Age 55–64

Person	Odds
Smoker A	4–1
Smoker B	5–1
Smoker C	6–1
Non-Smoker	9–1

8

Respiration System

Smoking greatly reduces the efficiency of the lungs, especially in those who inhale.

In a normal lung, glands in the interior lining are constantly producing mucus. This captures dirt and bacteria, and the mucus and its contents are then forced out of the lungs by the action of cilia. These are small, hair-like projections that are constantly moving, pushing the mucus up into the throat, where it is swallowed. Inhaled smoke hinders the action of the cilia, whilst stimulating mucus production. As a result, mucus, tar, dirt and bacteria collect in the lungs in festering pools, encouraging tissue degeneration and hindering gas exchange. Inhaled tobacco also tends to irritate the air passages, and to reduce air flow in the bronchi and bronchioles by making them contract.

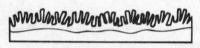

Bronchial cilia

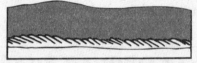

Cilia immobilized by mucus

Smoker's cough The constant cough that attends regular smoking is an attempt by the lungs to rid themselves of the tar and phlegm. Healthy lungs do not collect such phlegm, and only need the normal action of the cilia.

Bronchitis and emphysema Bronchitis is often triggered off by the irritation caused by cigarette smoke, and by the presence of bacteria in the lungs of smokers. Once established, it can progress rapidly from just a troublesome cough to a chronic condition which can kill. Emphysema is also made more likely by the damage smoke and tar do to the lungs. Smokers, especially of cigarettes, run a much higher risk than non-smokers of contracting and dying from either of these.

Cardiovascular System

Reduced oxygen intake

Carbon monoxide is the most concentrated gas in tobacco smoke. Its affinity for blood hemoglobin is greater than that of oxygen (i.e. it combines with it more readily than oxygen does). The greater concentration of carbon monoxide in a smoker's lungs means that hemoglobin which should be carrying oxygen to the tissues is now carrying useless carbon monoxide. The amount of oxygen in the bloodstream can be

reduced by up to 8%. At the same time, the effects of smoking
on the respiratory system also reduce the efficiency of oxygen
intake. All this makes heart-strain a danger, as the heart works
harder and harder to keep up the body's oxygen supply.

Atherosclerosis and thrombosis
Atherosclerosis and thrombosis are more common in smokers
than in non-smokers. Smoking raises the level of fatty acids
and cholesterol in the blood, and encourages blood platelets
(clotting bodies) to adhere to each other and to the blood vessel
walls. Carbon monoxide in the bloodstream also seems to
favor atherosclerosis.

Coronary heart disease
All these factors greatly predispose the smoker to coronary
heart disease of all kinds. Coronary heart disease occurs, on
average, up to seven years earlier in smokers than in non-
smokers.

Cancer

Smoking is a direct cause of much cancer, because tobacco
smoke contains carcinogens and these can set off cancer
wherever in the body the smoke reaches. As a result, cigarette
smokers are 70 times more likely to have lung cancer than non-
smokers. Smokers in general are also more likely to suffer from
cancer of the mouth and pharynx (4 times more than non-
smokers), larynx (5 times more) esophagus (2 times more),
stomach (1½ times more) and bladder (1½ to 3 times more).
Cancer of the mouth, pharynx and larynx are the main forms
in pipe and cigar smokers.
Lung cancer remains, however, the major type of cancer
directly caused by smoking. Lung cancer rates in men have
risen steadily since 1930 and by the mid-1980s it was causing
almost three times more male deaths than any other type of
cancer. By the mid-1980s, it had become the principal cause of
death from cancer in women.
The risk of developing lung cancer is twice as high in men who
began smoking before the age of 24 than in those who began
later, and 5 times as high in men who began smoking before
the age of 19. The risk of cancer is also considerably increased
in smokers also subjected to other forms of air pollution – at
work or in the environment. Great Britain, which has the
highest rate of deaths from lung cancer in the world, has
abnormally high levels of air pollution.

8

Other Risks

Smoking reduces fertility in men and women. Fertility clinics report a higher number of dead or abnormal sperm in the semen of men who smoke. This reduces the chances of conception occurring, and it raises the possibilities of a child being born with birth defects. Smoking also depresses libido and can affect potency.

The unborn child Pregnant women who smoke may retard the growth of the fetus - the babies of smokers average 6oz (170.1gm) lighter than those of non-smokers. They are also more susceptible to miscarriages, still births, and the death of the child soon after birth. Children regularly exposed to tobacco smoke within the home have a greater tendency to suffer from respiratory illnesses and infections. Evidence is emerging that the incidence of cot death or sudden infant death syndrome (SIDS) is slightly higher in households with one or more regular smokers.

Ulcers Those who smoke are five times more likely to suffer from gastric ulcers, and twice as likely to suffer from duodenal ulcers. This may be partly due to personality differences between non-smokers and smokers, but it has also been shown that smoking hinders the healing of these ulcers.

Smoking, Illness and Death

The risk to smokers

Not only do smokers have a higher death rate than non-smokers, but the death rate is generally higher the more cigarettes smoked. These graphs show this for two age groups in two different surveys.

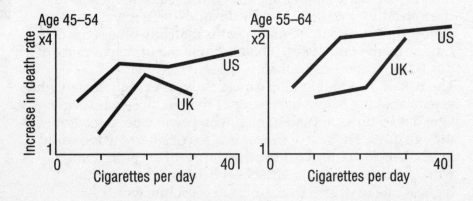

All lines below the first show mortality rates for smokers

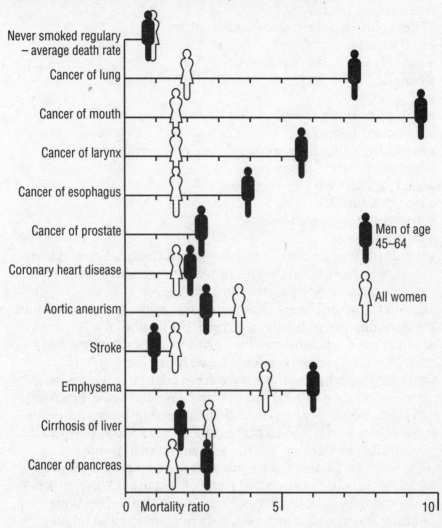

Never smoked regulary
– average death rate

Cancer of lung

Cancer of mouth

Cancer of larynx

Cancer of esophagus

Cancer of prostate

Coronary heart disease

Aortic aneurism

Stroke

Emphysema

Cirrhosis of liver

Cancer of pancreas

Men of age
45–64

All women

0   Mortality ratio   5   10

8

Secondary Smoking

Secondary smoking is the inhalation of air polluted with
cigarette smoke by others. During the late 1980s the results of
many studies first proved that people who regularly inhale
other people's cigarette smoke but do not smoke themselves
may be affected by smokers' illnesses. One study showed that
women who were married to men who smoked two or more
packs of cigarettes a day, or who were exposed to passive
smoke from at least 20 cigarettes a day, were twice as likely to
die from lung cancer as women who did not smoke and did
not inhale air polluted by smokers. The US Environmental
Protection Agency has estimated that secondary or

'sidestream' smoke causes the deaths of some 5000 American nonsmokers every year.

'Sidestream' smoke causes non-smokers:

- eye irritation;
- sore throats and hoarseness;
- coughs;
- headaches;
- asthma and other severe allergic reactions;
- increased heart rate;
- breathing difficulties in people suffering from chronic obstructive lung diseases;
- heart and circulatory diseases;
- lowered fertility rates;
- bronchitis and emphysema;
- lung cancer;
- low birth weight, fetal distress, perinatal mortality and birth defects in the unborn babies of women who are forced to inhale secondary cigarette smoke.

Smokers have become a persecuted minority. About 45 million US smokers quit in the decade 1985-1995 and of the 25 per cent of Americans who still smoked, around 90 per cent wanted to quit. In recent years the effect of passive or 'sidestream' smoking (i.e. inhaling the smoke from cigarettes, cigars or pipes smoked by others) has become a heated issue. Smoking has fast become a career hazard, as some employers refuse to employ smokers. Even in places where smoking is permitted, non-smokers will often ask (or tell) smokers to put out a cigarette. Most states have some sort of non-smoking laws banning smoking in specified parts of restaurants and in work areas and other public places. Smoking is banned on most public transport such as buses, subways, trains and on all domestic flights. In most cities smoking is also prohibited in public restrooms, stores, banks, hotel lobbies and elevators. Smoking is usually banned in movie and other theatres. Bans are likely to be (or have been) extended to indoor sporting venues, shopping malls and school properties. Coupled with the ban on advertising tobacco products on radio and television, and the increased taxation on tobacco products, public opinion and mounting legislation are conspiring to make the smoker's habit increasingly difficult to maintain.

Giving Up Smoking

Just stop! If you really want to you can.
But if you don't believe in yourself enough, then do make the
change from cigarettes to a pipe or cigars – and stop inhaling.
If even that is impossible, at least be sure to: smoke fewer
cigarettes; inhale less; take fewer puffs on each cigarette (but
not longer ones); leave a longer stub at the end, avoid leaving a
lit cigarette in your mouth; and change to a brand with a low
concentration of tar and nicotine. Also buy, and use, a
detachable filter.

Giving up is an act of self-determination, not self-denial. The
benefits to your health – and your finances – far outweigh the
possible discomfort of a week or two.

Ways of giving up There are four main paths.

1 Group sessions, where the new ex-smoker gives and receives
support in his attempt to stop. Some groups are organized on a
voluntary basis. Others are operated by medical and health
organizations. A doctor, library, or local information service
can advise you on these.

2 Individual medical care, in which the ex-smoker receives the
personal attention and help of a physician.

3 Psychotherapy, psychoanalysis, and hypnotism work with
some people by reinforcing their desire and resolve to stop.

4 An act of will and self-assertion.

Breaking any habit is difficult and success depends on real
determination, planning, and willpower – cravings take time to
die down. Plan to stop by following these rules. Then join a
self-help group to reinforce your resolve to quit:

● Analyse your smoking habits. Keep a record.
● Decide that you want to stop smoking. Think of the benefits.
● Then stop. Change your habits. Avoid trigger situations.
● Spoil yourself with a positive reward from money saved.
● Give yourself time. It takes time to break a habit.
● Extra help: nicotine chewing gum or patches applied to the
skin, which provide nicotine by slow release to help cut
down the craving; dummy cigarettes, which may give some
comfort by satisfying the need to hold something in the
mouth, or pseudocigarettes (herbal cigarettes). These contain
no nicotine, but they do produce tar and are not a safe way of
smoking, although they can be useful for helping smokers
overcome addiction. Support groups, clinics run by health
organizations, and groups of friends all giving up at once and
supporting each other all show a high rate of success among
smokers. In the hands of a skilled and experienced

8

practitioner, a course of acupuncture is reputed to decrease both the physical and psychological craving to smoke.

Caffeine

This stimulant of the central nervous system is present in or added to many foods and drinks, including coffee, tea, cocoa and cola drinks. It is a relatively mild drug, acting to relieve fatigue. It is also a diuretic, i.e. it increases the urine output of the kidneys. It is often included in headache pills to counteract the dulling effect of the painkilling ingredient. Abuse of this drug is rare because such large quantities are needed, but it has recently been discovered that some people are especially sensitive to it. They, and people who drink large amounts of coffee, may experience shakiness, heart palpitations, nausea and indigestion. Feelings of tiredness are often experienced when the stimulation wears off.

Amphetamines

The amphetamines ('pep pills' or 'uppers') generally stimulate the sympathetic nervous system, which mobilizes the body for action with the 'fight or flight' syndrome. They increase the production of epinephrine (adrenaline), the heart rate, the blood sugar, and muscular tension.

Effects

The user experiences a sense of well-being and, with strong doses, euphoria. Alertness, wakefulness and confidence are accompanied by feelings of mental and physical power. The user becomes talkative, excited and hyperactive.

Accompanying physical symptoms include sweating, trembling, dizziness, insomnia and reduced appetite. Mood effects are probably due to stimulation of the hypothalamus, and sudden shifts to anxiety and panic can occur.

Dependence

Amphetamines create tolerance, but are not considered physically addictive. However, psychic dependence is easily produced. The extra energy is 'borrowed' from the body's reserves: when the drug's action has worn off, the body has to pay for it in fatigue and depression. This creates the desire for more of the drug to counteract these effects.

Medical usage

This has become rarer since realization of the dangers. But amphetamines are still used for some purposes, e.g. to prevent sleep in people who have to be alert for long periods; to treat minor depression; and to counteract depressants.

Abuse of amphetamines is common because of the feelings of euphoria and alertness they give. The dangers include not only psychic dependence, but also physical deterioration due to hyperactivity and lack of appetite; induced psychotic conditions of paranoia and schizophrenia, resulting from prolonged overdose; suicide due to mental depression following large doses; and death from overdose.

Amphetamine	Description (appearance varies with dose and source)		Nickname
Benzedrine	▣	Red/pink	'Bennies'
	♥	Pink	'Bennies'
Dexadrine	▣	Orange	'Dexies'
	♥	Orange	'Dexies'
Methadrine	○	White	'Speed', 'Meth', 'Crystal'
Biphetamine	▭	White	'Whites'
Edrial	○	White	
Dexamyl	♥	Green	'Christmas tree'

Cocaine

Cocaine (often nicknamed 'coke' or 'snow') is a white powder obtained from the coca plant, *Erythroxylon coca*, found in South America. Synthetic derivatives are also available.

Effects

Cocaine stimulates the central nervous system, dispelling fatigue, increasing alertness, mental activity and reflex speed. Local application has anesthetic effects. It is used as a local anesthetic in minor operations on the eye, ear, nose, and throat, and may be injected into the spinal fluid to anesthetize the lower limbs.

Abuse

Cocaine when inhaled induces euphoria. After an initial 'rush', the effects steady. Accompanying physical symptoms include dilation of the pupils, tremors, loss of appetite and insomnia. Psychic dependence easily develops for the same reasons as with amphetamines. As a powder, it is inhaled, which

8

eventually results in deterioration of the nasal linings and finally of the nasal septum separating the nostrils. Injection of a liquid form is an alternative, but using cocaine alone is unpopular, because of the violence of the sudden effects, so heroin and cocaine are often injected together. Cocaine is a short-acting drug and must be taken repeatedly to maintain the 'high'.

Cocaine narrows the blood vessels and reduces the blood flow to the heart. Dangers of prolonged use include inflammation of the heart and disturbances in heart rhythm, collapsed lung caused by the formation of crystals after inhaling, plus insomnia, paranoia, hallucinations in the sense of touch, called 'cocaine bugs', loss of weight, and malnutrition through loss of appetite. An overdose causes convulsions, and a single dose of 121g (7.8gm) or more causes death by respiratory failure.

Crack

A purified form of cocaine sold as pellets which are heated and smoked. Crack reaches the brain rapidly, producing a brief, intense 'rush', followed after about 10 minutes by an equally intense 'down'. Addiction deadens basic human emotions and can lead to psychosis.

Hallucinogens

The best known of these drugs is LSD (lysergic acid diethylamide). Other hallucinogens include mescaline (derived from the desert peyote cactus, *Lophophora williamsii*), psilocybin (derived from a mushroom), and the seeds of the morning glory flower, which contain lysergic acid. All these drugs are illegal in the US and many European countries.

Physical dependence on hallucinogens is thought unlikely; there is little evidence to show long-term damage. Very disturbing reactions can occur, however. Hallucinogens have strong effects on the brain: the limbic system, influencing mood and emotions; the reticular formation, making the user acutely aware of sensory input; the visual centers, producing visions ranging from flashes of light to complex scenes; and the memory centers, which are suppressed, affecting perception and judgement. The interpretation of incoming sense stimuli is radically affected, and this produces hallucinations, delusions, and extraordinary reactions to normal situations and events.

Serious accidents and fatalities have resulted from people experiencing a 'bad trip'.

LSD

LSD (lysergic acid diethylamide) was originally obtained from the fungus 'ergot', which is found in certain cereals. It is now produced synthetically. Nicknamed 'acid', it is the most widely used hallucinogenic drug. LSD can be injected, but is usually taken orally, either as a pill or as a drop of liquid on another substance (such as a sugar cube or a small square of blotting paper). Upon absorption, it concentrates mainly in the liver, kidneys and adrenal glands. Only about 1% is found in the brain.

Physical effects LSD causes an initial tingling in the extremities, goose pimples, and sometimes nausea and muscle pain. The user feels cold and numb, and looks flushed. These effects soon wear off, leaving dilated pupils and increased heart rate, blood pressure, blood sugar level and body temperature. Muscle co-ordination and pain perception are reduced.

The LSD 'trip' The psychological effects begin with the user becoming extremely emotional. This passes but the senses are increasingly affected. Perception is enhanced and distorted: colors are more vivid, sounds more audible, inert objects seem to move. Synesthesia may occur, and orientation in time and space may be lost. Hallucinations varying in intensity and involvement are often experienced. At the same time, normal mental processes are impaired, and acquired modes of thought and behavior are disrupted. Emotional barriers are broken down, the past may be seen in a new light, and repressed experiences may be released and relived.

Dangers In the panic of a 'bad trip', the user may cause himself and others physical harm. The mental impact can also be long-lasting: the release of repressed emotions and experiences may produce psychotic conditions in a previously unstable or neurotic person. Paranoia, schizophrenia, and acute depression have all been caused through use of LSD. In addition, the power of the hallucinations can produce harmful actions; eg a belief that he can fly may cause the user to leap to his death. 'Flashbacks' are spontaneous recurrences of sensory disruption at a later date. They may occur at any time up to 18 months after the drug's use. They are especially dangerous where sudden loss of orientation may cause an accident (e.g. driving a car, or crossing the road). It is possible that LSD can cause chromosomal damage, but this is not yet certain.

8

Marijuana

This is the dried leaves, flowers, stems or pollen of hemp grass, *Cannabis*, of which there are several species. The drug is usually smoked in cigarettes called 'joints' or 'spliffs', or in pipes to produce euphoria and an apparent intensification of sensory experience. However, the cannabinoid tetrahydrocannabinol in cannabis resin also slows reflexes and distorts perception, especially of dimensions and distance. Anxiety and panic attacks may occur, and persistent use of the drug may result in psychosis, mania, feelings of depersonalization, apathy and loss of motivation.

Designer Drugs

Chemical substances engineered to have similar effects to illegal drugs are not in themselves illegal at the time of manufacture, but are usually rapidly scheduled. Synthetic versions of heroin (e.g. MPPP and 'China White') are drugs of abuse; each illustrates the dangers inherent in the abuse of such 'designer drugs'. With MPPP, a substance similar to meperidine (Demerol), a contaminant (MPTP) was frequently present, affecting nerve cells and linked to cases of Parkinson's disease. Powerful 'China White' has caused overdoses in heroin users. MDMA ('Adam' or 'Ecstasy') has features of both psychedelics and amphetamines; hallucinations occur with high doses; there are feelings of greater empathy, sensuality and euphoria; physical effects include tension of jaw muscles, nausea, dizziness, then fatigue and insomnia; negative effects include panic attacks during a 'high,' and, with repeated use, psychological effects, dependence and nerve damage. 'Angel dust' is the popular name for Phencyclidine, or PCP, an analgesic and anesthetic drug. Used as a recreational drug, it is extremely dangerous, as it can cause muscular rigidity, convulsions and death.

Treatments for Drug Addictons

Treatments for all types of addiction are similar. They are long-term, and success depends on the individual's desire to be cured.

Detoxification

This first stage of treatment takes place in a clinic or hospital.

The patient is deprived of alcohol or other addictive drug. This results in severe withdrawal symptoms: sweating, vomiting, body aches, running nose and eyes, convulsions, and hallucinations. Sedatives give relief, but must be withdrawn before new addictions are formed. Any physical problems are treated and the alcoholic encouraged to eat a balanced diet.

Therapies

While supporting the patient's motivation, self-confidence and trust, healthcare workers try to identify the psychological reasons for addiction and treat them. The most common treatments are:

Psychotherapy aimed at bringing the reasons for addiction to light and helping the patient to accept and face up to them.

Group therapy aimed at giving the patient objective outside views of himself and helping him to come to terms with them; and helping him to overcome his isolation by developing personal relationships by contact with others.

Support groups such as Alcoholics Anonymous and Cocaine Anonymous, run by former addicts, provide group therapy and guidance outside the hospital situation in regular meetings. These provide essential support for continued abstention and rehabilitation.

8

MALE SEX ORGANS

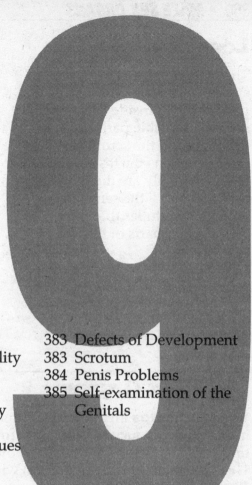

9

Location

The male reproductive
system is partly visible and
partly hidden inside the
body. The visible parts are
the penis and the scrotum,
which contains the testes.
Inside the body are the
prostate gland, the seminal
vesicles, and tubes that link
the different parts of the
system.

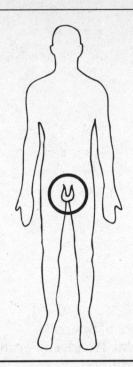

Male Sex Organs

The two testes are the male reproductive glands. They hang
in an external pouch of skin, the **scrotum**, below and behind
the penis. Each testis is a flattened oval shape, about
1¾in (4.4cm) long and 1in (2.5cm) wide.

The scrotum is divided into two compartments, called
scrotal sacs, each containing one testis. (Usually the left testis
hangs lower than the right, and its scrotal sac is slightly
larger.)The scrotum normally keeps the testes at a little below
body temperature - the optimum temperature for healthy
sperm.

The testes make:

● a male sex hormone called testosterone;
● sperm cells, the male cells of reproduction, which fertilize the
  egg in the female body to produce a baby.

The epididymes are triangular structures on top of each
testis and connected to its testis by a number of tubes. The
young sperm cells (spermatocytes) produced by the testes
travel along the tubes into the epididymes, where they are
stored, and develop into mature sperm.

The vasa deferentes are two muscular tubes, each about 16
inches long, which wind upward from the scrotum into the
pelvic cavity. Each vas deferens leads from its associated
epididymis into an ejaculatory duct. The ejaculatory ducts are

two short tubes that pass through the prostate. During sexual excitement the mature sperm pass along them to be mixed with semen from the seminal vesicles prior to ejaculation.

The prostate is a gland that surrounds the junction of the vasa deferentes and the urethra. Here, the sperm cells are mixed with its secretions – seminal fluid: an alkaline liquid in which the sperms are carried out of the body, and which enables them to swim. The prostatic secretions (35% of the seminal fluid) also help prevent the semen from coagulating immediately after ejaculation.

The seminal vesicles are two small sacs that lie at the junction between the vas deferens and the prostate. They secrete 65% of the seminal fluid as a thick alkaline solution containing fructose, a sugar, a source of energy that helps the

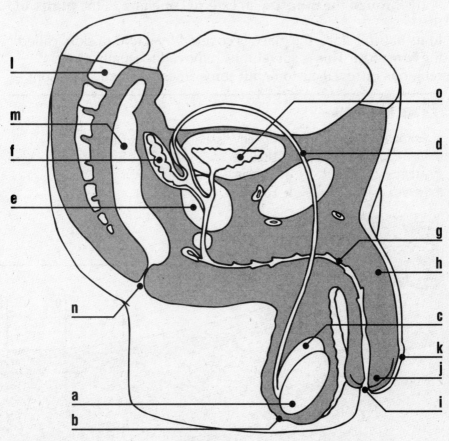

a Testes	**f** Seminal vesicles	**k** Foreskin
b Scrotum	**g** Urethra	**l** Pelvis
c Epididymis	**h** Penis	**m** Rectum
d Vasa deferentes	**i** Meatus	**n** Anus
e Prostate	**j** Glans	**o** Bladder

sperm to move.

The urethra is an S-shape tube, about 8in (20.3cm) long, which leads from the bladder, along the penis to the exterior. It passes through the prostate gland, where the ejaculatory ducts open into it. It has two functions:

- it carries urine from the bladder to the exterior;
- it is the route by which semen reaches the penis from the prostate and passes into the female vagina during copulation.

The penis is an organ made of spongy tissue containing many blood vessels, covered with loose skin The urethra enters the penis from the body and passes through it to the tip. The penis is capable of lengthening and increasing considerably in overall size during sexual arousal. Urine and semen leave the body through the **meatus** an external opening in the **glans** or tip.

In its natural state, the glans is covered by a fold of skin, called the **foreskin**. This is sometimes removed – usually as a religious or social custom, but sometimes for medical reasons –

The Penis

a Fibrous tissue   **e** Spongy tissue   **i** Glans
b Vein   **f** Urethra   **j** Shaft
c Artery   **g** Meatus
d Nerve   **h** Foreskin

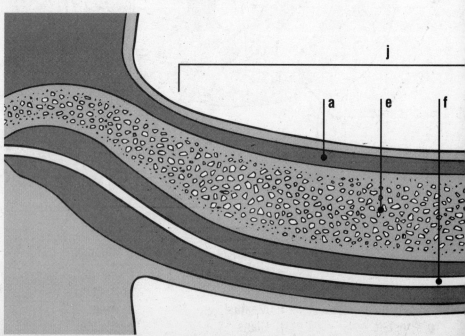

Erection

When a man is sexually aroused, blood flows into the many blood vessels within the spongy tissue inside the penis, making them swell. At the same time, the veins that normally carry blood out of the penis are compressed. From being 'floppy' and hanging down, the penis becomes stiff, lengthens, and juts out from the body. This is called an 'erection'. It sometimes takes as little as 5 to 10 seconds.

Erection is an involuntary process, controlled by the parasympathetic nervous system (which controls functions such as the opening and closing of the pupils in the eye). A man cannot, therefore, have an erection at will. It occurs when the parasympathetic nerves are stimulated by sexual arousal.

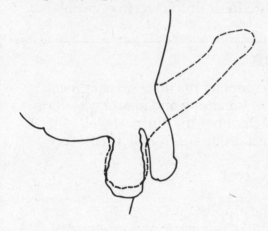

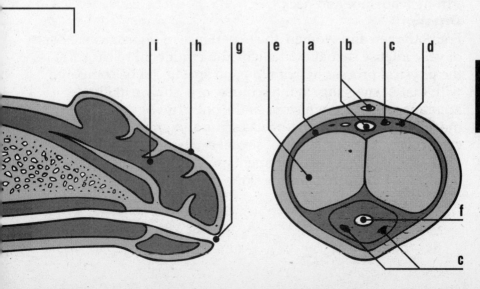

Sexual Arousal

The sexual process takes the male sexual-system from its unaroused state to orgasm. On orgasm, semen is discharged from the penis.

The stimulus that first arouses the system can be purely psychological – the thought of sex. But the system normally needs physical pressure on the skin surface of the penis to reach orgasm. In copulation this is provided by the contact of the penis with the female genitals. For both arousal and for orgasm, conditions need to be right. The system can be inhibited, or the process reversed, by:

- adverse physical conditions in the surroundings (e.g. cold);
- psychological distractions (e.g. worry, or sudden disturbance);
- adverse body states (e.g. tiredness or too recent orgasm).

Bodily Responses

The following responses accompany the male sexual process:
- blood pressure, and rates of breathing and heart beat, all rise often, on orgasm, to about 2½ times the normal level.
- muscular spasms may affect groups of muscles in the face, chest, and abdomen;
- contractions of the rectum occur.

In some men there is also:
- swelling and erection of the nipples
- flushing of skin color around chest, neck, and forehead
- perspiration from soles, palms, and body, and sometimes from head, face and neck.

Orgasm

For both men and women, the experience of orgasm can be one of very intense sexual excitement and emotional release. Yet the physical process of irritation and spasm can be compared with that of sneezing. In intercourse, orgasm is usually accompanied by convulsions of the body, involuntary movements, and sounds such as sighs and groans. But orgasm can occur at various levels of sexual excitement. Evidence, in men, of a high level of excitement are very high rates of breathing and flushing of the skin.

1 Heart rate quickens rapidly
2 Heart rate levels off
3 Sharp rise as orgasm
 approaches
4 Gradual return to normal

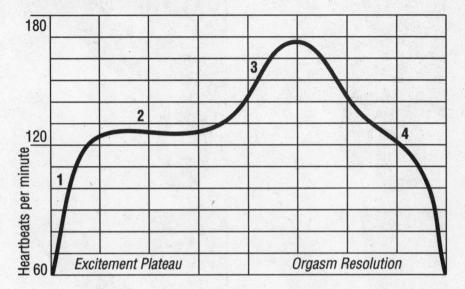

a Penis erects
b Scrotum thickens
c Testes rise
d 'Sex flush' appears
e Penis tip and testes swell

f Ejaculation, heavy breathing, and
 muscular spasms
g 'Sex flush' disappears
h Loss of erection
i Penis returns to normal state

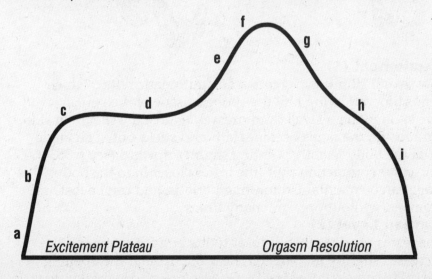

9

Behavior of the penis

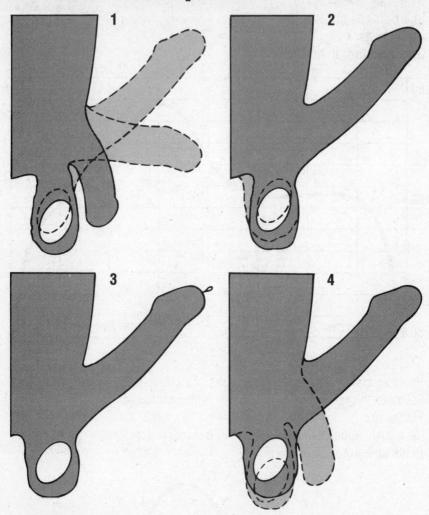

Excitement (1)
The sexual stimulus triggers off an automatic reflex, which
sends blood flowing into the spongy tissue of the penis.
The spongy mass swells and presses against the sheath of skin.
As a result, the penis becomes stiff and sticks out at an angle
from the body usually pointing slightly upward (see p 363).
Muscular contraction pulls the testes closer in to the body. This
stage can be maintained for long periods, and can be lost and
regained without orgasm, many times.

Plateau Level (2)
The testes are drawn still closer to the body. The penis
increases slightly in diameter, near the tip, and the opening in
the tip becomes more slit-like. The tip may change color, to a
deeper red-purple.

Orgasm (3)

The muscles around the urethra give a number of rapid involuntary contractions. This forces semen out of the penis at high pressure (ejaculation). There are usually three or four major bursts of semen, one every 0.8 seconds, followed by weaker, more irregular, muscular contractions.

Resolution (4)

Often there is: first, a very rapid reduction in penis size, to about 50% larger than its normal state; followed by a slower reduction back to normal.

But each of these stages may be prolonged, eg if the penis remains inserted in the female genitals.

The response pattern shown here and in sexual arousal were first described WH Masters and VE Johnson in "Human Sexual Response" (1966).

Circumcision

In its natural state, the glans or tip of the penis is covered by a fold of skin called the foreskin (see p 362). When rolled forward, the foreskin is like a hood around the glans, but it can also be pushed back along the shaft.

In many societies, ritual or religious custom dictates that the foreskin be removed – cut away – in a minor surgical procedure called circumcision, usually carried out shortly after birth or during puberty. Male Jews and Moslems are circumcised as a religious requirement.

Until recently, many hospitals in the USA routinely circumcised all baby boys, and 60% of American babies are circumcised every year. But the value of routine circumcision is debatable. Good hygiene is one argument in favour of it. When the foreskin is intact, white secretions called 'smegma' can accumulate underneath it. Unless these are regularly washed away, the foreskin can become smelly, dirty, and possibly inflamed. Men who allow smegma to accumulate may also accumulate papilloma viruses, which can cause tumors to develop in the bladder. However, this is easily prevented by regular washing. Men who allow smegma to accumulate may also papilloma viruses, which can be passed on to their sexual partners. Papilloma viruses have been implicated in the development of cervical cancer women. However, build up of smegma under the man's foreskin can be readily prevented by regular washing.

9

In rare cases there are medical reasons for circumcision. Boys can suffer pain from a foreskin that does not expand as the penis develops, and in adults the foreskin can become tight and difficult to move.

The value of routine circumcision is, however, debatable. Some doctors argue that there is no clear evidence that the presence or absence of a foreskin makes much difference to sexual sensitivity, or pleasure, or time taken to reach orgasm. However, others accept that the surface of the circumcised glans, which has a greater concentration of nerve endings than the shaft of the penis, becomes gradually toughened and less sensitive as a result of keratinization. The exposure of the skin of the glans to pressure, abrasion and urine causes the fibrous keratin of the outermost layer of skin to thicken, becoming more like skin on the outer surfaces of the body and less like the mucous membrane tissue on the inside of the lips, for example.

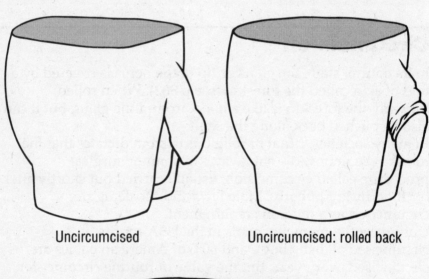

Uncircumcised   Uncircumcised: rolled back

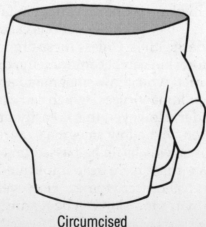

Circumcised

Foreskin Regeneration

Since the 1970s, some American men have experimented with ways of recreating the foreskin. Recently, a Californian psychologist, Dr. J. Bigelow, reported having recreated a skin covering for the glans by gently stretching the skin on the shaft of the penis and holding it in place with tape. After some years of such gradual stretching, the skin partially covers the glans. The skin covering created by such methods does not, however, cover the glans tightly like a natural foreskin. A more natural foreskin can be made by skin grafts in cosmetic surgery procedures.

Reports of these and other attempts to regenerate the foreskin have been received with sympathetic interest by men who resent the fact that they were circumcised. Some retrospectively experience the operation as a form of abuse.

Erect Dimensions

The longest erect penis for which there is reasonable scientific evidence measured 12in (30cm) The smallest recorded with testes and normal functioning has been under ½in (1.3cm) in length. In other abnormal cases the penis can, of course, be totally absent.

Body size is no guide to penis size: the erect penis has a less constant relationship to body size than any other organ. Nor is flaccid size decisive: penises which hang longer when flaccid tend to gain less when erect. A short penis can gain as much as 3¾in (9.5cm), and a long one as little as 2in (5cm).

There is no relationship between penis size and sexual prowess or female satisfaction: the female vagina accommodates its size to that of the penis, and stimulation of the female clitoris does not depend on penis length.

Flaccid Dimensions

In its normal state, the penis hangs down loosely. It averages about 3¾in (9.5cm) long, and most examples are between 3¼in (8.2cm) and 4¼in (10.8cm), though a few cases will fall well outside this range.

The penis gets temporarily smaller than usual in certain circumstances, such as cold temperatures, through immersion in cold water, in extreme exhaustion, or after a failed attempt at sexual activity. These circumstances also pull the testes and scrotal sac closer to the body.

The penis may get permanently smaller in old age, or after longish periods of impotence.

9

Angle of erection

This shows the variation
between different men.

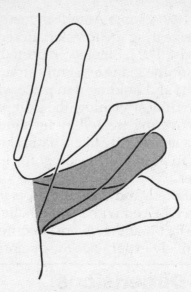

Appearance

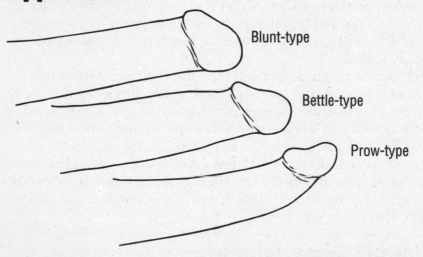

Blunt-type

Bettle-type

Prow-type

Potency

The characteristics of potency are sperm production, erection
and ejaculation.

Sperm production

Sperm cells are formed in tiny 'tubules' inside the testes, at the
rate, in maturity, of 10 to 30 billion a month. Each is about
$1/500$th of an inch long, and each takes about 74 days to
develop. They are stored during this time in the two
epididymides (muscular tubes which, if uncoiled, would

measure 20 feet (6m in length), and remain there until
ejaculated from the body during sexual arousal – or until they
disintegrate, being reabsorbed into the testes.

Sperm production can only occur at a temperature 3 or 4°F
(1 or 2°C) below normal body temperature. That is why the
testes are suspended below the body in the scrotum. High
temperatures not only prevent new sperms being formed, but
also kill those in storage. The effects may be temporary
(infertility) or – in extreme cases – permanent (sterility). Very
low temperatures also halt sperm formation, but do not kill
those in storage. Otherwise sperm production is continuous,
though there is some evidence of seasonal variations (the
sperm concentration seems to be lower in the warmer months).

Erection

Erection has been recorded at all ages – from baby boys a few
minutes after birth, to old men in their late 80s. But the ability
usually develops with puberty, and may be lost as old age
approaches. Erection can occur gradually, or in as fast a time as
3 seconds, and can also be lost rapidly or slowly. The length of
time for which erection can be maintained varies considerably,
and depends on circumstances, but tends to decline with age.

Ejaculation

On orgasm, a man usually ejaculates between and 1 and 5
milliliters of semen (an average range of 2 to 3 milliliter – a
small teaspoonful). The volume is usually within the average
range after two to three days of sexual abstinence; toward the
top end of the range after prolonged sexual abstinence; and it
usually diminishes with frequency of ejaculation.

The ejaculate is 90% water. It consists mainly of semen, of
which some 65% is contributed by the seminal vesicles and
35% by the prostate (which gives the semen its characteristic
smell). The remaining 5% consists of other fluids, and sperm.
The typical sperm count totals some 90 million sperm per
milliliter of semen. The sperm live for up to 21 days after
reaching maturity.

Ejaculation is preceded by an emission of 1 or 2 drops of a
clear, colorless, alkaline fluid from the Cowper's glands — two
small glands just beneath the prostate. This fluid neutralizes
any acidity remaining in the urethra from recent urination.
(This clear fluid is also sometimes released after the plateau
level (see p 364) has continued for some time, even if no
orgasm occurs. It is not semen, but its emission follows sexual
intercourse even if no semen has been ejaculated.

This emission of fluid is followed by ejaculation, which has
two phases:

9

1 The emission of a thin, milky fluid from the prostate, which usually contains some sperms.

2 The ejaculation of semen containing sperms.

The overall appearance of semen is milky, opalescent and opaque. The opalescence increases with the concentration of sperms. A forceful ejaculation, after prolonged sexual abstinence, may shoot semen, if there is nothing in the way, 3ft (0.9m) or more; but 7 to 10in (17cm - 25cm) is the average distance.

Repeated Ejaculation

The ability to have repeated orgasms with ejaculation in a short time varies enormously, and begins to decline almost immediately once puberty is complete. Kinsey records one man who had 4 to 5 orgasms a day, with ejaculation, for 30 years; and another man who had one ejaculation in all that period. Within a space of one or two hours, most men can manage one ejaculation, some a second, a few three to four. Kinsey records one achievement of about 6 to 8 ejaculations in a single session; but regular multiple ejaculation is typical of only a small number of men.

Impotence

There are great variations in normal potency, and almost all men experience some failure of potency at some time in their lives. Being impotent means being unable to acheive or sustain an erection firm enough to achieve normal sexual intercourse. More than 90% of impotence is the consequence of some psychological problem (see p 421). Anxiety about impotence is one of its major causes. The few physical causes of long-term impotence can be categorized either as stemming from impediments to physical development; or from changes in the adult body state.

Birth defects may result in impotence if they affect the sexual functioning of the genitals, and defects in physical development, due to hormonal failure, may mean that a boy fails to mature sexually. But such defects are rare.

In a person who has experienced normal sexual functioning, long-term impotence from physical causes can only arise from changes in the adult body state. These may include:

● some diseases of the genitals;
● some hormonal disorders;
● some general disorders, such as diabetes, debilitating illnesses, and infectious damage to the spinal cord;
● some surgery (e.g. for cancer of the prostate or colon);
● continual heavy drug or alcohol use; ànd
● heart disease.

However, none of these is certain to cause impotence. Physical causes of short-term impotence can include almost anything that lowers the body's vitality: immediate factors like great fatigue or heavy doses of alcohol or drugs, and more mild ones like poor health, poor nutrition and perhaps even lack of exercise.

(These things are also likely to affect sperm production. But poor sperm production does not itself cause impotence. A man can produce few sperm, but still ejaculate normally.)

Sperm Development

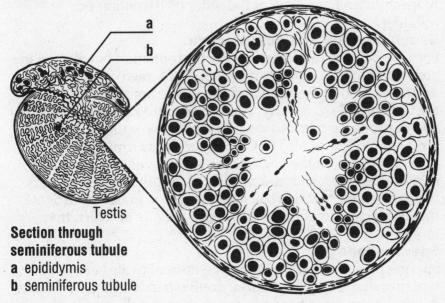

Testis

Section through seminiferous tubule
a epididymis
b seminiferous tubule

Stages of maturation

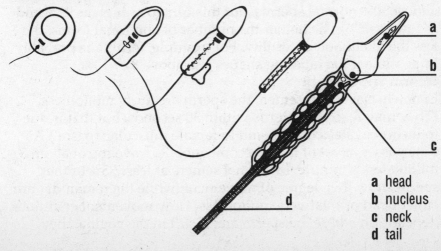

a head
b nucleus
c neck
d tail

Fertility and Infertility

Fertility is the ability to produce healthy sperm capable of fertilizing a female ovum. It takes an average 5.3 months for pregnancy to occur in a normal couple not using contraception; 25% will have conceived after 1 month and 63% after 6 months.

Sperm concentration

The 2 to 3 milliliters of semen a man usually ejaculates after sexual arousal typically contains some 300 million sperm. The lower limits for fertility are estimated at between 20 and 40 million sperm per milliliter, but sperm counts taken from men seeking sterilization by vasectomy after having fathered one or more children have been of the order of 10 million per milliliter.

Semen volume and composition

Fertility depends not only on sperm production but also on the amount of fluid – ie. the total volume of semen – and by its alkalinity. Both very small and very large amounts of semen are unfavorable to fertility. A small amount suggests that sperm production is also low. If its volume or its alkalinity level are too low, it also fails to buffer the sperm against the acidity of fluids in the vagina. Too great a volume of semen dilutes the sperm and makes it likely to spill out of the vagina. Normal semen contains fructose, a sugar, and other nutrients that energize the sperm and increase the rate at which they move.

Sperm shape

Sperm appear in several forms: the normal oval shape; tapering shapes; round shapes; double-headed shapes; double-tailed shapes; giant-headed shapes; pinhead shapes; and various other, amorphous shapes. In average semen, there are almost 90% normal sperms, but this can go as high as 99% and as low as 66%. The higher the number of abnormal forms, the less the likelihood of fertility. For example, fertility is probably impossible if the tapering shapes rise above 8 or 10%.

Sperm movement

In newly ejaculated semen, the sperm are fairly motionless. (They may reach the uterus within 30 seconds, but that is due to the force of ejaculation and to female muscular spasm.) As time passes, most of them become mobile, traveling at about 3 millimeters a minute. In normal semen, at least 75% of the sperm show this degree of movement, while the remainder are either dead or relatively motionless. How movement continues depends on where the sperm are. If still in the vagina, they stop moving after about an hour. In the uterus or cervix, they typically live for 24 to 48 hours.

The length of life of the sperm (as shown by their movement) is not only important because of the time they may need before encountering an egg to fertilize. For some reason not yet understood, sperm also need to stay for some time in the female reproductive tract, before they are capable of fertilizing an egg.

Healthy sperm production

From the concentration, shape and motility (movement) of sperm, it is possible to make a general estimate of the likely fertility of a man's sperm production. Causes of poor sperm production include:

1 Heat around the testicles, due, for example, to tight underpants or jeans.

2 Poor general health, inadequate nutrition and lack of exercise.

3 Emotional stress.

4 Excessively prolonged abstinence (this can increase the numbers of abnormal sperms in the ejaculate).

5 Infrequent copulation. Coitus between once and three times a week has been estimated to provide a 32 to 84% probability of conception occurring.

6 Too frequent ejaculation. Intervals of less than 12 hours or more than 7 days have been found to reduce the fertility of the ejaculate.

Types of Sperm

a Normal oval sperm
b Normal oval sperm with cytoplasmic appendages
c Abnormal sperm, tapering form
d Abnormal sperm, round form
e Abnormal sperm, duplicate form
f Abnormal sperm, giant form
g Abnormal sperm, amorphous form

9

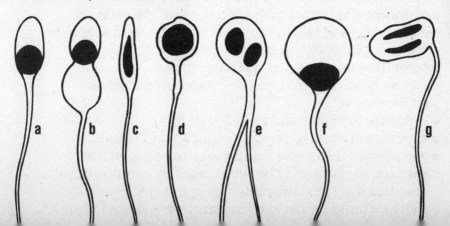

a   b   c   d   e   f   g

Recent Trends in Fertility

Fertility appears to have decreased in recent years. The number of couples seeking treatment at infertility clinics has grown from over 600,000 in 1988 to more than 2 million in 1992. However, this may not be because fertility is decreasing, but because people are no longer realizing their full fertility potential. There are several reasons:

1 The tendency to delay marriage and childbearing is a major factor, especially as fertility decreases markedly with age.

2 The proportion of couples who have delayed childbearing has increased dramatically.

3 The children of the 'baby boom' period have now aged beyond the period of optimum fertility. Because they make up a large part of the population, proportionally large numbers seek infertility advice and contribute to the infertility statistics. Improved health during the second half of the 20th century may have resulted in more fertile men and women of childbearing age, but some factors are known threats to fertility:

- syphilis and gonorrhea can sometimes lead to infertility.
- a suspected decrease in the quality of semen during the past 50 years.

Subfertility

Recent research in Denmark compared measurements of the density of sperm in samples of semen taken from men without a history of infertility between 1940 and 1990. The studies found a decline in semen quality over the past 50 years, below the normal range. Sperm count has a direct effect on male fertility. The researchers noted the parallel increase in abnormalities of the male urinary and reproductive systems over the same period, such as cancer of the testes. They concluded that environmental factors were more likely to be responsible for the decline than genetic factors.

Environmental factors that could have an effect on sperm production – and which can also cause abnormalities in an embryo if conception occurs – include:

- secondary inhalation of cigarette smoke;
- carbon monoxide and gasoline fumes in the urban environment;
- exposure to X-rays and radioactivity;
- exposure at work to certain chemicals and metals;
- ingestion of the female hormone estrogen, which recent research suggests may be synthesised by certain chemical mixtures used in some plastic food wrappings and can as well as a build up of excreted estrogens in recycled water.

Infertility

A practical indicator of infertility is a couple's failure to
achieve conception in 1 year or more of sexual intercourse, if
no contraceptives are used. Rates of infertility vary with age
group:

Age group	% of infertile couples
30-34	14
35-39	20
40-44	25

Incidence of infertility

On average, out of every 100 couples, 10 are unable to have
children and 15 have fewer children than they wish, so one-
fourth of couples are subfertile, or below normal fertility. The
infertility may result from a dysfunction in either or both
partners: in the female partner in 50 to 55% of cases; in the
male partner in 30 to 35%; and in both in about 15%.

Psychological factors

Infertility is often caused by physical malfunctions, such as
failure to ovulate in women or abnormal sperm in men.
However, there is an important psychological element in
reproductive functions. Premature ejaculation occurring before
full penetration reduces the likelihood of large numbers of
sperm reaching the ovum. Two studies have shown that more
than half the couples attending infertility clinics report marital
or sexual problems, and others have shown that female orgasm
increases the possibilities of fertilization.

Infertility in Men

In men, fertility is threatened if healthy sperm are not
produced and ejaculated into the vagina in sufficient numbers
to give them a good chance of reaching the ovum and
fertilizing it This can have several causes:
- certain birth defects impair the reproductive process - for
  example, the testes fail to descend into the scrotum before
  puberty;
- childhood illnesses, such as mumps, or accidents, damage the
  reproductive system;
- genital disorders of the urinary or reproductive system, such
  as varicocele or urethritis, cause blockages;
- unusually high or low production of the male hormones may
  cause low quantities of sperm to be produced;
- infrequent copulation. Coitus between once and three times a

9

week has been estimated to provide a 32 to 84% probability of conception occurring;

- too frequent ejaculation. Intervals of less than 12 hours or more than 7 days have been found to reduce the fertility of the ejaculate;
- normal sexual performance is impaired and there is no ejaculation, or ejaculation occurs outside the vagina;
- sexual function is normal but disorders of the ejaculate make conception unlikely.

Investigating Infertility

Many of the causes of infertility are treatable. Investigations in an infertility clinic can often reveal the cause and lead to successful treatment. About half the couples treated for infertility achieve pregnancy – just the knowledge that something is being done may help build an atmosphere in which fertility can occur. But success varies with reason for infertility. Finding the reasons and the right treatment for infertility is often a very long process, taking one or more years. It involves:

An initial interview: both partners initially discuss the problem with a physician, who assesses their needs and decides what investigations are necessary.

A medical checkup: the physician assesses the overall health of both partners and may recommend changes in diet, exercise and other aspects of lifestyle, and treatment for any general health conditions that may be necessary.

Keeping records: couples are asked to record the woman's basal temperatures, bleeding patterns and changes in cervical mucus, and occurrence of sexual intercourse for several months.

Semen analysis: the male partner is asked to produce a specimen of semen by abstaining from ejaculation for two to three days, then producing a sample of ejaculate by masturbation, ideally at the infertility clinic so that the sample can be stored immediately under optimum conditions. This is then analyzed to determine the volume and composition of semen produced, and the density and quality of sperm within it. Further analyses of ejaculate may be made as treatment progresses.

Postcoital test: this is usually made 6-18 hours after intercourse, and as near as possible to the day of ovulation. A mucus specimen is taken from the cervix. Microscopic study of this shows the quantity and quality of the sperm present – which depend on both the material originally ejaculated and the condition of the cervical mucus. The receptivity of the mucus to the sperm will be assessed, since infertility sometimes results from incompatibility between mucus and sperm.

Treatment by specialists: depending on the outcome of the above, either or both partners may be referred to any of the following:

● andrologist, specialist in disorders of the urinary tract;
● endocrinologist, who investigates disturbances in the hormones produced by the endocrine system;
● psychosexual councellor, a specialist in overcoming sexual difficulties and psychological barriers to fertility.

Treating Infertility

Several types of treatment may be tried before conception occurs:

Improving general health
Poor sperm production may be caused by malnutrition and vitamin deficiency, recurring fevers, chronic diseases such as pulmonary tuberculosis, and the action of drugs such as Salazopyrin (used to treat rheumatoid arthritis and a number of other diseases). Infections of the urethra, prostate and other parts of the urinary and reproductive system may cause swelling and obstruct the production or passage of semen. Initial advice and treatment concentrates on treating underlying illnesses or infections, investigating the effects of drugs taken regularly and possibly substituting others, and considering possible adverse effects of the working environment.

Timing of intercourse
Timing of sexual intercourse will also be investigated. The chances of conception may be improved by concentrating intercourse during the woman's fertile phase of each month. If the charts that she keeps show that she has regular 28-day periods, her fertile phase will usually lie between days 11 and 16. With irregular cycles of between 27 and 35 days, chances of pregnancy will improve if intercourse occurs on five alternate days, starting with the 13th day of the cycle. Intercourse on all the fertile days would exhaust the man's sperm output and so reduce the chances of conception.

9

Techniques of sexual intercourse

Sometimes infertility is due to poor coital connection. Positions that increase penetration may be recommended, for example, the woman hooking her knees over the man's shoulders (**1**), or squatting over the man as he lies on his back, and lowering herself onto his penis(**2**).

**Two positions likely
to result in conception**

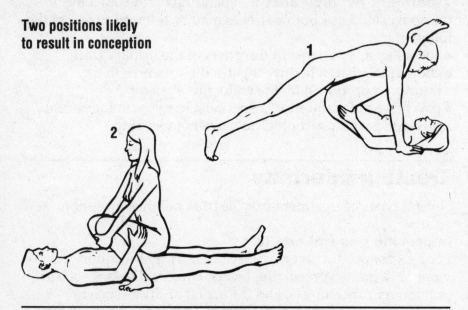

New Fertility Techniques

Several new methods of achieving fertility, many of them still largely experimental, have been developed in recent years. Those involving the donation and freezing of sperm, ova or embryos, bringing theoretical possibilities for genetic engineering within reach, have raised complex social and moral issues. As a result, certain research is now subject to legal restrictions.

Direct intraperitoneal insemination (DIPI)

However, new techniques for overcoming subfertility in men (the production of insufficient healthy sperm) are less controversial. These involve using a centrifuge to concentrate healthy sperm in a sample of ejaculate, and introducing them into the uterus of the female partner at the time of ovulation, thus bypassing 'hostile' cervical mucus. The success rate for this technique is up to 30%.

GIFT and POST

In a technique called **gamete intrafallopian transfer (GIFT)**, ovum and sperm may be mixed and injected into a Fallopian tube. In **peritoneal oocyte and sperm transfer (POST)**, a related technique, they may be injected into the space behind the uterus. These techniques also have a success rate of up to 30%.

In vitro fertilization (IVF)

When the male partner has a low viable sperm count, when sperm and mucus are incompatible, and when the female partner is healthy, but her Fallopian tubes are not functioning normally, a couple may be able to conceive by IVF. In this procedure, ovulation is induced and the ova collected by laparoscopy (using an endoscope, a narrow fibreoptic tube). The ova are mixed with sperm in a nutrient solution in the laboratory and allowed to develop into embryos. These are then transferred into the uterus. Unused embryos may be frozen for later transfer attempts.

IVF may be difficult to obtain as part of a public health program because it is very expensive and has a low success rate. There are problems with the timing of ovulation, fertilizing the ovum, encouraging it to grow under laboratory conditions, and in inducing the correct uterine conditions for successful implantation.

IVF is controversial because donor sperm, ova and embryos are also sometimes used, so that in theory a woman may become a surrogate mother and bear a child for another woman who is infertile. A woman may also bear a child from an ovum that developed after her partner's sperm was used to fertilize the ovum of another woman.

Intracytoplasmic sperm injection (ICSI)

When the male partner's sperm quality is too poor to qualify for use in IVF, or when standard IVF has been unsuccessful, ICSI may be a viable option. ICSI uses micromanipulation techniques to inject a single healthy sperm into the cytoplasm of a woman's ovum. The single sperm is selected from a sample provided by the male partner. The ovum is obtained by laparoscopy and the growth of the embryo and its placement in the uterus is essentially the same as for standard IVF. The hi-tech method increases the chances of successful fertilization compared to standard IVF.

9

Defects at birth

Displaced outlet

The outlet of the urethra should be at the tip of the penis.
Epispadias is the condition in which the urethra comes out on the upper surface of the penis, instead of at the tip.
Hypospadias is the condition in which it comes out on the under surface.

Both cause difficulties. During urination, the man may have to sit, or tilt his penis. During intercourse, he may be effectively infertile, because too little semen finds its way to the uterus. Both conditions can be dealt with by surgery. A new urethra can be formed, lined with epithelium tissue grown in a tissue culture from the man's own cells.

Undescended testes

The testes normally move down from the fetus' abdominal cavity to his scrotum during the eighth month of pregnancy. If they are still in the abdominal cavity at birth the condition is called cryptorchidism. It can be corrected surgically. If this is not done before puberty, sterility results. The probability of cancer developing in the abnormally placed organ also increases significantly.

Intersex

Otherwise normal people can be born with genitals that are intermediate between those of the two sexes: for example, an unusually short penis, perhaps surrounded with folds of skin, and a half or fully formed vagina. In such cases, the dominant hormonal activity that begins at puberty may well be different from that of the sex as which they have been brought up.

Other abnormalities

A very small number of boys are born with only one, or without, seminal vesicles, or vasa deferentes, causing infertility or sterility. Sexual development appears to be normal, but men with these defects tend to produce a low volume of ejaculate. Some are born with abnormally small testes, or poorly functioning semeniferous tubules – the sperm-producing structures inside the testes.

Sites of disorders

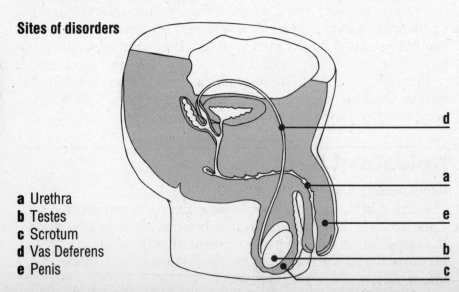

d

a

e

b

c

a Urethra
b Testes
c Scrotum
d Vas Deferens
e Penis

Defects of Development

Genetic abnormalities

Some people, from the moment of their conception, do not have the normal sex chromosomes of either a male (XY) or a female (XX). This occurs because of errors in cell division or fertilization, and the consequences generally appear at puberty. Among such people, those that appear to be male fall into two groups. The first group have an extra Y chromosome (XYY): they have normal male functioning, though they often have other, non-sexual difficulties. The second group have one or more extra X chromosomes, sometimes with extra Y ones as well: XXY, XXXY, XXXXY, XXYY, XXXYY. All these are male, but usually their genitals fail to develop at puberty, and they may also show some female secondary sexual characteristics. The first three types listed (with the single Y chromosome) are always sterile. The fertility of XXYY and XXXYY cases is not yet clear.

Hormonal abnormalities

People with normal sex chromosomes can nevertheless have hormonal defects. At puberty, normal sexual growth and functioning may be late or never develop, even though the genitals in childhood were the normal shape and size. Hormone treatment may be needed, with occasional pauses to see if the body hormones have started up yet.

Scrotum

Varicocele

This is a condition in which there is a collection of varicose veins around the scrotum. The blood carried in the dilated veins makes the testes warmer than they should be, and infertility can result. Regular bathing of the testes in cold water may be enough to counteract the temperature change. Also weight reduction will help prevent the veins getting worse if obesity has been one cause of the condition. If the problem continues, surgical removal or tying of the swollen veins may be needed. This does not interfere with the general blood supply to the testes.

Disorders of the seminal fluid

Hydrocele is accumulation of fluid in the layers of cells around the testes. It can cause overheating and infertility, and may require surgical drainage. Hematocele is a similar condition resulting from injury: blood is mixed in the fluid. Spermatocele is accumulation of seminal fluid.

9

Scrotal swellings
These can be caused not only by fluid accumulation, but also by cysts, tumors, inflammations and hernias in the area, or by an attack of mumps.

Blocked ducts
Blockage can occur in the vas deferens tubes, that carry sperm from testes to urethra. Infertility results. Infection, such as venereal disease is the usual cause. Corrective surgery bypasses the blockage, joining the unaffected part of the tube directly to the end of the urethra.

Swellings in the testicle
Lumps and swellings in the testicle can be a sign of tumors. Routine, regular self-examination for these is recommended (see p 385). If you notice any changes in one or both testicles, see a physician immediately. The tumors may be benign, but the earlier a malignant tumor is diagnosed, the more likely it is to be treatable.

Penis Problems

Pains
Pains in the penis can be caused by trouble either there or in some associated tube or organ as a result of inflammation, stones or growths. Report any pains to your physician without delay.

Skin disorders
Growths on the penis surface can include warts, ulcers, sores connected with sexual infections, and cold sores. None is especially hard to treat. Cancer of the penis may appear as irritation and discharge from beneath the foreskin, or simply as a pimple on the penis surface that does not heal. In most western countries, it accounts for only 2% of all male cancers, and usually responds well to radium treatment.

Priapism
This is non-sexual erection of the penis; it may be painful. It is most common in the elderly, when causes can include prostate enlargement, inflammation, piles, etc. In children, it may be due to penis inflammation, circumcision, over-tight foreskin, or worms. In adults, to drug abuse, gonorrhea, epilepsy, leukemia, back injury or convalescence from an acute illness. Continual priapism can be due to severe spinal injury, or to a clot in prostatic veins.

Crooked Erection
This can be due to short-term inflammation of the urethra,

especially from gonorrhea. Otherwise, usually in older men, it is linked with spontaneous formation of scar tissue along one side of the penis. In this case, it gradually stops being painful, and the condition itself may eventually disappear without treatment.

Self-examination of the Genitals

Examine your genitals once a month, standing (**1**), ideally after a warm bath or shower. Fully retract the foreskin and examine the end of the penis and urinary opening (**2**). Examine each testicle separately with the fingers by placing the index and middle finger underneath the testicle, and the thumb on top (**3**). Roll the testicle between thumb and fingers feeling for any small lump or abnormality. (The sausage-shaped lump at the back and top side of each testicle is normal – it is the epididymis.)
Look out for any change especially:
- swelling (which may not be painful)
- tenderness
- hardness or any lump
- weight gain in either testicle
- blood in urine or passing from penis
- back pain

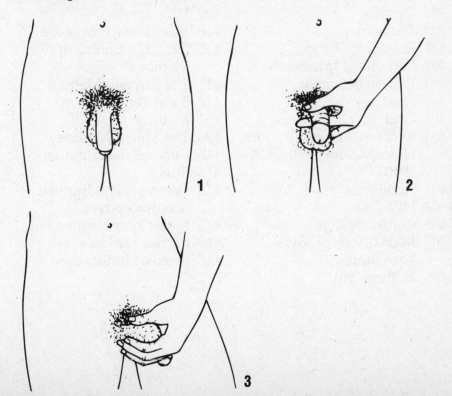

9

SEXUALITY

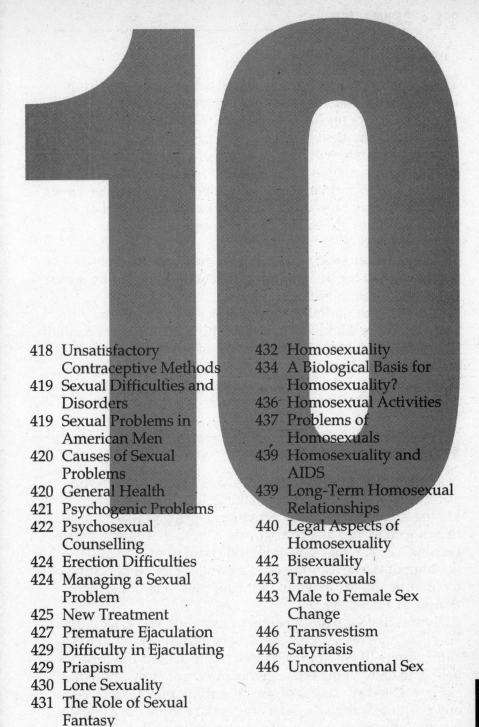

10

Sexual Activity

There is a broad spectrum of sexual activity, ranging from looking at and touching another person to penetration of the vagina by the penis (in heterosexual sex), and ejaculation of semen. In many societies, especially in the West, sex between a man and woman, with the intention of producing children, has long been regarded as normal, and other types of sex as deviant and abnormal. In many modern societies these views are increasingly regarded as unnecessarily rigid, and other sexual activities are gaining acceptance.

Some definitions:

Heterosexual sex: sex between a man and a woman.

Vaginal sex: the penetration of a woman's vagina by a man's penis or another object

Oral sex: stimulation of the genitals with the mouth.

Fellatio is the stimulation of the penis by the partner's mouth.

Cunnilingus is the oral stimulation of the female genitals.

Homosexual sex: sex between two men or two women.

Anal sex: penetration of the partner's anus by a man's penis – or, sometimes by another object, such as a hand.

Heterosexual Sex

Sexual arousal may occur suddenly as a response to sexual attraction, or gradually after looking, touching, stroking, kissing and other foreplay activities. During sexual arousal a man normally has an erection, and a woman's vagina may become moist. Other physiological changes may include flushing of the face and neck, the swelling and moistening of the mouth and the erection of the nipples in both partners.

Stage 1: Foreplay

Activities that take place before penetration and ejaculation. Foreplay enhances sexual enjoyment and makes a satisfying climax more likely. It may consist of the actions described below, usually in the order given, interrupted by removing clothes. The early stages of sexual activity may take place in any position, but by the later stages the couple have usually taken up the position in which penetration will occur. Foreplay varies from very gradual and gentle to rapid and forceful. It may be omitted altogether in hasty sex.

1 Touching, stroking, fondling, grasping parts of the partner's body. This often occurs in a sequence that begins with parts of the body that are not specifically sexual, the hands and arms,

face, neck and hair; and progresses to those that are – the
abdomen, buttocks, breasts and thighs, then the genitals.
2 Kissing, biting, and exploring the partner's body with the
tongue, usually beginning with the lips. A man may kiss his
female partner's breasts and suck her nipples.
3 Manipulation of the partner's genitals. The woman may
fondle the man's penis; the man may caress his partner's
labia (the lips at the entrance to the vagina); separate
the labia to expose the clitoris, which helps to arouse the
woman sexually; insert one or more fingers into the vagina,
and move them in and out of the vagina in imitation of the
movements of the penis.
4 Pressing and rubbing the genital areas against the partner's
genitals and against other parts of the partner's body. This
helps prepare the genitals for penetration:
penis: during sexual arousal, the penis becomes stiff (erect)
enough to enter the vagina. Erection may then develop only
slowly, or not at all. Both the female and male partners may be
able to stimulate the penis by hand until it becomes erect. If it
is only partially erect, it may be possible to give it enough
support by hand to allow entry
vagina: sexual excitement causes a woman's vagina to
prepare itself for penetration and ejaculation. Glands, called
the Bartholin glands, in the labia major, produce a clear
lubricating mucus. This may be spread over the outer genital
area during foreplay. The mucus membrane that lines the
vagina also becomes moist, facilitating entrance by the penis.
The muscles controlling the vagina relax, enabling it to expand
when the penis is inserted. During foreplay, the male partner
helps the vagina to relax further.
Stage 2: Penetration
The couple adopt a position that allows sexual intercourse to
take place. The man positions the tip of his penis at the
entrance to the vagina – or the woman lowers her vagina onto
the penis. Either partner might hold the penis to direct it into
the vagina. Alternatively, either partner might hold the
woman's labia apart to help the penis slide between them.
The penis might be inserted gradually, just the tip at first, then
progressively more of the penis is inserted in a series of small
forward movements and half retreats. This spreads the vaginal
lubricant over the penis, and enables the vagina to
accommodate itself to the penis's size.
Delaying entrance
The penis can be inserted into the vagina once it is erect, but a

10

couple may continue love-making without penetration for some time, reaching high levels of sexual excitement before penetration.

Difficult penetration

This depends on:

1 the relative sizes of penis and vagina;

2 the stiffness of the penis and the degree of relaxation and lubrication of the vagina.

The second set of factors is much more important. A vagina, however small, can normally accommodate a penis of any size providing that the vagina has become sufficiently relaxed. So problems of insertion usually arise because sexual arousal in the woman has not gone far enough.

A woman who has not had intercourse before will usually have a hymen; an unbroken ring of fleshy tissue just inside the vaginal opening. This may need to be stretched or broken to allow entrance. If so it is encountered by the penis as an obstruction, beyond the labia. Hymens vary greatly in strength and stretchability. If a hymen has to be broken, a more forceful pressure of the penis may be needed (or the fingers can be used). (In extreme cases, a minor surgical operation may be necessary.) But, today, hymens have often been stretched by physical exercise, use of tampons, and the 'petting' of boyfriends (i.e. insertion of fingers into the vagina). Often, in this case, a woman's first experience of intercourse will just take further the slow process of stretching and breaking down the tissue of the hymen. The normal techniques of insertion are all that is needed. This is especially true if entrance is not attempted until the woman is highly aroused and her vagina fully relaxed.

Positions for Sex

The 'missionary position'

The face-to-face position most often adopted by couples because it is reassuring and loving. But the man is very dominant and women often prefer a position that gives them more control.

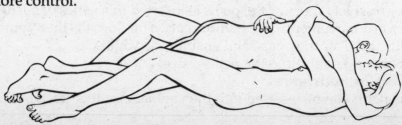

Variety is important to maintain sexual interest, especially in a long-term relationship. However, there are also practical reasons for adopting certain positions:

1 Each partner can move.
Ease of movement for both partners is important if sex is prolonged.

1

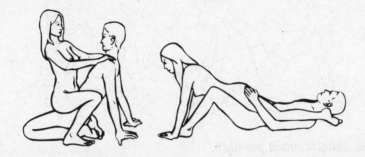

2 One partner bears the other's weight.
A couple may find it more comfortable if the heavier partner is underneath, especially if one partner is weak for any reason, or tired. Some women find it easier to reach orgasm in a woman-above position.

2

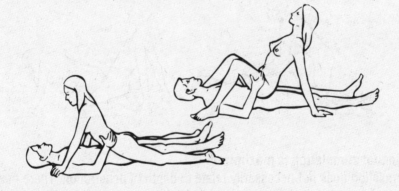

3. Each partner's hands have free access to the other's body.
Satisfying the sense of touch is an important part of the sexual experience for both partners.

3

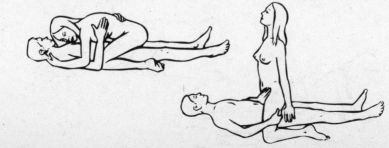

4 Each partner can look at the other's body.
Sexual excitement is heightened for many people by watching their partner making love. For this reason, they find rear-entry positions least satisfying. The position allows deep penetration.

4

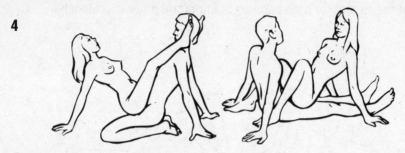

5 Deep penetration is possible.
Penetration can usually be deeper the greater the angle between the woman's body and her legs. In side positions, it is deepest where the angle between the partners' bodies is greatest: (i.e. they form a cross shape). In rear entry, deep penetration is difficult if either partner is overweight.

5

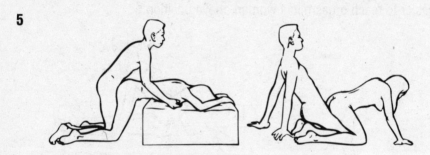

6 Genital stimulation is maximized
Stimulation does not necessarily relate to depth of penetration. There may be more pressure (between penis or pubic bone and clitoris) where penetration is more angled but less deep. However, direct contact between penis and clitoris usually decreases pleasure for a woman. Full penetration in a frontal position gives indirect stimulation because of pressure between the partners' pubic bones.

6

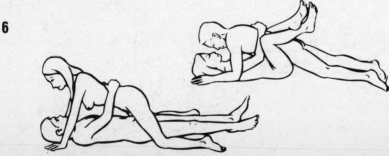

Positions Grid

How to use the grid
The grid illustrates corresponding male and female positions.
Every black circle at the intersection of two lines marks a
possible male/female combination (follow the lines back to the
figures to see which position each should adopt).

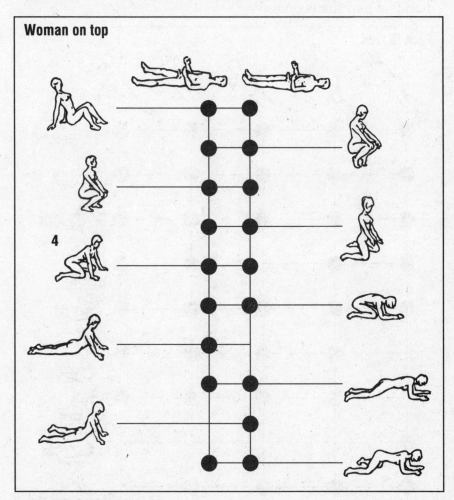

Woman on top

Changing positions
Adopting a variety of positions during sex is not essential,
either for emotional satisfaction or sensual pleasure. However,
moving and changing position is natural while making love.
Positions also fall into groups, with easy movement between
those in the same group.
This grid shows the main groups (only standing positions are
not shown; they depend on the relative height of the partners
and the available means of support).

10

Some points about positions

- for some of the more athletic positions, the woman needs good pelvic muscle control
- in positions in which the woman is on top, she should move with care and check that she is not hurting her partner. Uncontrolled movements could rupture his penis.
- the man can often help his partner's movements with his hands when she is on top

Face to face

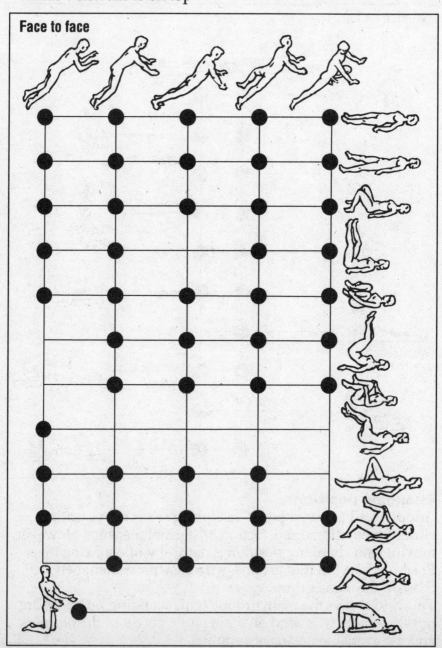

- when the female partner lies on her back, a cushion under her hips can help the man to increase penetration
- a man in a sitting position will be more comfortable if he leans against a wall or piece of furniture that will provide a backrest, instead of supporting himself on his hands. His arms are then free to embrace his partner.

Face to face

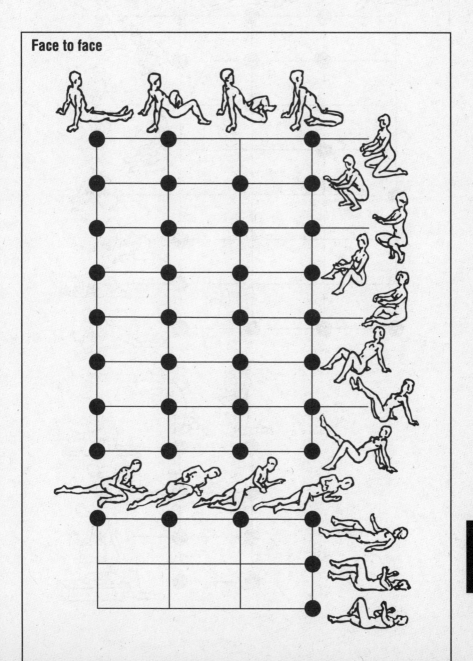

10

Rear entry

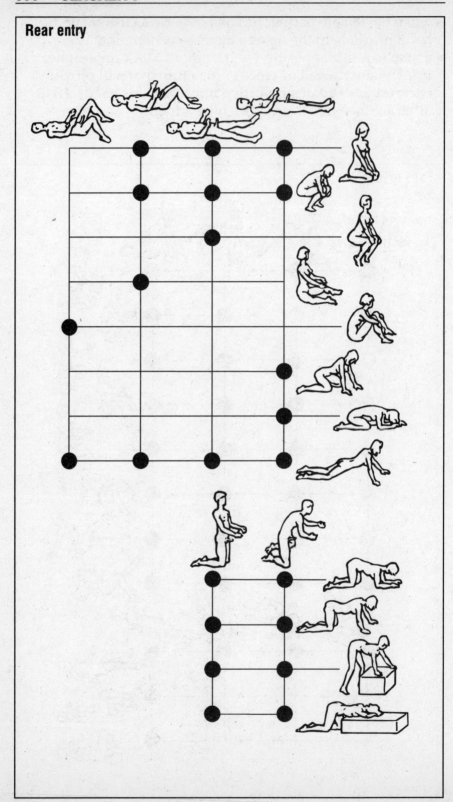

Rear entry

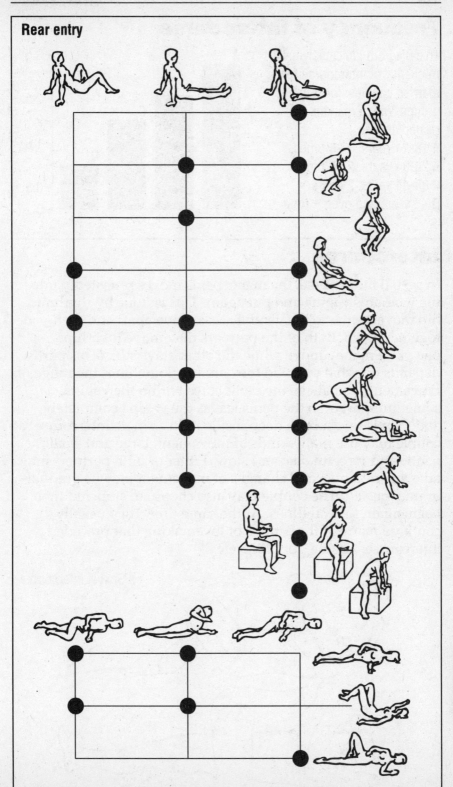

10

Frequency of Intercourse

This diagram indicates weekly frequency of intercourse for married couples, for four age groups, with a marked age-related decline.

A 18-24 years: 3.25 times.
B 25-34 years: 2.55 times.
C 35-44 years: 2 times.
D 45 years and over: 1 time.

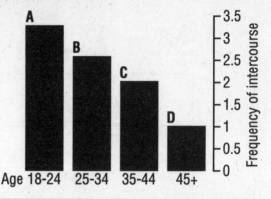

Intercourse

In sexual intercourse, the man's penis moves repeatedly into the woman's vagina and out again. This is done by rhythmic hip movements: so the genital areas move apart and then together again. Both of the partners may move their hips, or one of them may move while the other stays still. (This partly depends on what position they are in.) Sometimes the range of movement is small, so the penis stays within the vagina, sometimes large, so the penis leaves the vagina completely, and then is thrust back deep inside it. In a single intercourse, a couple may use many kinds of movement: large and small, gentle and forceful, fast and slow. Either or both partners may take the initiative, and changes of movement may be gradual or unexpected. The couple may also choose to stop and then begin again several times. At the same time, they usually continue many of the actions of lovemaking that preceded intercourse: kissing, fondling, etc.

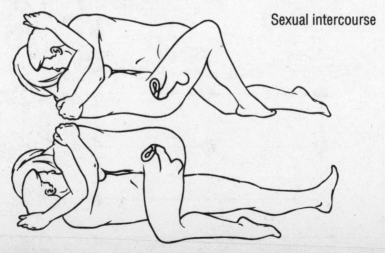

Sexual intercourse

Orgasm

Orgasm was defined in the 1950s Kinsey report as 'an explosive discharge of neuromuscular tension'. In men, ejaculation of semen containing sperm occurs during orgasm. In women, the function of orgasm has been unclear. However, research has recently confirmed a theory that has been controversial since the Kinsey report: that orgasm maximizes the possibilities of conception by 'sucking' the sperm toward the ovum in the Fallopian tube. Radiotelemetry (minuscule transmitters placed in the uterus) has recorded a change in pressure from +40 cm of water (i.e. the pressure of a column of water 40 cm high during contraction to -26 cm water when relaxed) were recorded every 0.8 seconds. This change in pressure supports the theory of insuck.

Male orgasm is but a complex experience, not entirely understood. After a period of time that may vary from a few second to several minutes, the man's pelvic thrusts become less voluntary, and other muscles of the body also begin to contract rhythmically. He becomes aware that he is about to ejaculate. During orgasm, the heart rate increases from 20 to 80 beats per minute; the blood pressure rises (systolic pressure from 25 to 120 mmHg; diastolic pressure from 25 to 50 mmHg). Respiration increases to hyperventilation levels – around 40 breaths per minute.

Orgasm is not just ejaculation. Subjectively, the experience varies. Some men say that they feel sensation mainly in the genital area; others say it is spread over more of the body, or felt all over the body. Some men maintain a greater degree of conscious control over the experience than others.

Ejaculation

Overleaf we show the genital coupling, and the route of the semen. Ejaculation occurs in two stages. Rhythmic muscular contractions begin in testes and epidymides and continue along the vas deferens also involving seminal vesicles and prostate. Sperm and seminal fluid collect in the urethra inside the prostate. Then a sphincter relaxes, letting this semen pass down toward the penis. Contractions along the length of urethra cause ejaculation. Inside the woman's body, semen passes from vagina into uterus and Fallopian tubes. For conception, sperm must find their way into a Fallopian tube containing a ripe ovum.

10

Ejaculation

Conception

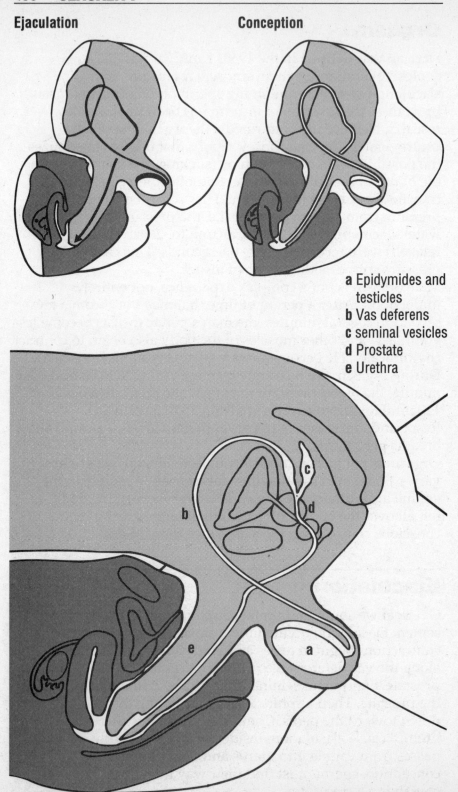

a Epidymides and
testicles
b Vas deferens
c seminal vesicles
d Prostate
e Urethra

Refractory Period

Ejaculation is accompanied by a discharge of tension, after which the rhythmic muscular contractions rapidly die down, the heart and breathing rate slow to normal, and a state of calm and stillness usually follows. Immediately after ejaculation, many men go through a 'refractory period', when they cannot respond to sexual stimulation or experience another ejaculation. During this period, which may last for only a few minutes in young men, and increases with age to several hours, replenishment of seminal fluid and sperms takes place. Since too frequent ejaculation reduces fertility in men, the refractory period may be the body's way of maximizing fertility potential.

Patterns of Intercourse

Mutual orgasm

Frequently, only one partner in the sexual act reaches orgasm during vaginal sex, and it may be necessary for the partner who has experienced orgasm to try to bring the other partner to a climax by stimulating the genitals orally, or with the hands. Simultaneous orgasm – both partners reaching orgasm simultaneously – is rare. Though it is undoubtedly extremely pleasurable, to concentrate on it as a goal can be futile and reduce both partners' pleasure.

Non-penetrative sex

Orgasm is not essential to sexual enjoyment and satisfaction. Research has shown that the repertoire of practices of heterosexual couples is wide, encompassing oral sex and sexual stimulation without penetration (commonly called 'mutual masturbation'). Research very recently carried out in Great Britain shows that after vaginal sex, non-penetrative sex was the most frequently reported activity.

This increase in non-penetrative sex results from a general relaxing of attitudes to sex during the 1970s and 1980s, and from its role as a form of 'safe sex', preventing the spread of HIV infection and AIDS.

10

Percentage of men reporting non-penetrative sex, by age group	
16-17; 1.2	35-44; 1.2
18-24; 1.4	45-59; 0.8
25-34; 4.5	

Brief intercourse

Men are capable of achieving ejaculation rapidly – Kinsey found that three-fourths of men studied could ejaculate within 2 minutes after intercourse began, and some within as little as 10 to 20 seconds. This, added to the male refractory period (see p 401) has caused many complaints from women of brief, unsatisfying sex. The man begins after few preliminaries, and reaches orgasm very quickly, usually leaving the women dissatisfied.

In recent years, however, better sex education and awareness of the emotional needs of both men and women has resulted in changed attitudes. Recent research has revealed fewer reports of this pattern of intercourse.

Brief intercourse pattern

——— Male level of bodily response

– – – Female level of bodily response

Intercourse

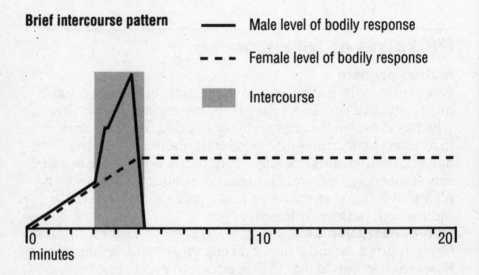

minutes

Prolonged intercourse

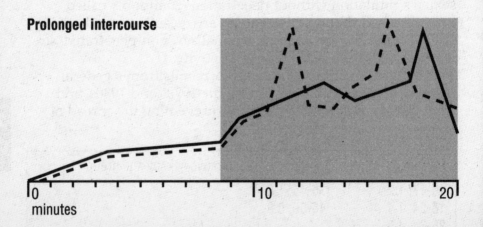

minutes

Withdrawal
The man withdraws just before ejaculation. This practice,
which was common in the past to avoid contraception, appears
to be infrequently practiced now. It is highly unsatisfactory as
a method of contraception, and has been superseded among
couples who do not use other forms of contraception by the
rhythm method. Men generally found it frustrating, and if the
woman has not reached orgasm when the man withdraws, she
may be left extremely dissatisfied.
Prolonged intercourse
The woman has one or more climaxes before the man
ejaculates. This usually results from conscious control by the
man – he may lie still for a while just after penetration, when
his excitement is beginning to peak. Recent research in Great
Britain indicates that this pattern of intercourse is increasing as
better sex education has made couples more aware of the
needs of the female partner.
Repeated male orgasm
With some – especially young – men, the 'refractory period'
after orgasm may be so brief that erection occurs almost
immediately afterwards, and intercourse may occur several
times within a short period.

Pattern of Sexual Practices

Recent research in the US and Great Britain has shown that the
pattern of sexual practice has changed in the generations since
the 1950s, when the Kinsey Report was produced, in the
direction of widened sexual experience. Vaginal sex is still the
form most commonly practiced. However, as well as non-
penetrative sex (mutual masturbation), oral sex is now a
common practice.

Oral Sex

The lips are extremely sensitive and one of the body's main
erogenous zones. Oral sex includes kissing the partner on the
lips, deep kissing (inserting the tongue into the partner's
mouth), and kissing and tactile exploration of other parts of the
partner's body with the lips. However, the term is used
generally to mean fellatio (exploring a male partner's genitals
with the tongue and lips) and cunnilingus (exploring a female
partner's genitals with the tongue and lips). All oral sex
involves kissing, sucking and licking. In fellatio, the penis is

10

moved inside the mouth in imitation of vaginal intercourse and the male partner may be brought to ejaculation in this way. Both partners may be stimulated to orgasm through oral sex.

Recent surveys suggest that oral sex – which was once a state offense in many parts of the US – is becoming a common practice, mainly as a result of more relaxed attitudes to sex, especially over the past two decades:

1950s: Kinsey data shows evidence of increasing experience of oral sex among American men and women born in the first 30 years of the 20th century, including 45% of women who had already had intercourse

1960s: a report on American teenagers showed that in 1967 about 80% of American women who frequently had vaginal sex also practiced oral sex

1980s: surveys of American teenagers showed that virgin teenagers experienced oral sex before vaginal sex.

Oral Sex Among Heterosexuals in the UK 1990s

	Men%
Cunnilingus and fellatio	46.5
Cunnilingus only	6.4
Fellatio only	2.7

Anal Sex

There is some evidence that the practice of anal sex is also increasing, though by a much smaller proportion of the population than oral sex. Various studies have concluded that between 8 and 10% of Americans practice anal sex with any regularity. A recent British survey found that the younger age group (18-24) showed greater levels of experience of anal sex; of those, approximately 8% practiced anal sex regularly.

HIV Risk

The HIV virus, which causes AIDS, can be transmitted through oral, anal and vaginal sex. Oral sex is the least threatening since the virus is present in very small concentrations in saliva. Studies have shown, however, that women who have vaginal and anal intercourse with HIV positive male partners are more likely to become infected than women who only have vaginal intercourse.

Contraception

For conception to occur, several conditions must be fulfilled:
- semen from the man must enter the woman's vagina
- the semen must contain enough healthy sperm to make conception likely
- the sperm must find conditions in the vagina in which they can survive
- the living sperm must make their way into the woman's uterus and (possibly) the Fallopian tubes
- they must find an egg there ready for fertilization
- the fertilized egg must implant in the wall of the uterus.

For contraception to be achieved, one of these conditions must be prevented. However, three factors weigh against the success of contraception:
- sperm may reach the vagina even if the penis does not enter it. Sperm ejaculated onto the vulva or surrounding skin can swim into the vagina
- the healthiest sperm can live in the vagina for 6 hours or more even if conditions are hostile – so any barrier to prevent sperm moving up into the uterus must last at least 6 hours after ejaculation
- once sperm have reached the uterus they can live 4 to 5 days or more. To avoid conception, there must be a time gap of at least 5 days between the arrival of sperm in the uterus and the arrival of the egg.

A normally fertile woman having sex regularly with a normally fertile man stands about a 60% chance of becoming pregnant in any month. For a couple who intend to have heterosexual intercourse but who do not want babies, effective contraception is essential.

Male Contraceptives Techniques

10

There is a wide variety of contraceptive techniques in use today – none of which is ideal. Most are designed for use by women. The only male contraceptive methods are the unreliable withdrawal method, the condom and vasectomy.

However, research is under way into a 'unisex pill' based on a hormone, inhibin, and into a 'male pill' based on Chinese drug called Gossypol, which is derived from a plant, and considerably reduces fertility in men who take it.

Although men have little choice in the use of contraceptives, they have a great responsibility in preventing the transmission of sexually transmitted diseases (STDs). The condom is the only device that gives effective protection against the transmission of the HIV virus, syphilis, gonorrhea and many other bacterial and viral infections during vaginal and anal sex.

Withdrawal

Coitus interruptus is one of the oldest but perhaps the least effective contraceptive technique. The man withdraws his penis from the woman's vagina when he feels he is about to ejaculate, to try to prevent semen from entering the vagina. The method can be effective only if all seminal fluid is kept away from the vulva and vagina, but:

- drops of fluid produced by the urethra containing a few live sperm may 'weep' from the penis before ejaculation
- in the excitement of orgasm a man may not be able to bring himself to withdraw properly. Many couples find prolonged use of the withdrawal technique frustrating.

The Condom

The condom (otherwise known as a 'sheath', 'rubber' or 'French letter') is still probably the most widely used contraceptive. It originated hundreds of years ago and has been used mainly as a protection against venereal disease. Now it is widely recommended as a protection against AIDS. When used carefully, preferably with a spermicide, it is an effective method of birth control.

Condoms are sold in pharmacists and many other outlets, in sealed packages of three or more. They have a maximum life of 2 years if kept away from heat. A condom is taken out of the package rolled up and is unrolled onto the erect penis just before penetration.

A condom consists of a thin rubber sheath, about 7in (18 cm) long, open at one end and closed at the other. It fits tightly over the man's erect penis. When he ejaculates, his semen is trapped in the sealed end. This prevents sperm from entering the vagina.

Types of condom include plain-ended and teat-ended. They can be of different colors and textures. Some men complain that they reduce sensitivity, and lubricated brands claim to be an improvement. Some have a lubricant impregnated with spermicide; others have a spermicidal solution in the teat.

Using a condom: the condom is taken out of the package rolled up, and is unrolled onto the erect penis just before intercourse. The female partner may roll the condom onto the penis as part of the sexual act.

Practice may be necessary before a condom can be put on and worn comfortably. The BMJ, Journal of the British Medical Association, reported that 25% of men have difficulty in putting on condoms, mainly because they are too tight. Of these, 73% had condoms come off during intercourse; and 52% of men who do not find condoms too tight have had them come off. A few men have had trouble with condoms splitting. More than one-third of British penises exceed the British Standard Institute's standard dimensions for condoms. As a result of these findings, there has been a call for a range of sizes.

Types of Condom

About 7 in (18 cm)

Plain ended

Teat ended

10

Damage and Failure

Used consistently from the beginning of every intercourse, the condom is an effective contraceptive. Failures are caused by condoms bursting due to a manufacturing defect, and bursting or slipping off after ejaculation due to 'user errors'. Sharp fingernails and rolling the condom onto the penis the wrong way can cause damage and result in failures. Few couples realize that baby oil, vaseline, and several vegetable- and mineral-based vaginal and rectal treatment creams and preparations can destroy the rubber within 15 minutes. These include: Arachis oil enema, Cyclogest, Ecostatin, Fungilin, Gyno-Daktarin, Gyno-Pevaryl, Monistat, Nizoral, Nystan cream, Ortho-Dienoestrol, Ortho-Gynest, Premarin cream and Sultrin.

Putting on a condom
Hold the condom with the rolled end towards the penis (**1**). Roll it over the tip of the penis, leaving the teat - or pinching about 1 inch at the end of a round-ended sheath (**2**). Roll the condom over the shaft of the penis until it is completely unrolled (**3**).

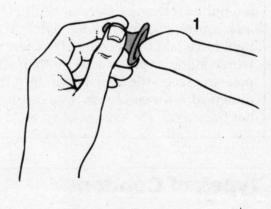

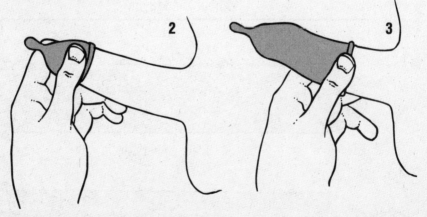

The Condom and STDs

The condom, used correctly and carefully, is an effective
barrier against many sexually transmitted diseases (see p 360).
It is especially effective if impregnated with a spermicide, since
many spermicides are known to deactivate the HIV virus.

American or Grecian Tips

These are short rubber condoms that fit over the tip of the
penis only. It is claimed that they increase sensitivity, but users
report that they do not. Their failure rate is high because they
tend to come off in the vagina.

Vasectomy

A vasectomy is male sterilization. It is a safe, simple, surgical
operation in which each vas deferens – the duct leading from
each testis to the penis is cut and tied off. As a result, the
semen a man ejaculates no longer contains sperm. Only
fertility is affected. Libido, erection, sexual excitement, climax
and ejaculation are unaffected.
Apart from rare instances when the cut tubes rejoin, the
operation is completely effective. It does not alter a man's
ability to have an orgasm or to ejaculate.
The operation is reversible, but this is not always successful in
restoring fertility, although new microsurgery techniques have
raised the success rate above the 50% rate achieved by the
older techniques. However, a man should be absolutely sure
he does not want children before undergoing a vasectomy.
The operation lasts under half an hour and is usually carried
out under local anesthetic. The man returns home and is back
at work within two or three days. After-effects may be soreness
and bruising but this will not be long-lasting.
Vasectomy is not immediately effective. Sperm remain stored
in the seminal vesicles above the cut. Barrier contraception
must be used until two successive follow-up semen tests over
two or three months show negative sperm counts.

10

Vasectomy Procedure

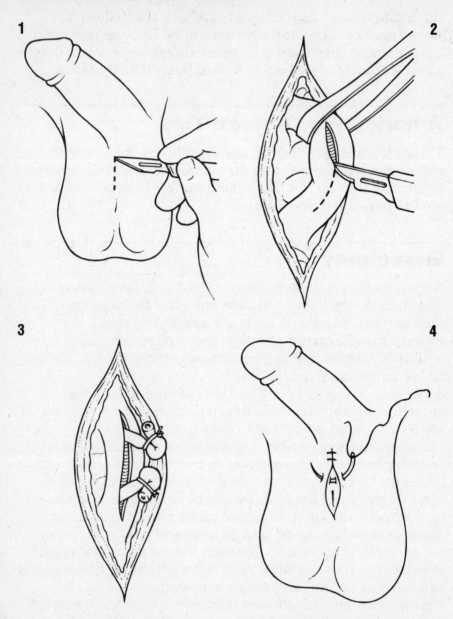

1 Local anesthetic is injected into the scrotum and an incision is made.
2 The spermatic cord is drawn out and cut, and the vas deferens drawn out of it.

3 A piece about one half inch is cut out of each vas deferens, and the ends are folded back and tied tightly.
4 The free ends of the vasa deferentes are put back through the wound, which is sewn up.

'Natural' Contraceptives Methods

Couples who prefer not to use barrier methods or
contraceptive drugs for religious reasons – or just because they
dislike them – should learn how to tell when the female
partner ovulates, and abstain from vaginal sex during that
fertile period. The rhythm method alone is unreliable, but it is
used as the basis for other, more accurate, techniques for
detecting ovulation.

The Rhythm Method

In 'natural' methods of contraception, a couple abstain from
intercourse through the few days of the woman's menstrual
cycle during which she can conceive, i.e. when a egg is
released from an ovary. An ovum is available for fertilization
for only about 24 hours following ovulation, which typically
occurs halfway between two periods – on about the 15th day.
To work out when ovulation will occur, a woman should count
forward 14 days from the start of her last period.
Working this out by the calendar tends to be unreliable, even if
a few days are kept free from intercourse around the likely
date of ovulation. This is because many women have irregular
periods. Even with regular periods, ovulation may occur
anywhere from 16 to 12 days before the start of a period –
indeed, it can be induced by the stimulus of sexual intercourse.
Sperm can live in the cervix for 72 hours or more, during
which time ovulation may occur. Also, it is possible to ovulate
more than once in a single menstrual cycle.

Basal Temperature Method

This is based on the fact that a woman's body temperature
normally rises by several degrees during ovulation, due to
increased progesterone production. You can see this if you take
your temperature every morning as soon as you wake up, and
record it on a chart.
By the time the temperature rise is recorded, the possible
fertilization period is normally over, and a post-ovulation 'safe
period' for sexual intercourse has begun, which lasts up to
(and including) the next menstruation (see chart overleaf.)

10

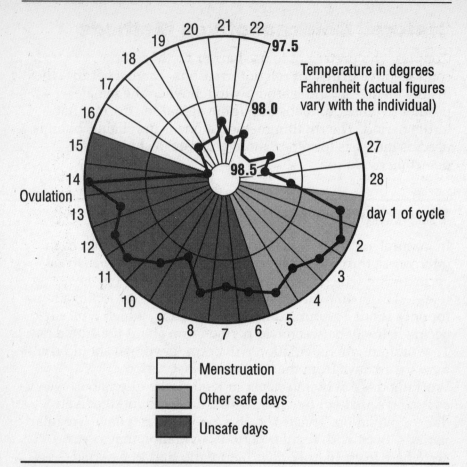

Temperature in degrees Fahrenheit (actual figures vary with the individual)

Menstruation

Other safe days

Unsafe days

The Mucus Method

A second change at this time of the month can help to pinpoint the beginning of the 'safe period' more accurately still. The release of progesterone causes changes in the mucus produced by the cervix, making it unfavourable to sperm. The 'mucus' method of contraception (also called the 'Billings', and 'sympto-thermal' method) monitors the amount, appearance, and feel of the cervical mucus.

During the fertile part of the menstrual cycle, more mucus is produced than during the non-fertile half. It is cloudy-looking at first, gradually becoming clearer, thinner, and more elastic. It stretches out if you put some between your finger and thumb and draw them apart. Ovulation occurs at the point of peak production of this clear, elastic mucus. A daily temperature chart usually shows the period of fertile mucus corresponding with the last five or six low readings. A couple should abstain from sexual intercourse until two or three high-temperature readings have been taken.

Cervical Examination

These 'natural' methods of contraception can be highly accurate – equal to barrier contraceptives – if the body is examined for other signs of fertility. The condition of the cervix is an accurate gauge of fertility, and it may be easiest for the man to examine his partner's cervix. When a woman is fertile, her cervix is softer and higher up in the vagina, and its opening is not so tightly closed as usual.

In addition, women learn to recognize certain personal symptoms of ovulation: an abdominal pain, tenderness in the breasts, slight bleeding, perhaps, or a bloated tummy. Couples should bear in mind, however, that symptoms of ovulation are not reliable shortly after stopping the pill, after having a baby, and shortly before the menopause – usually during the late 40s in most women.

Pills

No other form of contraception has been as revolutionary as 'the Pill'. It is easy to use, reversible, and nearly 100% effective, provided a woman remembers to use it.

The contraceptive pill uses synthetic forms of the hormones estrogen and progesterone, which are produced naturally in the body for a few days in each menstrual cycle, and continuously during pregnancy. In each case, they have the effect of inhibiting the output of FSH and LH hormones. FSH and LH are needed if follicles are to ripen for ovulation: this is why no ovulation occurs during pregnancy. The contraceptive pill has a similar effect; and, as no ovulation occurs, no ovum is available for fertilization by sperm.

The combined pill is the most widely used and effective type. It contains both estrogen and progesterone. The woman takes the standard pill each day for 21 days, starting on the first or fifth day after menstruation, and ending on the 21st or 25th. There is a gap of 7 days, during which withdrawal bleeding occurs; some brands include seven inactive pills to be taken during this period. As well as preventing ovulation, the combined pill affects the uterine lining, so implantation cannot occur; it also causes the cervical mucus to thicken, forming a barrier to sperm.

The continuous mini-pill pack contains 28 pills, all active and all containing synthetic progesterone only. One is taken

10

every day, even during menstruation. They work mainly by their effect on the uterus lining and cervical mucus, rather than by preventing ovulation.

Taking the pill is quite easy; the problem is to remember to do so. Combined pills come in packages of 21 that are labeled with the days of the week to aid memory. The first day of a period counts as day 1. Pill-taking begins on day 1 or day 5, whether bleeding has stopped or not. 'First day start', however, is currently recommended in the United States because the woman is then protected for her entire cycle. It continues until day 21 when the last pill is taken. A gap of 7 pill-free days follows before the next course, during which withdrawal bleeding occurs. For women who have difficulty remembering this sequence, combined pills are available in packs of 28 - the extra pills are dummies.

The progesterone-only mini-pill (also called the continuous mini-pill) comes in packages of 28, all of which are active. The first package of pills may not give complete protection, and for the first two weeks additional methods of contraception should be used.

Side effects

Most women experience some side effects on the contraceptive pill. There may be headaches, nausea, swollen or tender breasts, heavier periods (although menstruation is generally lighter) and vaginal discharge. But not all women experience these, and most symtoms disappear within the first few months. If they do not, a change of brand may alleviate any unpleasant side effects.

No woman should take the contraceptive pill without consulting a doctor. All high-estrogen pills especially carry a risk of blood-clotting. The resulting thrombosis, more likely in women over 35, may be fatal. Other disorders a doctor might consider before prescribing the Pill include heart and circulatory problems, hepatitus, diabetes, migrane and epilepsy. Opinions vary over whether the contraceptive pill increases the risk of breast and cervical cancer. The length of time a woman should stay on the Pill is a matter of dispute. The average tends to be 3-4 years.

NOTE: Both types of pill can become ineffective if medication is being taken, particulrly antibiotics. Also, note that after the age of 35, a woman who smokes is well advised to switch from the pill to another form of contraception.

The 'morning after pill'

This method, which should only be used in consultation with a doctor, tends to be used only in emergencies, such as after a rape or in cases where a couple's normal method of contraception is unavailable or has failed. It contains large doses of synthetic estrogen and must be started within 72 hours of unprotected intercourse. Two pills are taken twelve hours apart. It is 98% effective; it can cause nausea but the risk of dangerous side effects (e.g. blood clots) is low.

Copper IUD

The insertion of a copper-containing IUD within 5 days of unprotected intercourse can achieve effective contraception.

Injectable and Implant Contraceptives

Injectable contraceptives and implants are based on similar hormonal principles to those of the Pill. Injectables are used in more than 80 countries, but have not been approved in the United States for use as contraceptives. Implants, such as Norplant, are available for use in the United States; they are inserted under the skin and release progestogen into the bloodstream. They remain effective for 5 years.

Both methods are very effective but they have possible side effects and links with disease. Symptoms may include disruption of menstrual bleeding – perhaps prolonged, heavy, unpredictable or absent – vomiting, dizziness, moodiness, headaches and weight gain. There are established links with blood-clotting disorders, and unproven ones with breast and cervical cancer (similar to the Pill).

Tests have shown that for every 100 women using implants, fewer than two will get pregnant in a year. This method is most suitable for women who cannot take the contraceptive pill or other methods. Fertility returns once the implants are removed.

Male Contraceptive Pill

A search for a male contraceptive pill has centered on substances that stop sperm production or hinder sperm maturation. Sperm production in the testes is controlled by a cocktail of hormones. Altering this hormonal balance can inhibit sperm production or maturation. Unfortunately, countering the effects of these hormones – using estrogens and progesterones, for example – also has the effect of reducing libido (sex drive) as well as altering secondary sexual characteristics such as beard growth. New, alternative approaches to a male pill, combining low doses of several hormones or using synthetic analogues, are currently being

10

tested and evaluated. Gossypol, a chemical derived from cottonseed oil, has been used by the Chinese as a male contraceptive. The chemical blocks the motility of sperm. However, gossypol appears to effect kidney function and has several other deleterious effects. Research is examining the possibility of developing analogues of gossypol which do not have serious side effects. A reliable male contraceptive pill, free of marked side effects, has yet to be developed.

Barrier Methods

The diaphragm

Various devices can be placed in the vagina to cover the entrance to the uterus, and so prevent sperms passing through. Examples include sponges that can hold spermicide, and small plastic caps that fit tightly over the cervix. But by far the most commonly used – and the most reliable – is the large rubber cap called the 'diaphragm' or 'Dutch cap'.

A diaphragm, covered with a spermicide, is folded for insertion into the vagina, and placed in position by hand (or sometimes with a plastic inserter), so that its bottom edge rests against the rear of the vagina, and its upper edge against the vaginal wall behind the bladder. When released, the diaphragm regains its circular shape, under the tension of a circle of flexible metal concealed in its rim. The vagina stretches to accommodate it, and so the diaphragm is held in place, covering the cervix. Diaphragms are available in various sizes. The size number represents the diameter in millimeters. The size needed must be decided by a physician on examination. A physician should also instruct a woman in its use. A re-examination for size is needed every two years and after each pregnancy.

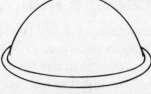

Diaphragm

As long as a diaphragm is correctly positioned, a woman cannot feel it when it is in place. Its advantages are that it can be put in position several hours before sex. It should not be removed until 6 hours or more after intercourse, but can be left in position for up to 24 hours. Some women complain, however, that it reduces sensation during vaginal sex, and some men complain that they can feel it – the tip of the penis sometimes pushes against the outer rim.

The female condom

This is a rubber bag, which is inserted into the vagina before intercourse to prevent semen from touching the cervix or vaginal walls. It is held in place by rings. Used correctly it should give protection against pregnancy and sexually transmitted diseases. Several new female condoms have been developed; one is a latex panty with a built-in 'condom'.

Spermicides

These are chemical products that are inserted into a woman's vagina before sexual intercourse. They act by killing the sperm, or by creating a barrier of foam or fluid through which sperm cannot pass into the uterus. Spermicides come in various forms: creams, jellies, aerosol foams, foaming tablets, suppositories and C-film, a spermicide-impregnated plastic. But used by themselves, none of these is a reliable contraceptive. Each should be combined with another method, such as the diaphragm or the condom. Used in this way, some are doubly useful since they have been shown to deactivate the HIV virus. Some women find, however, that spermicides irritate their genitals.

Female Sterilization

This is the most effective form of birth control – but it is unpopular because it is permanent. As we write, no effective method has been found of restoring fertility in a sterilized woman. Nevertheless, about 33% of all couples practicing contraception do so through female sterilization.

Female sterilization is a small operation, in which the Fallopian tubes are cut and tied, or are all or partly removed. Thus, the eggs cannot pass from the ovaries to the uterus, and the sperm is unable to reach the eggs. If the operation has been done correctly, tubal sterilization is virtually 100% effective. There is, however, a failure rate of between 1 and 6 per 1000. What causes failure is not clear.

Sterilization can be carried out in hospital or private clinics. Rarely is hospitalization necessary. In some centers, operations are performed under local anesthetic with sedation. This shortens recovery time considerably.

After sterilization, sexual interest remains unchanged and the menstrual cycle continues normally.

10

Unsatisfactory Contraceptive Methods

Withdrawal (see p 406), the 'safe period' without temperature or mucus checks (see 412-13), and spermicides used on their own, all have high failure rates, as do the following methods:

Breastfeeding mothers

If women breastfeed 'on demand', lactation is an effective method of contraception. It becomes less so if the mother does not breastfeed on demand or regulates and lengthens the time between feedings, and other contraceptive methods are needed.

Douching

This is washing out the vagina after intercourse, and it is a completely ineffective contraceptive method. Sperm can reach the cervix within 90 seconds, and fluid squirted into the vagina could help the sperm on their way.

Rehability of contraceptive methods

Pregnancies per 1000 women
Vasectomy ● 1
Tubal ligation ●○○ 1-3

Pregnancies per 100 women in one year

With careful use		With less careful use, where applicable
1 ●	combined pill	●●● 3+
1 ●	progester one-only pill	●●● 4+
1 ●	injections	
1 ●	implant*	
1-2 ○●	IUD	
2 ●●	condoms	●●○○○○○○ ○○○○○○○○ 2-15
2 ●●	rhythm methods	●●○○○○○○○ ○○○○○○○○○ 2-20
4-8 ●●●●	injections diaphragm and spermicide	●●●●●○○○○ ●●●●●○○○○ 10-18
10 ●●●●●●●●●●	sponge	●●●●●●●●●●● ●●●●●●●●●●●● 25

In first year of use. Over five years, the life of the implant, the rate rises to 2 per women.

Sexual Difficulties and Disorders

People's perceptions of sexual difficulties and disorders depend on their expectations. One man might normally want to have sex at least once or twice a week, and might worry about suffering some disorder if at any time he found himself sexually unresponsive for as long as a month. Another might expect to want sex once every two to three weeks, and would scarcely notice a month go by without feeling any particular desire for sex.

While it is important to keep this perspective on sexual difficulties, it is also necessary to recognize that sexual dysfunction is a common problem in men, and that it often goes untreated because many do not seek advice. However, treatment centers and facilities have multiplied in recent years, and there are new and effective treatments for such dysfunctions as failure to have or sustain an erection, or to ejaculate.

There is a shortage of accurate statistics about sexual dysfunction, partly because treatment clinics are a relatively new phenomenon. However, reports from such clinics indicate that almost all men pass through a period of sexual dysfunction at some stage in their lives; and that at any one time probably as many as 1 in 10 men experience difficulty in getting or sustaining an erection.

Sexual Problems in American Men

A 1980s study of predominantly white, well-educated, happily married American couples* established that approximately 7% of men experience erectile dysfunction. This figure has been borne out by some other recent surveys.

The 1950s Kinsey reported stated that 1.6% of men interviewed had 'more or less permanent erectile impotence'. The report showed a rapid increase in erectile dysfunction with age – but such data are unreliable in view of the very few elderly men in the samples of men that were questioned.

10

Disorder	%
Erectile or ejaculatory dysfunction	40
Difficulty in getting an erection	7
Difficulty in sustaining an erection	9
* mean age of male subjects: 37.4	

Causes of Sexual Problems

Some physical causes of sexual dysfunction are described in Chapter 2. These days, however, physicians are always wary of diagnosing sexual problems as having specific physical causes. Physicians are increasingly aware that sexual problems tend to have multiple causes, and researchers believe there are psychological factors – such as anxiety – even in clearcut physical problems. Men often report the spontaneous disappearance of a problem, especially when some underlying anxiety is relieved.

As a result of this new awareness, both physicians and psychologists refer to a pattern of physical and psychological factors, which interact as a vicious cycle to bring about sexual dysfunctions:

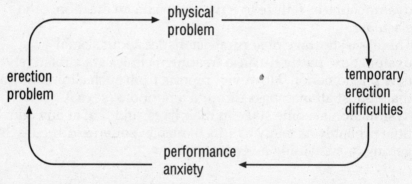

This vicious cycle can lead to loss of confidence and long-term sexual function.

General Health

It is worth reiterating here, however, that so many illnesses affect sexual interest, potency, and enjoyment of sex that a general checkup on physical health is the first step every physician takes when consulted about any functional problem that might arise.

● smoking, diabetes, and high blood pressure can all affect the ability to have and sustain an erection
● illnesses that affect libido include common infections, such as the flu and inflammations of the urinary tract (see pp 145-6), as well as serious illnesses, such as diabetes and heart disease.
● drug treatment for illnesses also have side-effects resulting in lowered libido or sexual function. One report of men (mean

age 58.4) attending a medical outpatient clinic found that
34% experienced erection problems. In 35% of these men,
their medication was found to be the cause.
If you have problems with erection while ill or on medication,
deal with the illness and forget about sex until the body feels
ready again.

Pain during intercourse

This is one physical problem that obviously has a radical effect
on sexual performance. It can also have psychological
repercussions, in that a man may semi-consciously begin to
fear penetration or ejaculation, setting up a vicious cycle.
Disorders that may cause pain in the penis are described on p
384. They are summarized below. If you experience pain
during sex, you must not try to continue, nor should you wait
and try again after some time. See a physician urgently, and
forget about sexual intercourse until the condition has cleared
up.

- overtight foreskin (common during first sexual intercourse
  and after inflammation and infection)
- inflammation of the foreskin (due to friction, injury or
  infection)
- tears in the foreskin (due to vigorous intercourse or
  masturbation; often become very painful)
- chronic prostate infection (see p 147)
- scars in the urethra (usually caused by untreated gonorrhea,
  see [p 157)
- herpes infections (see p 161)
- allergy of the penis to vaginal fluids or contraceptive
  chemicals
- deformities of the penis (e.g. hyperspadias)
- hypersensitivity of the glans after orgasm and ejaculation
  (often extremely painful)
- sexual stimulation without ejaculation may cause aching in

Psychogenic Problems

It used to be thought that deep-rooted psychological conflicts
are a major cause of sexual dysfunction, but more recent
research shows that this is unlikely. In the study of men
attending an outpatient clinic, only 14% of those with sexual
dysfunction were thought to be of psychogenic (mental) origin.
Physicians now believe that the vicious cycle described above
(see p 420) is a major factor in producing permanent sexual
dysfunction (what used to be called 'impotence').

10

Depression, anger, worry and tensions with the female partner can all cause sexual interest to fail on occasions or over a stressful period. Only if the sexual dysfunction occurs regularly, or lasts a long time, can it be thought of as a problem.

Sexual problems often create anxiety, which is likely to prolong the problem, so it is better to open up to outside influences by talking about them than to worry alone. Talking to the female partner, and dealing with any contributory physical disorders, also help.

Anxieties which might themselves be the cause of difficulties in having an erection might be:

- fear of the consequences of sexual intercourse: pregnancy; an STD, such as AIDS
- resentment, disgust or dislike of the partner
- fear of sexual failure – the feeling that you are on trial
- trying too hard to 'perform' impressively or please the female partner
- the female partner's obvious disappointment or frustration
- fear of premature ejaculation, and of losing the erection.

Such fears may be set off by a single incident, by a situation, or by the effect of your own sexual difficulties or those of your partner.

Deep-seated psychogenic problems are usually due to early experience, including the relationship with one's parents, or to traumatic sexual experiences. They can result in distaste for sexual activity, a general resentment of women; an inability to reconcile sexuality with an idealistic image of women, and other psychological effects. Psychosexual counseling and – although rarely – in-depth psychoanalysis are used to help the very small percentage of men who have deep-seated problems of this nature.

Psychosexual Counseling

Management of a sexual problem that is thought to have a psychogenic basis or component usually consists of sensitive counseling, which aims primarily at helping men to deal with immediate stressful life situations, and in preventing or breaking into the vicious cycle referred to above. The therapist might encourage a man to explore and question current thinking about and attitudes to sex, sex roles and performance. There might be emphasis on using new sexual techniques and new ways of giving and receiving pleasure – and on having fun.

Very tense and anxious patients might be guided toward
relaxation exercises and other ways of reducing anxiety.
There is a great emphasis in all therapy on bringing a female
partner into the treatment, and encouraging the couple to
discuss problems together and with the therapist. Easing and
promoting effective communication between the couple is one
of the therapist's most important aims.

Sensate focus exercises

These simple exercises, which help therapists to diagnose
sexual problems and help couples to resolve them were
devised by Masters and Johnson, who researched into human
sexual biology in the 1960s, and published their findings in
their book *Human Sexual Inadequacy*. The philosophy of Masters
and Johnson is that sex is a form of communication, and that
treatment of sexual problem can only occur in the context of a
sexual partnership. Successful therapy depends on the
goodwill of both partners, their ability to learn to relax, and
their realization that sex is not primarily a matter of successful
performances. Their aim in sensate focus therapy is to redirect
the emphasis of sexual activity from ejaculation and orgasm to
mutual exploration, and giving and experiencing pleasure in
other aspects of sexual activity. The exercises are carried out in
private, and at fairly regular intervals. What happened during
each session is discussed and analyzed at intervening therapy
sessions.

Very briefly summarized, sensate exercises begin with the
couple together and naked, stroking and feeling each other's
bodies, but not the breasts or the genitals. Vaginal intercourse
is not permitted. The couple learn to relax and experience
sensual pleasure free from any demand (of release, self-
explanation, reassurance or immediate return of pleasure
received). At first, clumsiness, self-consciousness and
embarrassed humor are likely, but usually genuine enjoyment
soon begins. This undermines the crippling tendency to sexual
self-evaluation. As therapy progresses, the couple begin
touching each other's breasts and genitals, guiding each other
and explaining what is most pleasurable.

During the exercises the couple use a lotion for lubrication,
where necessary, and to help them overcome any distaste for
genital excretions. It was found that couples who rejected the
lotion tended not to benefit from therapy.

Those who did benefit would eventually go on to techniques
for managing specific sexual problems, such as difficulty in
reaching orgasm or achieving an erection.

10

Erection Difficulties

Difficulty in having or sustaining an erection – a response that is not under voluntary control – is one of the main reasons for men seeking treatment at sex therapy clinics. Men tend to diagnose themselves as 'impotent', but the term is imprecise. Men commonly mistake erection difficulties for:

- lack of sexual desire and arousal. This often results from concern about a female partner who is going through a period of loss of desire, or experiencing pain or other difficulties during intercourse. In these circumstances a man may simply feel reluctant inside about having an erection.
- failure to understand the body's need for time to recover between ejaculations. Men sometimes report erection problems when, in fact, they are still in the refractory period (see p 401) between ejaculations.
- ejaculatory problems: the erection subsides rapidly after premature ejaculation and this can be mistaken for failure to sustain an erection.

However, fatigue, drinking, smoking and drug abuse are often the cause of sudden, short-lived erection difficulties. Mild illnesses, such as flu, and more serious diseases, such as diabetes, high blood pressure, and heart disease can all affect erectile potency. It is also reduced by damage to the blood vessels supplying the penis, and by damage to the central nervous system – which may be caused by disease, such as diabetes.

Managing a Sexual Problem

The first thing a doctor does to investigate the cause of sexual problems, such as erection problems, is to look for signs of physical illness, checking blood pressure, size and shape of the testes, the liver and, in patients over 60, hormone levels. The second is to ask careful questions to establish whether the man is in fact experiencing erectile difficulties or some other problem. On the basis of these checks, his problem will be assessed against a scale of four major 'risk factors'. These are:

- **psychological**: he may be experiencing a crisis in his marriage, or reveal during questioning that he might benefit from practicing new love-making techniques
- **vascular**: he may have a blockage in the main artery supplying blood to the penis, high blood pressure or a heart condition

- **eurological:** he may be suffering from some degree of nerve damage due, e.g. to diabetes
- **hormonal**: a man over 60 may have reduced levels of testosterone (a male hormone) in the blood.

To make the assessment, the physician will consider 10 to 15 points under each of these four headings.

Management of the problem is likely consist of a spectrum of treatments, ranging from medical treatments for conditions such as infection or diabetes, to surgery and hormone replacement combined with relaxed psychosexual counseling (see pp 422-3). This will aim at helping the man to resolve any problems he may be experiencing in everyday life, while attempting to prevent the loss of confidence which may set in motion the kind of vicious circle described on p 420.

In the Masters and Johnson therapy for this problem, the female partner stimulates the man's genitals, with him guiding her hand. If erection occurs, it is allowed to die down, then re-establish itself. Gradually, erections become more and more easily obtained. Eventually, vaginal intercourse is attempted, with the woman astride the man. She first tries to keep the erect penis inside her vagina. Later, she begins, gentle, non-demanding thrusting. Eventually the man joins in slow thrusting, but with no goal of ejaculating or satisfying his partner. Orgasm, if it occurs, is accepted as an equal part of the other sexual activity also taking place.

Single men are at high risk of developing chronic erection problems, since they have no partner to help them overcome their difficulties, yet haven't the confidence to find them. Sensate focus exercises using masturbation allied with sexual fantasy have been devised to help them relearn to induce an erection. Group therapy often provides the support men need to find a partner.

New Treatment

Erection-inducing drugs

New treatments have recently been discovered for men with serious erectile inadequacy (inability to have an erection) due, for example, to nerve damage. Drugs used in laboratories to induce an erection in men during scientific investigations of sex are now more and more commonly used to help men suffering from erection problems.

The drugs used are smooth muscle relaxants. In the penis they relax the smooth muscle of the veins and arteries. This dilates

10

(expands) the arteries and compresses the veins – which has the effect of increasing the amount of blood flowing into the penis and restricting the amount flowing out.

At first, these drugs were only given to men with erection problems caused by nerve damage. The majority were able to inject themselves at will in their homes, and to have vaginal intercourse. Later, the drug was tried out on people with a high psychogenic element to their erection problems. These men were also found to benefit, and it was found that being able to inject themselves at home, at will, helped them to break the 'vicious cycle' deadlock .

Priapism – prolonged erection – is a side-effect of this treatment. An erection that lasts for 6 hours or more can

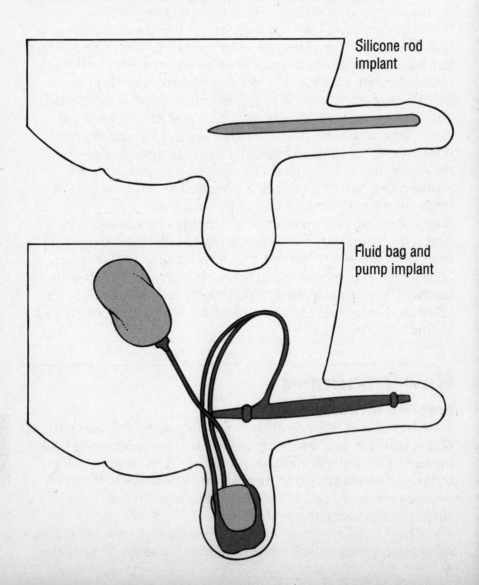

Silicone rod implant

Fluid bag and pump implant

damage the penis permanently, and needs to be treated is an
emergency clinic.

Surgery

Men experiencing erection problems because of obstruction or
damage to the main arteries in the penis can now be helped by
microsurgery, in which the path of an unaffected artery is
redirected to bypass the damaged or blocked artery, restoring
normal blood flow to the penis.

Penile implants

Men with irreversible erection problems caused by injury to
the spinal cord, the pelvis or radiation damage, and men who
do not respond to counseling or drug treatment, sometimes
benefit from penile implants. There are three types:

- a rod made of silicone is implanted in the penis, which is
  kept semi-rigid
- a bag containing fluid is embedded in the abdomen, and a
  pump is implanted in the scrotum. The pump forces fluid out
  of the receptacle in the abdomen, into two chambers inside
  the penis. This stiffens and lengthens it. After intercourse,
  pressing a valve returns the fluid to the bag in the abdomen.
  Follow-up trials show satisfaction with the implants, which
  appear to work well, and so increase confidence
- two inflatable silicone cylinders are implanted in the penis, a
  receptacle of fluid is implanted in the abdomen behind it,
  and a pump is implanted in the scrotum. All are connected
  by silicone tubing. Repeated pressure on the scrotal pump
  transfers the fluid into the scrotal cylinders, which increases
  the length and girth of the penis, and makes it stiff.

Men have declared themselves satisfied with all three devices.
The third is most realistic, but far from natural.

Premature Ejaculation

This is the second most common problem that men report:
ejaculation occurs so early in sexual intercourse that neither
partner achieves satisfaction.

Causes of premature ejaculation

Young men often experience premature ejaculation during
their first sexual experiences, as a result of over-excitement.
The longer the period between ejaculations, the more likely it is
to occur again. As young men gain sexual experience, and
experience regular sex, it is believed that they learn to control
their sexual responses by recognizing when they are close to
ejaculation, and learn to lower their arousal level temporarily.

10

In fact, men of all ages should expect to experience premature ejaculation now and again, especially when extremely aroused, or after a prolonged period without sex.

However, some researchers into human sexuality believe that men who have problems with premature ejaculation did not learn this control, some because of over-excitement, and others because of anxiety. Anxiety – perhaps over the obvious dissatisfaction of the female partner – appears to exacerbate the problem, leading to more and more rapid ejaculation, and inhibiting orgasm. In extreme cases, this can lead to severe premature ejaculation, which seems uncontrollable, in which the man produces an emission (continuous flow) of semen, rather than an ejaculation. This condition is, however, rare.

It is also important to consider that when asked to help with this sexual problem, sex therapists begin by trying to establish what the patient understands by the term. Some men who seek help for premature ejaculation in fact have a female partner who takes a very long time to reach orgasm, so that it is impossible for a man to prevent his sexual excitement rising to the heights of ejaculation before she reaches orgasm. Some couples expect to reach orgasm simultaneously, and blame sexual performance instead of misplaced ideals when they are unable to achieve their goal.

Any man whose enjoyment and satisfaction is consistently impaired by too rapid ejaculation – and whose partner is also frustrated as a consequence – has a problem that can usually be dealt with by simple techniques. These include:

● learning self-distraction to control ejaculation
● concentrating on foreplay that does not involve touching the man's genitals but concentrates on stimulating the female partner to a state of high arousal
● Masters and Johnson therapy.

In the effective therapy derived by Masters and Johnson, the woman, in a sitting position, leans against something and the man sits with his back to her, between her legs, leaning back against her. The woman stimulates the man's penis until he reaches the point when ejaculation feels inevitable (usually 2 to 4 seconds before ejaculation. He warns his partner, and she squeezes the penis immediately behind the glans (tip) between her thumb and first two fingers for 3 to 4 seconds. The man loses the urge to ejaculate. This is repeated 4 or 5 times in a single session.

After thorough practice (the 'squeeze' needs to be learned and practiced to be effective), the couple attempt vaginal intercourse with the woman above. In the first attempts they remain motionless, with the man's penis inside the woman's vagina. If necessary, the woman can intervene to control the man's response by the 'squeeze' maneuvre. Should the male partner lose his erection, he may thrust to retain it. As the couple succeed in controlling their sexual response, they adopt the lateral position. The 'squeeze control' is, however, maintained for as long as is necessary.

Difficulty in Ejaculating

This is a rare disorder, which a man has no problems with erection, but is unable to ejaculate inside the vagina. The problem causes anxiety, self-consciousness and, eventually, impotence.

Failure to ejaculate can have physical causes: damage to the nervous system, and certain drugs used in treatment can cause this condition. It may also be the result of a deep-seated psychological problem, often a traumatic incident in the past, associated with a sexually restricted upbringing. The result is an attitude that sees the female partner as repulsive, contaminating or threatening.

Treatment initially concentrates on establishing and, if possible, eliminating, any physical cause. An effective therapy introduced by Masters and Johnson begins with masturbation of the man's penis by the woman, discovering what the man finds stimulating and gradually raising his levels of excitement, at his own pace. Once the man's ability to ejaculate after manual stimulation is restored, the couple resume vaginal intercourse, but step by step, progressing only when the man feels ready for the change.

Priapism

One of the side-effects of drug treatment for erection problems (see p 384) is priapism, the name for a prolonged, painful erection of the penis. This condition can also, but rarely does, occur as a result of prolonged sexual activity, in men who suffer from sickle cell anemia, and in men with blood-clotting disorders and as a result of treatment with a drug, prazosin. Priapism is a medical emergency. If it persists for more than 6 hours, it causes internal damage to the tissues of the penis. In time, the body lays down thick fibrous tissue in place of the damaged tissue, and this results in permanent inability to achieve erection.

10

Priapism is treated in a number of ways: surgically by draining blood from the penis, but now more often by injecting a drug called metaraminol and massaging the penis, which contracts the smooth muscles of the blood vessels in the penis, allowing blood to escape along the veins. At the same time, blood is drawn off from the penis.

Lone Sexuality

People exhibit sexual responses and behaviour from infancy. Erections are common in male babies. Researchers have reported sexual self-stimulation in the form of genital play in boys from about 6 months and in girls from about 10 months. Infants under 1 year old have been observed to masturbate to orgasm. It appears that social restraint causes children to conceal or stop overtly sexual behaviour as they grow older. Later, pre-pubertal children – aged 8-9 years – resume masturbation and engage in sex play with other children of the same or opposite sex.

Attitudes to self-stimulation

Strongly negative attitudes to masturbation – self-stimulation of the genitals in order to reach orgasm – are evident in ancient writings from the Middle East to China. In the East it was thought to be injurious to health. In Western religions it was regarded – along with all non-procreative sex – as a sin. Attitudes to sexuality have changed radically during the last century. At the end of the 19th century male masturbation was regarded as abnormal behaviour in many Western societies; in Victorian Britain it was severely punished, and in extreme instances people who had been caught masturbating were made to wear mechanical devices to prevent them from repeating the act.

During the 20th century, through the influence of psychology and improved medical knowledge, people have come to accept not only that masturbation (also called auto-eroticism) is neither physically harmful nor a cause of mental deterioration, but that self-stimulation combined with sexual fantasy has therapeutic value.

Doubtful and negative attitudes persist, nevertheless. For example, research on sexuality in Great Britain published in the mid-1990s omitted to include surveys of masturbation on the grounds that the formulation of questions on the subject was distasteful to the question planners.

For these reasons, while it is estimated that 90% of men and

75% of women have masturbated at some time in their lives,
and that the frequency may vary from three or four times per
week in adolescents to twice a week in adults, there is a
paucity of more accurate and detailed data.

One reason for the persistence of negative attitudes at the end
of the 20th century is the implication that an adult who needs
to indulge in lone sex has difficulty in establishing
relationships with people of the opposite sex, or that existing
sexual relationships are unsatisfactory.

Available research suggests that the frequency of masturbation
depends on the existence of alternative sexual outlets. Teenage
men who have not yet established relationships with women
show the highest frequency of masturbation. In other age
groups, frequency of masturbation is indeed highest among
unmarried men and women, and those who have infrequent
sex with other people. However, surveys in different countries
suggest that devoutly religious men and women masturbate
less than those who are not religious; and in other
socioeconomic groups, masturbation is believed to be
unnecessary or undesirable during marriage.

Techniques of masturbation

Most men masturbate by stimulating the penis manually until
ejaculation occurs. A small number attempt to reach orgasm by
imitating vaginal sex with objects that resemble the vagina,
and a very few men have reported being able to achieve self-
fellatio (sucking their own penises).

Women stimulate the clitoris, usually with the fingers, but
sometimes with another object, such as a vibrator. A very small
number try to achieve orgasm by inserting a vibrator or other
object into the vagina and imitating the movements of the
penis.

The Role of Sexual Fantasy

Many people say they fantasize about the sexual act while
masturbating. Since the 1970s, researchers and writers have
begun to explore the nature and function of sexual fantasy and
its association with masturbation and sex with other people. By
interviewing many subjects about the types of fantasies they
have, their need to fantasize, and the satisfaction fantasizing
gives them, they have concluded that fantasy – a powerful tool
of the human imagination – enables people to explore their
sexual reactions, overcome inhibitions, come to terms with and
perhaps resolve sexual difficulties and so realize aspects of

10

their potential as sexual beings that might otherwise never be developed.

As an example, a man who is normally sexually assertive might fantasize about being ravished by a dominating woman. Such a fantasy could well be a safe and personal way of expressing a need to relax from daily responsibilities, or to accept being cared for by someone else. The fantasy, translated into reality with a partner, could therefore help the man to rediscover the childish or the feminine parts of himself, or another aspect of his personality that had previously been repressed.

The value of self-stimulation

In several books published during the 1990s, psychotherapists have pointed out the value of masturbation allied with sexual fantasy in the modern world. Satisfying self-stimulation is an excellent antidote to self-denial when one partner is temporarily absent, when a relationship is passing through a period of emotional or sexual difficulties, when one partner has a prolonged illness and the other wants to remain faithful. It is also a valid sexual activity for anyone recovering from a broken relationship, who feels a need to spend time alone for a while before entering into new relationships. Above all, when the threat of HIV infection and AIDS necessitates a reduction in the number of sexual partners, masturbation – and mutual masturbation - are the safest of safe sex practices.

Homosexuality

Homosexuals are men and women who are emotionally and sexually attracted to their own sex. Homosexual women are also called lesbians. Hetrosexual women are also called lesbians. Hetrosexual people tend to classify homosexuals as exclusively attracted to people of their own sex, but many people tend to have both homosexual and heterosexual instincts. Recent anthropological studies have shown that exclusive homosexuality tends to exist only in societies in which homosexuality is repressed.

In history, for example in ancient Greek society, and in many present-day cultures, homosexual relationships have been and are considered normal. In Europe, the US, Australia and other societies strongly influenced by European culture, male homosexuals in particular have for centuries been considered by heterosexual males as abnormal or sinful, and have been repressed, often savagely. Lesbianism has tended go unrecognized.

In modern western societies, unsubstantiated conventional images of male homosexuals still hold that they are more feminine than masculine, and that their influence makes them a danger to children, especially boys. Lesbians are still largely ignored.

In reality, homosexuals are not identifiable by body type, mannerisms, dress or occupation. Most heterosexual people may, without realizing it, have friends and relatives who are homosexual. However, in contemporary Western culture, many homosexuals have felt able to declare their sexual preferences openly, and refer to themselves as 'gay'. In American and some European cultures, they are now able to formalize their personal relationships by religious services in which their union is blessed. Lesbian couples have borne children by AID, and some homosexual couples have been able to adopt children.

Incidence of homosexuality

Homosexuals are a minority in any human society. It is estimated that between 2% and 6% of any population are homosexual. It is difficult to calculate the numbers of homosexuals in any population since, because of guilt and secrecy, surveys cannot be considered accurate. Also, it is difficult to define true homosexuality, since many largely heterosexual people have an occasional homosexual incident in their lives, especially during pre-pubertal sex play. Strong feelings toward a person of the same sex, perhaps accompanied by some sexual activity, is typical of one stage of emotional development during adolescence.

It is estimated that perhaps one-third of all men have at least one homosexual experience to orgasm during or after adolescence. But only perhaps 2% to 4% of adult males are exclusively homosexual. Between these extremes are individuals who have varying degrees of adult experience of both heterosexuality and homosexuality, some contiguously and some at different periods in their lives. Many such individuals marry and bear or father children.

The incidence of homosexual activity is higher in all-male cultures, such as the armed forces, or all-female cultures, where opportunities for heterosexual relationships are reduced.

10

A Biological Basis for Homosexuality?

In Western society, attempts have been made over centuries to explain homosexuality. With the development of psychology, for example, it was explained as the product of deep-rooted emotional conflicts in childhood. Since understanding of genetics has increased, the occurrence of homosexual men in families has been investigated, and attempts have been made to discover a genetic basis for homosexuality.

In 1991, researchers working on sexual dimorphism (differences between men's and women's brains) discovered that a minute group of cells near the front of the hypothalamus (a gland, the meeting place of the body's nervous and hormonal systems) is twice as large in male as in female brains. The medial prioptic area, where these cells are located, is involved in the generation of sexual behaviour in males. Later research showed that in homosexual men the cell group is two to three times smaller than in heterosexual men, and comparable, after adjusting for overall brain size, with the size of the cell group in women's brains.

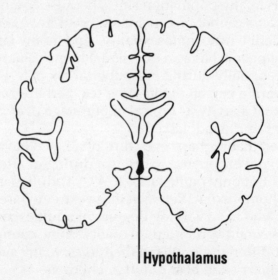

Hypothalamus

It was subsequently found that the many of the cells in the group receive stimuli from the sex hormones. In male fetuses, around the time of birth, a surge of androgens, the male hormones, stabilizes the population of these cells. In females, this surge does not occur and the receptors for testosterone die. This and other factors indicate that this structural difference related to sexual orientation is present at birth. It may be that fetuses destined to become lesbian or gay individuals have unusually high or low levels of androgens respectively, or that some difference in the fetal brain causes differing responses to androgens.

Since these findings, researchers have discovered that a bundle of fibers which help transmit information running from one side of the brain to the other, called the anterior commissure, is larger in gay men and women than in heterosexual men.

Genetic link

Twin and family tree studies for homosexuals were first carried out in 1985, and have demonstrated a degree of what geneticists call 'family clustering'.

Men

57% of identical twins of gay men)
24% of fraternal twins of gay men) are also gay
13% of brothers of gay men)

Women

50% of identical twins of lesbians)
16% of fraternal twins of lesbians) are also lesbian
13% of sisters of lesbians)

Geneticists have since established that there is:
- a 14% likelihood that the brother of a gay man will be gay, compared with a 2% likelihood that the brother of a heterosexual man will be gay
- a 7% likelihood that the maternal uncle of a gay man will be gay, whereas fathers and paternal uncles showed no correlation.

These findings indicate to geneticists that the trait, if genetically influenced, is inherited through the mother via a gene on the X chromosome. To find out more, in 1993 researchers at the National Cancer Institute embarked on a linkage study of the X chromosomes in gay men. This is based on the fact that if a trait is genetically influenced, relatives who share it will share the gene more often than probability would indicate; and that genes that are close together on a chromosome are usually inherited together, so any gene that influences sexual orientation will be 'linked' to a DNA marker. The researchers studied the genes of 40 families with two gay brothers, but no gay father-gay son pairs.

The results showed that a region labeled Xq28, at the tip of the long arm of the X chromosome, was shared by 33 pairs of brothers, whereas in a control group of randomly selected pairs of brothers, the Xq28 markers were randomly distributed. The interpretation is that a gene exists that influences male sexual orientation.

10

X-Chromosome   **Xq28**

Commentators on the significance of this result point out that
they are currently inconclusive. First, the results of this
experiment must be obtained in a repeat experiment by a
second team. Second, the gene has yet to be found. Third,
researchers have to find out how the gene interacts with other
genes, the brain and the environment to influence a trait as
complicated as human sexuality. Fourth, it has to be
investigated why 7 pairs of gay brothers in the group did not
inherit the marker. Lastly, hypotheses that other behavioural
traits – notably manic depressive psychosis – are X-linked,
supported by much clearer evidence than that available for a
genetic basis for homosexuality, have not been borne out by
subsequent research.

Analyses of the research carried out so far point out that what
the results available so far have most clearly shown has been
our lack of knowledge about how sexual orientation is
determined. The genetic basis of homosexuality has not yet
been established, and it is extremely possible that subsequent
findings will disprove the hypothesis. For example, one
analysis has pointed out that in the genetic study outlined
above, it is possible that the subjects' heterosexual brothers
also carried the genetic marker Xq28. As this book goes to
press, no further information has emerged.

Homosexual Activities

In expressing their attraction or affection for another, and in
sexual foreplay, homosexual and heterosexual practices are
identical. After sexual arousal, techniques used by gay men
and lesbians include mutual masturbation. Men practice
fellatio and interfemoral intercourse (the penis is stimulated by
being moved between the partner's thighs), and anal
intercourse. Women practice cunnilingus and vaginal sex,
using the fingers, a vibrator or sometimes a dildo, a penis-
shaped object made of rubber.

Many heterosexual people believe that homosexuals and
lesbians take on exclusively passive (traditionally female) or
active (traditionally male) roles. However, these roles are

blurred, alternated and interchanged in homosexual as in heterosexual life.

Anal sex

This is inserting the penis into the partner's anus, normally with the aid of an artificial lubricant. Two rings of muscles, called sphincters, are sited at the opening to and inside the anus. They are normally closed, to prevent faeces from being expelled involuntarily. The outer sphincter can be relaxed or tensed at will, but the inner sphincter is not altogether under conscious control. Homosexual men learn to relax both muscles to avoid pain during anal intercourse. A dilator can be used, which gradually stretches them, but most men find that both muscles relax if they are at ease with their partners during anal sex. When the penis has passed through the two sphincters it reaches the rectum, which is wide and does not register pain.

The passive partner often experiences intense pleasure in anal intercourse. This is because of the erotic sensitivity of the anus (a sensation enjoyed by many heterosexuals), and because the sexual thrusting stimulates the prostate through the wall of the rectum. Stimulation of the prostate seems to produce an especially prolonged and intense orgasm. During orgasm the anus automatically tightens and puts pressure on the penis inside, it, so intensifying the pleasure of the active partner. There are objections to anal intercourse on hygienic grounds, since the rectum, though empty of waste matter for much of the time, contains bacteria that can be harmful if spread to the genitals. The genitals should be washed thoroughly after anal intercourse and especially before any further oro-genital contact (fellatio).

In additional to anal intercourse, many homosexuals have practiced 'fisting' – inserting a hand or fist, or other objects, into the anus as a form of sexual stimulation. Experience has shown, however, that this practice should be avoided, since it can cause gay bowel syndrome – fissures and other damage to the walls of the rectum.

Problems of Homosexuals

10

These mainly arise because much of society still treats homosexuality as abnormal. Many young gay men and lesbian women have difficulty in recognizing, coming to terms with, accepting and admitting their sexual preference. It can take years from the first feelings of homosexual attraction to outright admission of homosexuality, and some may avoid it for a lifetime, suffering instead loneliness or a lingering dissatisfaction with heterosexual life.

Frequently, admission to oneself is followed by acute depression and shame, sometimes leading to suicide attempts and periods of psychiatric treatment. Homosexuals who are self-aware often fear that heterosexual peers, parents and people in authority over them may find out their sexual preference. 'Coming out' (declaring one's homosexuality openly) is a brave action, still beset with dangers, for homosexual men and women. And it does not mark the end of repression. Open flirting and other homosexual behaviour is still not accepted in heterosexual society.

Nevertheless, a number of clinics dealing with sexual problems reported in the late 1980s that the numbers of people seeking help for problems associated with homosexuality, especially for treatment for homosexuality, had decreased over the preceding 10 years. However, homosexuals were unlikely to received satisfactory help from heterosexual doctors, and were often refused treatment because of their sexual orientation. Consequently, as we write, comprehensive data on the numbers of gay men and lesbians seeking help for psychosexual problems within their relationships is not available.

Homosexual relationships

Even now, gay men and lesbians often find it hard to meet others like themselves. Networks exist in the cities to help people integrate, but elsewhere many individuals remain isolated.

In the decades since homosexuals first 'came out', in the 1960s, their alliances have in many cases tended to be fragile and transient (although AIDS has had an effect on this, see below). This may have been partly due to the newness of an open gay and lesbian society and a conscious decision by some of its members not to imitate heterosexual behaviour, allied to the mutually protective role such a society had to adopt against many hostile elements in outside society. In addition:

- the inability to reproduce removes the binding purpose of raising another generation, and leaves an empty sexuality
- the relationship, unsanctioned by society at large, may cause the partners to feel insecure
- the partnership suffers in time, since the partners' separate roles are undefined.

Homosexuality and AIDS

The appearance of HIV infection and AIDS (see p 121) in the 1970s has had a profound effect on relationships between gay men, one of the two groups most heavily affected. Cruising — visiting clubs and bars and picking up casual partners for sex — is one of the reasons why AIDS spread so quickly through the homosexual community. Since the mid-1980s, when awareness of AIDS spread, the emphasis among homosexual men has been on stable, long-term relationships, as well as on safe sex.

Safe sex rules for homosexuals

In addition to the safe sex procedures described on p 151-2

● always use a condom with a water-based lubricant. Lubricants prevent the sensitive anal canal from being injured, as well as protecting the condom from splitting

● never use an oil or fat-based lubricant – they make condoms porous and destroy the rubber (see p 406)

● during oral sex, never ejaculate into your partner's mouth

● take care when playing with toys – the HIV virus can be transmitted through cuts and scrapes

● do not share toys which have been inserted in another person or use a condom with them

● do not lubricate the penis before putting on a condom or it may come off during sexual intercourse

● put the condom on before any entry takes place

Long-term Homosexual Relationships

The legal position of homosexuals varies widely from criminalization of all male homosexual acts (lesbianism is largely ignored in prohibitive legislation) in some countries to laws which protect the rights of homosexuals and recognize formalized same sex partnerships giving them almost parallel rights to those of heterosexual marriage. Social attitudes do not necessarily match the legal situation and neither determine sexuality, though both can make life difficult for homosexuals. In some localities, or in certain professions, tolerance of homosexuality made it possible for same sex couples to acknowledge their relationship among close friends and associates but it is only in recent years that changes in law in some countries have made it possible for gay men to 'come-out' and declare their sexuality. While marriage gained public endorsement for an heterosexual pairing and brought social pressures against its dissolution, with the raising of children

10

placing further emphasis on a stable household, homosexuals usually had to hide a relationship and might often be limited to casual encounters for fear of discovery, nevertheless there were many homosexual couples who established lasting relationships. The development of the gay liberation movement saw many gay men, especially in the USA, seeking to establish lifestyles which were not dominated by the pattern of 'straight' society's marriage and supposed sexual monogamy. Others, especially since the threat of AIDS has put

Legal Aspects of Homosexuality

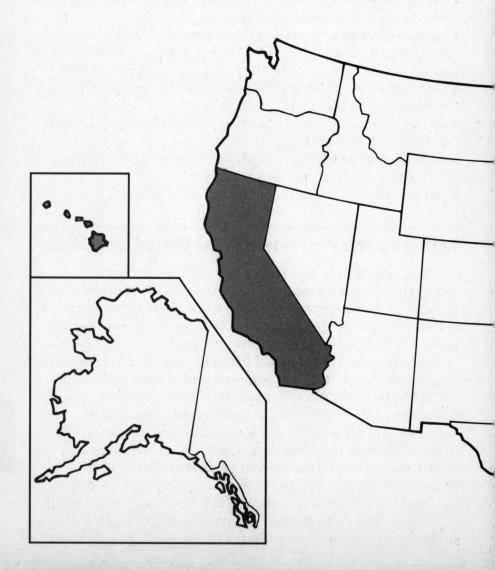

monogamous relationships in a different perspective, have sought state and religious recognition of formally committed homosexual partnerships and legal rightsfor partners to match those of heterosexual couples in terms of property, inheritance, taxation, the right to adopt, etc. Such legal changes might help to change public perception and decrease homophobia, as well as encouraging the stability of gay relationships. Within the gay community there are already counselling services to aid homosexuals with relationship and sexual problems.

The states of California, Wisconsin, Vermount, Massachusetts, Connecticut, New Jersey and Hawaii all ban discrimination against homosexuals in some or all of the following areas: employment, accommodations, education, housing, credit and union practices.

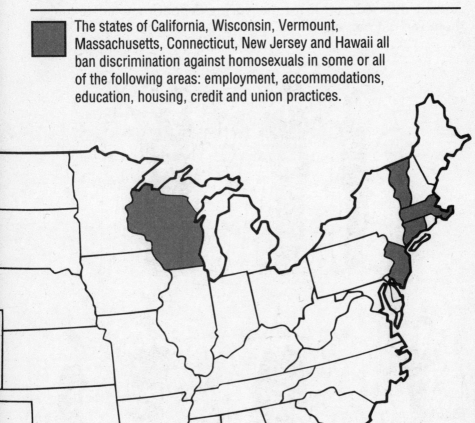

10

Bisexuality

Men who are bisexual engage in sexual activity with members of both sexes. Some men combine equal amounts of heterosexual and homosexual activity throughout their sexual lives, others may vary the degree to which they engage in bisexual activity and may appear to be exclusively heterosexual or exclusively homosexual at different periods in their lives.

Kinsey devised a scale for measuring the entire heterosexual-homosexual range.

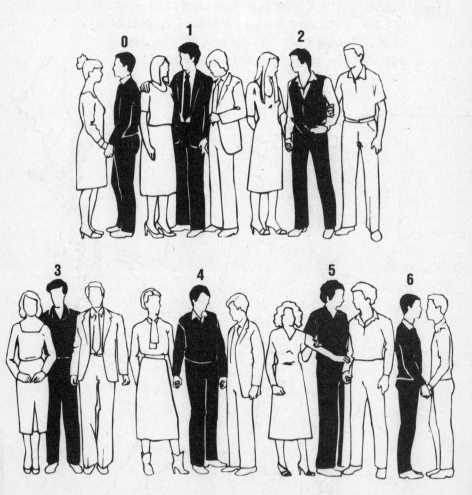

0: Exclusively heterosexual, all psychosexual responses and all overt sexual activity is directed toward women.

1: responses and activity are almost entirely heterosexual, but with incidental homosexual responses or activity.

2: Psychosexual responses and/or overt sexual activity are mainly heterosexual, but responses to homosexual stimuli are rather definite and/or homosexual activity is more than incidental.

3: At the middle of the scale, about equally heterosexual and homosexual in psychosexual responses and/or overt activity.

4: Responses and activity are more often homosexual, but responses to heterosexual stimuli are rather definite and/or heterosexual activity is more than incidental.

5: Responses and activity are almost entirely homosexual, but with incidental heterosexual responses and/or activity.

6: Exclusively homosexual, with all psychosexual responses and all overt sexual activity directed toward other men.

Transsexuals

Some babies are born with ambiguous genitalia and may be assigned a sex determined after considering all factors, surgery and hormonal treatment being given as appropriate and in rare cases this may occur later in life. However, there are also those who, automatically of one gender, grow up with an increasing conviction that they are really of the opposite gender. This is quite different from homosexuality or with transvestism (dressing in the clothes of the other sex) which can be an addiction of happily heterosexual males. A completely biological male may feel that he is a woman trapped within a man's body. If counselling and psychiatric investigation show that the person is unable to adjust to their biological sex and that they are capable of living life as the opposite gender, surgery can make a superficial change of sex. The patient may be required to show that they can live and pass as the other gender before the surgeon will agree to operate.

10

Male to Female Sex Change

Counselling and hormone therapy, which reduces male characteristics such as growth of beard and alters body shape, precede any surgery. Prosthetic breasts may be implanted to supplement growth resulting from hormone treatment.

Surgery removes and refashions the genitalia, excising the erectile tissue of the penis, repositions the urethra, forms a vagina from the perineum and lines it with skin from the penis, using scrotal skin to make the labia. Continuing hormone therapy may be necessary to maintain secondary sexual characteristics as a female. While intercourse will be possible with the constructed vagina it is impossible for the male to female transexual to conceive. The transexual is not permitted to marry in most countries and similarly many countries insist that birth-certificates and passports must continue to bear the gender assigned at birth. While some transexuals make a complete adjustment to their new genital sex there are others who still have considerable psychological problems.

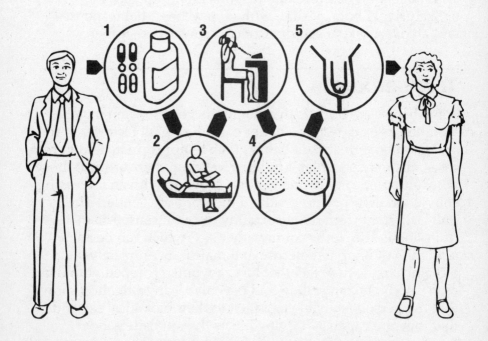

Stages in the male to female sex change

The first three stages shown here are preconditions of a legal sex change operation.
1 Taking female hormones.
2 Psychiatric counselling.
3 Living full-time as a female, usually for at least one year.
4 Breasts may be surgically augmented with silicone pads.
5 Sex change operation in which the genitals are remodeled.

The male to female sex change operation includes the following procedures:

1 Skin is partially removed from the penis; testicles are removed.
2 The penis and urethra are cut through.
3 A tunnel is made for the vagina using the penile skin.

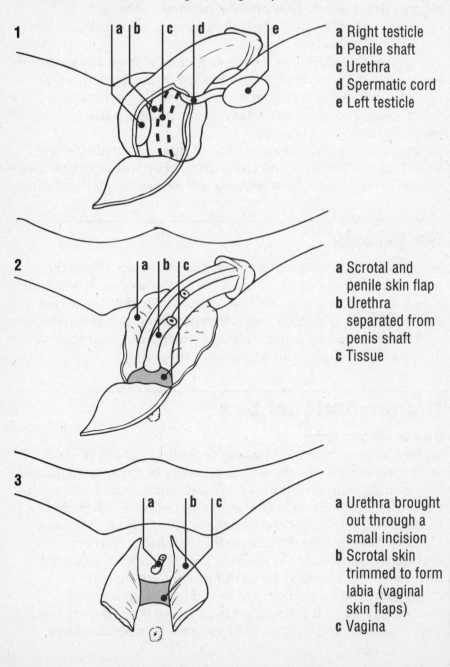

1

a Right testicle
b Penile shaft
c Urethra
d Spermatic cord
e Left testicle

2

a Scrotal and penile skin flap
b Urethra separated from penis shaft
c Tissue

3

a Urethra brought out through a small incision
b Scrotal skin trimmed to form labia (vaginal skin flaps)
c Vagina

10

Transvestism

Transvestism is also known as cross-dressing. For some men, it is a sexual activity in which emotional and physical pleasure are derived from dressing in women's clothes. It is wrong to assume that transvestites are homosexual – most are heterosexual with fairly conventional sex lives and many are married with children.

Patterns of cross-dresing vary considerably. Some transvestites reject male clothing completely and wear female clothing all the time. Some dress as women occassionally or frequently, whilst others have a more fetish-like approach, perhaps involving a single garment.

Some transvestites develop a form of dual personality – one male and one female – and cross-dress in order to express their female personality whilst remaining fundamentally masculine.

Satyriasis

Also known as Don Juanism or sexual addiction, this is the male equivalent of nymphomania, a psychological disorder in which the man is dominated by an insatiable dire for sexual relationships with numerous different partners. It is sometimes said to be caused by intense narcissism and the need to control feelings of inferiority through sexual success.

Unconventional Sex

Sadomasochism

Sadism – named for the Marquis de Sade (1740-1814) – is the term used to describe the sexual pleasure or excitement gained by inflicting pain on a partner. Masochism – named for another infamous writer about sexual exploits, Leopold von Sacher-Masoch (1836-1895) – describes the wish to receive pain and the obtaining of sexual pleasure through being hurt or humiliated (physically or verbally). Sadomasochistic sexual activity is characterized by techniques involving extreme doimination and submissiveness and by the giving and receiving of pain. It is so-called because all practitioners have both a sadistic and a masochistic side to their personalities.

Fetishism

A person may be aroused by one particular part of the body or by an object (such as a piece of underwear) but for most people these are just stimuli; they may form the basis for fantasies or they may enhance lovemaking but they are not the substitute for more conventional sexual activity. A true fetishist is someone who is unable to enjoy sex without the presence of a fetish. The fetish might be a part of the body (the buttocks, for example), an inanimate object (such as a pair of boots or shoes) or a fabric (such as rubber). In extreme cases the object may become a substitute for a real human partner.

Exhibitionism

Exhibitionism is when a person obtains sexual pleasure and gratification from exposing their sex organs to an unsuspecting person and is classed as a crime. For the exhibitionist, gratification comes from the other person's reaction, which is wrongly believed to express sexual excitement. Later this forms the basis for masturbatory fantasies. Research suggests that exhibitionists have an inadequate or immature approach to sexuality combined with a profound need to be noticed.

Voyeurism

Voyeurism is a crime and involves the gaining of unusual sexual pleasure and gratification through the surreptitious observation of naked persons in sexual acts. The typical 'peeping Tom' goes to considerable lengths to observe others when he has no right to do so, and the act of observation is usually an end in itself. By just looking, the voyeur is able to maintain a feeling of sexual superiority without running any risk of failure or rejection by a real partner.

10

AGING

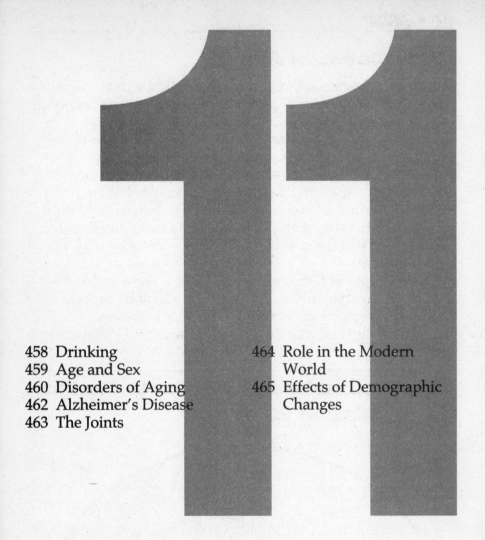

11

The Process of Aging

The human lifespan is thought to be genetically determined, but environmental factors and lifestyle have a greater effect on the length of time people live. In the US, Mormons and Seventh Day Adventists live considerably longer than the average American. People are living longer as medical advances and a rising standard of living overcome many illnesses that cause early death. Life expectancy has risen steadily in industrialized countries in this century. So, with declining birth rates, their populations are increasingly older. In the US, 13% of the population is 65 or over: at least 34 million people.

Everyone grows old, though some people show – and feel – their age more than others. And aging is a lifelong process. Children have many capabilities — such as better eye accommodation and more elasticity in the joints — that are lost

Projected Ratios of Women to Men in US Population 2000

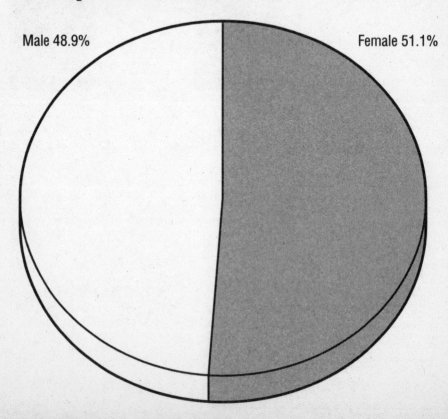

Male 48.9%   Female 51.1%

by adolescence. A father in his forties may lose a test of strength against his teenage son.

However, the aging process becomes apparent much later in life, when physical changes accelerate. Medicine can prolong the lifespan and repair some of the damage caused by aging, but it cannot stop the aging process.

Why Aging Occurs

Aging is believed to be caused by a number of factors that bring about a reduction in cellular energy and metabolism, causing a decrease in the production of proteins necessary for the manufacture of enzymes and for tissue repair.

Cell mutation

This is thought to be the main cause of aging. Most cells in the body reproduce to replace cells that have died. They do so by 'somatic division' (i.e. by dividing in two), so the exact characteristics of the original cell are preserved. However, the chromosomes, the code system built into the cell, which determines how it operates, may be damaged.

When a chromosome, or part of a chromosome, is damaged, a cell may become inactive, or do its job badly, or be actively dangerous (as in the case of cancer). Because the damage affects a chromosome, the distortion is passed on whenever the cell reproduces. This is mutation. Somatic division means that the numbers of mutated cells increase in geometric progression (1, 2, 4, 8, 16, 32, 64), so aspects of the body's functioning become inefficient or disrupted.

Mutation can be caused by exposure over a lifetime to natural radiation (from the sun or from naturally occurring isotopes). It may also be caused by disease, chemicals, or radiation from nuclear activity, exposure to X-rays, and so on.

Collagen theory

Aging changes in collagen, the chief protein of connective tissue, causes loss of elasticity in cartilage and other connective tissues, resulting in stiffness in many parts of the body.

Hormone theory

Aging is thought to be initiated by hormones. Research is currently taking place into thymosin and other hormones produced by the thymus gland, which is thought to have a significant role. The thymus, which is active until maturity and then atrophies, is important in the development of the immune system.

11

Changes in the Body

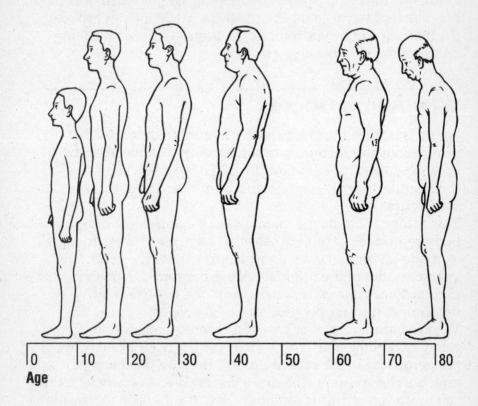

| 0 | 10 | 20 | 30 | 40 | 50 | 60 | 70 | 80 |

Age

Childhood: peak of physical development reached at 12.

Teens: eyes begin to lose flexibility of accommodation, joints become less elastic.

Young adult: total brain weight peaks at age 25-30, nerve cell loss from the brain and spinal cord begins.

Midlife: (30s-50s): fertility continues, but incidence of children born with birth defects rises after age 35. The basal body temperature (body temperature at rest) falls by about 2°F (1°C) between age 30 and 60. High blood pressure and heart disease are common in over-50s.

Over-60s: decrease in testosterone production. Osteoarthritis common in over-60s.

Elderly: total brain weight decreases one-sixth between age 70 and 90. Experience and wisdom increase. Vital signs, reflexes and senses, and sensitivity to pain, decline. Osteoporosis (bone loss) causes loss of height and curvature of spine. Immune system becomes inefficient.

Aging takes place gradually. In addition to the signs described as left:

a neuron loss from the brain results in loss of motor ability and short-term memory impairment.

b loss of accommodation in the eye causes long-sightedness.

c gradual damage to the inner ear results in increasing deafness.

d the teeth are gradually lost and dentures become necessary.

e the skeleton becomes thinner and more brittle as calcium lost from the bone tissue is not replaced.

f the heart valves become more rigid and the heart pumps less blood. The arteries become narrowed by atherosclerosis.

g the lungs become less effective, making respiratory infections more likely.

h changes in the stomach secretions may cause frequent indigestion.

i the liver's ability to metabolize some drugs is impaired. The number of filtering units in the kidneys decreases.

j the bowel may lose muscle tone, causing chronic constipation.

k sexual responses gradually diminish.

l in sedentary people, muscles may lose much of their strength, shape, and size.

m the joints may become worn and lose some of their ease of articulation.

n bunions, ingrowing toe nails and other foot problems occur.

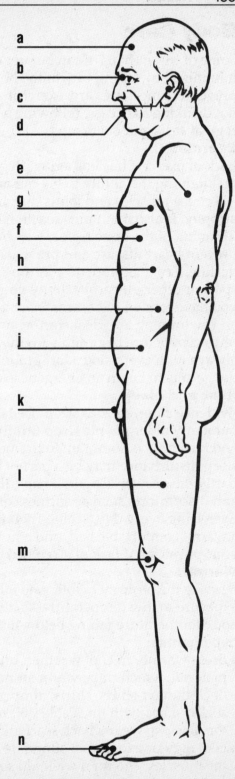

11

Body Care

Some of these changes can be prevented, others delayed or minimized by taking care of the body. The most important preventive measures are: exercising regularly, not smoking, not drinking to excess, following a healthy diet and getting regular tests and check-ups.

Exercise

Lack of exercise hastens aging. Regular exercise is crucial for maintaining the ability to get out and about – crucial in old age – because muscles and joints that are under-used stiffen and atrophy. It also maintains reactions, prevents osteoporosis (thinning of the bone tissue, which causes fractures), helps prevent heart disease and prevents other forms of physical decline. Try, therefore, to continue into middle and old age any sport or other physical activity you have always enjoyed. If you have tended to become inactive, gardening, walking, golf, and swimming are ideal start-again activities. Check with your physician before beginning anything more strenuous, and, as always with exercising, start gradually and build up. It can be dangerous to begin an energetic exercise regime suddenly.

Rest and sleep

Evidence suggests that sleep needs do not decline with age, but many older people sleep fitfully and shallowly at night, and insomnia is common. Retirement is a major life event, and sleep disturbance may be a part of adjusting. Keeping busy is partly the answer. Daytime naps, illness, anxiety, loneliness, and discomforts such as stiffness of the limbs, all contribute. Exercising every day, seeing friends and meeting new people, a warm, comfortable bed, and a hot milky drink, all help. See your physician if lack of sleep becomes a problem.

Warmth

Because the basic metabolic rate falls (see p 252), prolonged exposure to low temperatures can result in hypothermia (the body temperature falling below normal). To prevent hypothermia:

- dress warmly in cool weather: underwear made of thermal material, which traps warm air next to the skin; wear layers of clothing: t-shirts, shirts, jumpers, jackets, thin and thick socks, shoes with thick soles. 30% of body heat is lost through the head, so wear a neck scarf and a woollen hat.
- take regular exercise to stimulate the blood circulation and the muscles – go for a walk, do something around the house, go swimming.

- check your living space for drafts and damp and stop them as well as you can, or contact a help organization. Install roof insulation if you can. Put up curtains lined with thermal material to stop cold coming through windows, and keep warm air in.
- central heating is the best and safest heating system. Open gas or electric bar heaters and free-standing stoves can be fire risks, and solid-fuel fires (coal, etc.) can be difficult to maintain. Good ventilation and regular safety checks are essential for gas and oil heaters.
- take a warm bath or shower before you go to bed, and a warm drink before you sleep. Dress warmly – wear pyjamas, bedsocks, a woollen bed jacket – perhaps cover your head. A duvet filled with feathers traps warm air around you. Plenty of blankets will have the same effect.
- a hot water bottle is a cheap option – do not overfill it, put a cover over it, and never switch an electric blanket on if you have one in your bed. Use an electric overblanket, not an underblanket, and switch it off before you get into bed.

The Spine

Deterioration of the vertebral discs may cause a slight reduction in the length of the spine.

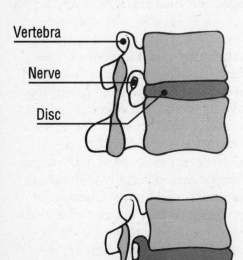

Vertebra

Nerve

Disc

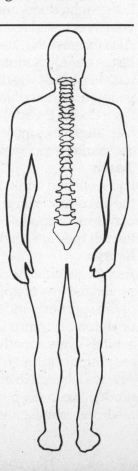

11

Feet

See a chiropodist about corns, calluses, bunions, or toenails that
have become too thick to cut – feet problems will restrict your
mobility and prevent you getting essential exercise. You can
prevent feet problems if you regularly soak your feet in warm
soapy water, brush the nails, and massage hand cream into the
skin. Change socks and stockings daily and wear well-fitting shoes
that give your feet good support.

Bladder and bowels

Report any change in your daily routine to a doctor immediately
you notice it. Such changes can be signs of illness, and should be
investigated. Drink 3 to 5 pints (1.7–2.8 liters) of water every day –
old people become dehydrated, and this causes chronic
constipation. Loss of bowel or bladder control is also common, and
distressing but usually temporary. See a physician, who may
recommend treatment, or a change of diet. Eating high-fiber foods,
switching from drinks that have a diuretic effect, such as tea and
coffee, to mineral water.

Sight and hearing

Long-sightedness and hearing loss occur as you get older. Have
your eyes tested annually and change your glasses if necessary.
Also increase the strength of the lighting in your home.
Listen out for symptoms of hearing loss – the ear and brain
together adjust so efficiently to overcome hearing problems that
people are often unaware that their hearing is becoming impaired.
See a doctor if your family complain, or if people accuse you of not
listening. New, more efficient electronic hearing devices appear on
the market every year.

Teeth

Bad teeth and badly fitting dentures may result in poor nutrition:
the discomfort causes elderly people to select comfortable instead
of nutritious foods. See a dentist every six months, have dentures
fitted if they are needed, and have them checked regularly.

Illness

As you get older, watch out for symptoms of illness. Notice
prolonged loss of appetite, sudden weight loss, blood in the urine
or the sputum, sudden or persistent pains, especially in the chest
or abdomen, unusual skin discoloration and lumps. Check your
genitals every month. Report symptoms if they appear – but also
see your doctor regularly, at least three or four times a year.
Always label medicines clearly, and dispose of any that are not
needed. Keep sleeping pills, relaxants and tranquilizers in a
medicine cabinet, not by your bed, in case of mistakes.

Safety in the Home

If you have difficulty moving around, or if your balance is affected by illness, you may need to some changes to make your home especially safe. Check:

electrical sockets and corded appliances
Contact a help organization for a professional assessment and perhaps help with repairs. Make sure electrical appliances are positioned where they are not easily knocked down.

lighting
People need better lighting as they get older. Halogen bulbs and lamps give more light and use less electricity than tungsten lights. Upgrade the lighting in kitchens and bathrooms, and on stairs.

worn floor-covering
Frayed carpet, especially on stairs, frayed linoleum edges, highly polished floors, loose stair carpet and treads on stairs. Remove worn carpeting and linoleum — it is dangerous. Tape rugs to highly polished floors and wear rubber-soled shoes in the house. Non-slip tiles are best in the kitchen and bathroom.

banisters, baths, toilets
Contact a help organization for professional help with loose banisters, and to get grips fitted in the bathroom and near the toilet.

security
Your local law enforcement or social welfare agency may have a home security officer who will come round and assess the security of your home. Many devices, such as window locks, are cheap and easy to fit, and more efficient devices appear on the market all the time. It is a good idea to buy an alarm to keep by you in case of an emergency. Neighbours are the best home security, so get to know yours.

Diet

Nutritional needs
The body's food requirements remain constant through life. With age, decreasing physical activity and falling metabolic rate often result in lower food energy needs. Although it is important to keep food intake and energy expenditure in balance to prevent obesity, it is equally important to remain active as you grow older, so energy output should not fall very much. It is as important when older as when young to follow a healthy diet, high in

11

fiber and polyunsaturated fats and low in saturated fats. A high fiber diet helps prevent incontinence.

Men suffer from osteoporosis, although to a considerably lesser extent than women. To prevent bone loss, which causes back pain and fractures, eat calcium-rich foods, including calcium supplements and foods providing daily vitamin D.

Several small meals a day, including a light breakfast, are better than one or two large meals, which may cause digestion and bowel problems. A large meal late at night may cause indigestion and insomnia. A light supper and a hot milky drink before bed is better.

Poor nutrition

Many old people eat badly. The lonely, impoverished and neglected may do so through apathy, poverty, inadequate cooking facilities, poor understanding of their nutritional needs, bad dietary habits or general physical or mental disability. Local senior citizens' clubs can help by providing low-cost meals, information, help with learning to cook, cooking facilities and shopping, or cut-price ingredients.

On the other hand, people who are unrestricted economically and practically may overeat foods rich in sugar and saturated fats, and meals low in protein and fiber, through ignorance or indifference.

Bad teeth, which prevent people from chewing, may cause people to buy foods that are easy to eat but not nutritious.

Drinking

Old people easily become dehydrated. A dry mouth (which impairs good taste), dry hair and skin, and reduced sweating are common. A liquid intake of 3-5 (US) pints a day is essential to maintain fluid balance and help prevent kidney damage, thick mucus forming in the lungs, chronic constipation and disorders of the urinary system. Drink more water, fruit juices, and milk, and fewer drinks containing diuretics and stimulants.

Alcohol drinking should be moderate. Over-consumption of alcohol promotes thinning of the bones and makes fractures and other injuries more likely. Regular heavy drinking causes liver disorders, erection and ejaculation problems, and confusion. But regular moderate drinking (see p 328) is now known to be beneficial: it stimulates the heart and helps prevent heart disease.

Age and Sex

Data published in the 1950s Kinsey report and in subsequent research has shown a steady decline in sexual activity with age. This has led to a belief that old people lose interest in sex. However, the effects of aging on sexual abilities has never been investigated and are not known, and recent research and surveys of sexual behavior are questioning assumptions about age and sex.

All research has shown a steady decline in the frequency of sexual activity. In a late-1970s study of Danish men aged 51-95, sexual interest and morning erections were shown to decline together. Studies have shown that masturbation declines much more slowly than sexual intercourse, and that men continue to masturbate well into their eighties. It may be that sexual activity declines because of falling opportunity, not falling potency.

However, research shows that in older men:
- erections take longer to develop, sometimes require more stimulation, and can be sustained for shorter and shorter periods as age progresses.
- less pre-ejaculatory mucus is produced and ejaculation is less powerful, with a reduced volume of semen and fewer contractions.
- the refractory period following ejaculation lengthens into days.

Studies carried out during the 1980s and early 1990s revealed interesting trends. A study of Baltimore men showed that:
- those who had experienced a high level of sexual activity early in adult life tended to continue to be sexually active in later life and showed the least decline. This was also found in a 1993 study of sexual behavior in Great Britain.
- men who had not been very sexually active when young were more likely to have erection problems in later life.

A further important finding in the US, which has parallels in the 1993 UK study, is that in the older age group, whereas well over 50 percent of married men aged 70 and over were sexually active, only 60 percent were sexually active with their partners.

To explain this, it is assumed that post-menopausal problems in the female partner caused joint sexual activity to cease, but that the men continued masturbating. However, the British study found that in couples of all ages, sexual activity declined with length of relationship. Moreover, people of all ages

11

experience an increase in sexual activity if they begin a new relationship.

Male hormones

There is a decline in the levels of testosterone, the male hormone, circulating in the blood, from around the age of 50. However, this decline differs markedly in different individuals. Researchers believe that individual men differ in the levels of testosterone they need to sustain libido. Hormone replacement therapy for men is by no means so widespread as it is for women. Evaluation of its effects on libido and sexual practices will throw light on the role of the male hormones in creating or maintaining sexual interest. Men remain capable of fathering children into old age, but it is believed that fertility declines with age.

Enjoyment of sex by American men aged over 50

Percentage of men sexually active in age group:

	Fifties	Sixties	Seventies
Married men	98	98	81
Unmarried men	95	85	75
All men	98	91	79

A study taken from respondents to a questionaire published by an American magazine, Consumer's Report, one of few reports to give a substantial amount of information about the older age groups.

Disorders of Aging

There is no escaping from the fact that aging reduces the body's efficiency, increasing the likelihood of malfunction. The body is susceptible to all the disorders that affect young people, but its maintenance and repair processes, and its defense – immune system – are weaker. Bone fractures and recovery from illnesses is slower in old people than in the young. Nevertheless, most people know a healthy and happy old person, and it can be valuable to bear in mind:

- that although there are many disorders of old age, you will not necessarily suffer from all of them, or even the most serious;
- that the younger you begin taking preventive measures in terms of following the healthiest possible lifestyle, the less likely you are to be ill when you are old.

Regular exercise and a good diet are part of the treatment of
the most feared disorders of old age, such as incontinence,
Parkinsonism (trembling due to degeneration of the nerve cells
in one part of the brain) and arthritis.
Aging reduces the body's efficiency, increasing the likelihood
of malfunction. With advancing age the body is still
susceptible to most of the disorders that affect young people.
However, the body's maintenance and repair processes, and its
defenses – the immune system – have become weaker. With
advancing age come associated physical changes: bone
fractures more easily, the skin is less elastic, muscles are less
poweful. Some biomechanical and physical changes may result
in characteristic disorders, among them:

- hardening and narrowing of the arteries (atherosclerosis)
  increases the likelihood of heart and circulatory disorders
  such as coronary thrombosis and strokes.
- severe mental impairment in the elderly (senile dementia) is
  associated with progressive degeneration of areas within the
  cerebral cortex
- the gradual build up of cell mutations, and lowering of the
  efficiency of cell repair mechanisms and immune responses,
  makes certain cancers more likely
- erosion of the cartilage inside joints contributes to
  osteoarthritis
- loss of calcium and other minerals from bone may result in
  osteoporosis
- biomechanical changes in the pancreas may result in late-
  onset diabetes
- impairment of the efficiency of the immune system may
  result in autoimmune responses leading to conditions such as
  rheumatoid arthritis, or may allow dormant diseases to re-
  emerge, as in the case of German measles flaring up in the
  form of shingles.
- decreasing elasticity of lung tissue with age may impaire
  breathing and makes respiratory conditions such as pleurisy
  more likely.

The causes of aging are still relatively poorly understood.
What is known, however, can be usefully applied to delay
many of the obvious signs of aging, and to lessent the chances
of getting an age-related disorder. Among the factors known to
accelerate various aspects of body aging are: an unsuitable
diet, lack of exercise of body and mind, smoking and excessive
alcohol intake.
With increasing age, recovery from an illness takes longer and

11

a special rehabilitation regime is more often necessary to get the person to recover their previous abilities. Secondary complications are also more likely. Among older people, multiple pathology (several diseases or disabilities present at once) is more common, and therefore correct diagnosis and treatment is more problematic. Often the successful treatment of disease or disability in older age requires a range of community resources. The successful rehabilitation of an elderly person is more likely to require a team working together: a doctor, a nurse, an occupational therapist, physiotherapist and social worker, for example, in the case of an elderly person with a fractured femur.

It is commonly assumed that the gradual loss of capacity – both mental and physical – is an inevitable feature of old age. This is not so. Frequently the decline in health is the result of unsuspected physical disorders that go undiagnosed and untreated. Regular medical examinations are at least as important in old age as at other times of life. Often, because of the low expectations of other people, the elderly present physical and mental symptoms which could otherwise be treated or counteracted if efforts were made on their behalf. Evidence to date strongly supports the view that achieving an active and healthy old age is not just about avoiding illness. It is at least as much to do with placing mental and physical demands on the body – engaging in physically and mentally demanding activities – so that the mind and body have to react adaptively to these demands. This results in a much wider repertoire of function. With changing circumstances, brought on perhaps by illness or changing home background, the mind and body are much better able to cope with these changes.

Alzheimer's Disease

A disease of the elderly in which nerve cells in the brain degenerate progressively, causing dementia. Its cause is not yet known. Diagnosis is positively confirmed by examination of the brain by biopsy after death. Awareness of the disease has developed with the increase in the numbers of the elderly, who in previous times might not have survived to suffer from it. It is rare before age 60 but up to one-third of people over 85 are affected; one recent study found that nearly half of those subjects over 75 had probable symptoms. Those with a family history of the disease being more likely to become victims.

The Joints

It is the constant wear and tear the joints receive through life
that causes degeneration. Injuries may accentuate and
accelerate any disorders. Yet it is essential to exercise to keep
the joints moving.

Osteoarthritis occurs to some degree in 80 to 90% of people
over 60. It originates from loss of elasticity in the cartilage of
the joints. Fragments of cartilage may loosen, be deposited in
the joint, then grow and become calcified, causing great
discomfort. Men are more prone to this illness than women,
who tend to suffer from rheumatoid arthritis. The tissues of the
joints thicken, so the cartilage becomes ulcerated and is
destroyed. Overproduction of connective tissue swells the
joint, which may become fused solid. The muscles waste with
disuse.

Treatment consists of painkilling drugs, special exercises, and
rest. Cortisone gives temporary relief, but may cause problems.
Replacement of worn-out hip joints is most effective and is
now a common operation. An artificial hip joint has a
chromium head attached to a titanium shaft, lined with acrylic
plastic. It replaces the ball part of the ball and socket joint,
which gives the leg its great mobility.

Osteoarthritis

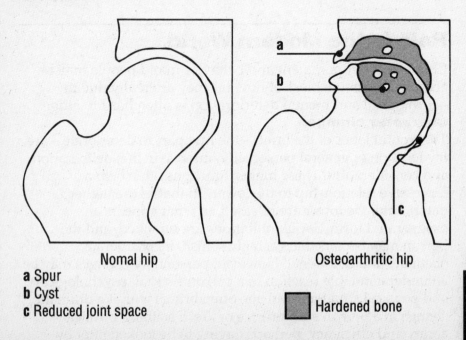

Nomal hip   Osteoarthritic hip

a Spur
b Cyst
c Reduced joint space   ▨ Hardened bone

11

Rheumatoid arthritis usually begins in middle age, but its severity increases with age. It affects more women than men. The tissue of the joints thicken, so the cartilage becomes ulcerated and is eventually destroyed. There is overproduction of connective tissue, and ultimately the joint is swollen and may be fused solid. The muscles waste with disuse. Special exercises, and rest in serious cases, are the main forms of treatment. Use of the drug cortisone is now thought to cause many problems, though it does give temporary relief.

Contractures are deformities of the joints due to shortening (contraction) of the surrounding muscles and ligaments. They can be caused by arthritic or neurological disorders or by prolonged inactivity.

If untreated, they become permanent and cause severe disability. Treatment is with muscle-relaxing drugs and physical manipulation.

Osteoporosis is increased porousness of the bone, usually from unknown causes, but sometimes due to severe nutritional deficiency of calcium salts. The skeleton becomes brittle and prone to fracture. The vertebrae are the bones most affected. They may collapse as they become weaker, and as they lose weight and size the vertebral discs expand, producing increasing curvature of the spine. The condition may be triggered off by prolonged immobilization in bed. It is more common in women than in men.

Role in the Modern World

Changes in temperament and behavior in old people may be accepted as inevitable. But how far they are really due to neurological and mental deterioration is often hard to judge.

Character changes

The frontal lobes of the brain – the first part to deteriorate – are the location of general personality, interest in life, deliberation and consideration. These higher functions often bear a repressive relationship to the lower, so that as the higher deteriorate, the lower are released, in what appears an exaggerated form. Social inhibitions are removed, and the person may become increasingly selfish, inconsiderate, obstinate and emotional. However, personality changes may be an understandable reaction to a person's social, psychological and physical situation. Old age often brings with it a dramatic change in a person's experience of life. Declining physical ability and efficiency, perhaps having to be looked after by others; the end of working life; and isolation, due to family mobility, disappearance of work contacts, and deaths of friends – all these can affect self-esteem and lead to depression and melancholia. Many old people keep up a wide range of active interests – but for others it is difficult, due to lack of finance, isolation, physical incapacity and lack of mental stimulation. The rate of change in 20th-century society adds to the sense of disorientation; and the life in many old people's homes does little to help.

All this can result in apathy, listlessness, resentment and mental stagnation, which others then dismiss as inevitable senility.

Effects of Demographic Changes

Because they live longer, there are more retired women than men – and more living alone. Over 60% of over-65s in the US are women. Elderly women often keep their self-respect better than men. A man's identify faces a severe crisis when he retires from work. Men who did not bother to learn to cook, sew and keep house when they were younger are often unable to look after themselves when they are left alone by the death of a female partner, for example.

It is important to realize the potential of middle and old age. For a working person, post-retirement can be up to one-third of the lifespan, and the majority of old people are not lonely, poor, incapacitated, neglected or ignored. With longevity and experience, values change, and the experience of middle and old can be rewarding in a way that is incomprehensible to a young man. Nevertheless, old people today can count it as individual good fortune or good planning if they are able to find growing old a rewarding experience. Western society does not have a good record for its treatment of the old. There is insufficient provision for their physical welfare; little or none for their self-esteem. After a lifetime of work, elderly people too often find they have no role to fulfill, and no social label but that of 'old person'. Physical and financial difficulties can reinforce this. Society's subtle message can often seem to be: you are no longer really useful, and although you are enjoying the deserved fruits of your labor, your difficulties and incapabilities are something of a problem for us. As, in the early years of the next millennium, the population of the US, Great Britain and other Western countries reaches a level of more than 50% of over-50s, of whom the majority will be experiencing the benefits of advanced medical science, and many again will have lived a far more healthy and active youth than their parents, these attitudes and experiences will go through a period of revolutionary change.

11

INDEX

INDEX